METHODS IN MOLECULAR BIOLOGY™

Series Editor
John M. Walker
School of Life Sciences
University of Hertfordshire
Hatfield, Hertfordshire, AL10 9AB, UK

For other titles published in this series, go to
www.springer.com/series/7651

Reverse Chemical Genetics

Methods and Protocols

Edited by

Hisashi Koga

Laboratory of Medical Genomics, Department of Human Genome Research,
Kazusa DNA Research Institute, Chiba, Japan

Humana Press

Editor
Hisashi Koga
Laboratory of Medical Genomics
Department of Human Genome Research
Kazusa DNA Research Institute
Chiba
Japan

ISSN 1064-3745   e-ISSN 1940-6029
ISBN 978-1-60761-231-5   e-ISBN 978-1-60761-232-2
DOI 10.1007/978-1-60761-232-2
Springer Dordrecht Heidelberg London New York

Library of Congress Control Number: 2009933592

Cover illustration: Adapted from Figure 5 in Chapter 14

Cover design: Karen Schulz

Printed on acid-free paper

Springer is part of Springer Science+Business Media (www.springer.com)

Preface

Reverse chemical genetics, in which specific small molecules are used for the analysis, has become a major approach to identifying the functions of certain gene products. It was brought about not only by the discovery of small molecules but also by the advancement of fully characterized genomic resources, such as genome sequencing, cDNA library generation, and siRNA libraries. The availability of complete in silico information through databases is also accelerating research in this field. Reverse chemical genetics corresponds to reverse genetics against forward genetics. In forward chemical genetics, phenotypic changes by molecules precede the identification of genes targeted by specific small molecules. Conversely, in reverse chemical genetics, the identification of target genes precedes phenotypic changes by specific small molecules. We allocated several chapters for the introduction of these fundamental resources, including databases for reverse chemical genetics. In subsequent chapters, we also discuss the modification of these cDNA resources by the most recent molecular technologies.

Recent innovations are dramatically changing the analytical platforms of established methods such as in situ hybridization, surface plasmon resonance, and 2D electrophoresis. We therefore have to emphasize the advancement of several scientific technologies including molecular biology, biochemistry, materials science, nanotechnology, optics, and several branches of engineering that may be applicable to reverse chemical genetics. In this book, we introduce newly established methods in addition to potentially applicable techniques that make use of specific small molecules, as well as functional assays utilizing these molecules. Especially in these techniques, we focus on methods that make feasible the functional discovery and comprehensive knowledge of particular target genes.

Especially, we asked each author to describe the method by which they arrived at their discoveries with consideration of the reader's merits. We hope that these methodological processes might lead readers to conduct further experiments on their own. Most of the authors were selected from among the participants to the International Symposium on Advanced Functional Genomics (October 11–12, 2007, Kazusa, Japan). We thank all authors for sharing their invaluable expertise in each specific field. We also acknowledge the invaluable editorial expertise of Dr. John M. Walker.

Tokyo, Japan *Hisashi Koga*

Contents

Contributors

TAKESHI AKASAKA • *Burnham Institute for Medical Research, Del E. Webb Neuroscience, Aging and Stem Cell Research Center, La Jolla, CA, USA*

EIJI ANDO • *Life Science Laboratory, Analytical and Measuring Instruments Division, Shimadzu Corporation, Kyoto, Japan*

HIROSHI ASAHARA • *Department of Systems Biomedicine, National Research Institute for Child Health and Development, Tokyo, Japan*

JUTTA BACHMANN • *Bachmann Consulting, Nesoddtangen, Norway*

TORU EZURE • *Life Science Laboratory, Analytical and Measuring Instruments Division, Shimadzu Corporation, Kyoto, Japan*

WATARU FUJIBUCHI • *National Institute of Advanced Industrial Science and Technology (AIST), Tokyo, Japan*

MINAKO HANASAKI • *Mitsubishi Chemical Group Science and Technology, Inc., Yokohama, Japan*

KIYOTAKA Y. HARA • *Consolidated Research Institute for Advanced Science and Medical Science and Medical Care, Waseda University, Tokyo, Japan*

ATSUNORI HIRATSUKA • *Research Center of Advanced Bionics, National Institute of Advanced Industrial Science and Technology (AIST), Tsukuba, Ibaraki, Japan*

SETSUO HIROHASHI • *Proteome Bioinformatics Project, National Cancer Center Research Institute, Tokyo, Japan*

HSIN-YUN HSU • *NMI Natural and Medical Sciences Institute at the University of Tübingen, Reutlingen, Germany*

KAZUKI INAMORI • *Biotechnology Development Department, Toyobo Co., Ltd., Osaka, Japan*

SHINICHI INOUE • *Laboratory of Human Gene Research, Department of Human Genome Research, Kazusa DNA Research Institute, Chiba, Japan*

MASAAKI ITO • *Life Science Laboratory, Analytical and Measuring Instruments Division, Shimadzu Corporation, Kyoto, Japan*

THOMAS O. JOOS • *NMI Natural and Medical Sciences Institute at the University of Tübingen, Reutlingen, Germany*

KUMARAN KANDASAMY • *Institute of Bioinformatics, Bangalore, India, McKusick-Nathans Institute of Genetic Medicine and Departments of Biological Chemistry Pathology and Oncology, Johns Hopkins University, Baltimore, MD, USA*

HYERYUNG KIM • *National Institute of Advanced Industrial Science and Technology (AIST), Tokyo, Japan, Tokyo Medical and Dental University, Tokyo, Japan*

HISASHI KOGA • *Laboratory of Medical Genomics, Department of Human Genome Research, Kazusa DNA Research Institute, Chiba, Japan*

TADASHI KONDO • *Proteome Bioinformatics Project, National Cancer Center Research Institute, Tokyo, Japan*

MOTOKI KYO • *Biotechnology Development Department, Toyobo Co., Ltd., Osaka, Japan*

AKIHISA MATSUYAMA • *Chemical Genetics Laboratory and Chemical Genomics Research Group, RIKEN Advanced Science Institute, Saitama, Japan*

TAKAHIRO NAGASE • *Laboratory of Human Gene Research, Department of Human Genome Research, Kazusa DNA Research Institute, Chiba, Japan*

HIDEKAZU NAGAYA • *Katakura Industries Co., Ltd., Saitama, Japan*

KAREN OCORR • *Burnham Institute for Medical Research, Del E. Webb Neuroscience, Aging and Stem Cell Research Center, La Jolla, CA, USA*

OSAMU OHARA • *Department of Human Genome Research, Kazusa DNA Research Institute, Chiba, Japan, Laboratory for Immunogenomics, RIKEN Research Institute for Allergy and Immunology, Yokohama City, Kanagawa, Japan*

KIMIHIKO OHTSUKA • *Summit Glycoresearch Corporation, Chiba, Japan*

YOSHIFUMI OKADA • *National Institute of Advanced Industrial Science and Technology (AIST), Tokyo, Japan, Muroran Institute of Technology, Muroran, Japan*

EIJI OKAMOTO • *Summit Glycoresearch Corporation, Chiba, Japan*

YUKITERU ONO • *Computational Biology Research Center (CBRC), National Institute of Advanced Industrial Science and Technology (AIST), Tokyo, Japan*

AKHILESH PANDEY • *McKusick-Nathans Institute of Genetic Medicine and Departments of Biological Chemistry Pathology and Oncology, Johns Hopkins University, Baltimore, MD, USA*

T.S. KESHAVA PRASAD • *Institute of Bioinformatics, Bangalore, India*

NICOLE SCHNEIDERHAN-MARRA • *NMI Natural and Medical Sciences Institute at the University of Tübingen, Reutlingen, Germany*

MASAMITSU SHIKATA • *Life Science Laboratory, Analytical and Measuring Instruments Division, Shimadzu Corporation, Kyoto, Japan*

KIYO SHIMADA • *Laboratory of Medical Genomics, Department of Human Genome Research, Kazusa DNA Research Institute, Chiba, Japan*

HIROHITO SHIMIZU • *Department of Systems Biomedicine, National Research Institute for Child Health and Development, Tokyo, Japan*

TOSHIFUMI SHIROYA • *Mitsubishi Chemical Group Science and Technology, Inc., Yokohama, Japan*

HIDEKO SONE • *National Institute for Environmental Studies, Ibaraki, Japan*

MAKIKO SUWA • *Computational Biology Research Center (CBRC), National Institute of Advanced Industrial Science and Technology (AIST), Tokyo, Japan*

TAKASHI SUZUKI • *Life Science Laboratory, Analytical and Measuring Instruments Division, Shimadzu Corporation, Kyoto, Japan*

HISAO TAKEUCHI • *Mitsubishi Chemical Group Science and Technology, Inc., Yokohama, Japan*

AKITO TANAKA • *Hyogo University of Health Sciences, Kobe, Hyogo, Japan*

HIROYUKI TANAKA • *Mitsubishi Chemical Group Science and Technology, Inc., Yokohama, Japan*

TAKEAKI TANIGUCHI • *Mitsubishi Research Institute, Tokyo, Japan*

KENTA UCHIBE • *Department of Systems Biomedicine, National Research Institute for Child Health and Development, Tokyo, Japan*

OSAMU WATANABE • *Toyota Central Research and Development Laboratories, Inc., Nagakute, Aichi, Japan*

KEI YAMAGUCHI • *Laboratory of Human Gene Research, Department of Human Genome Research, Kazusa DNA Research Institute, Chiba, Japan*

HISASHI YAMAKAWA • *Laboratory of Human Gene Research, Department of Human Genome Research, Kazusa DNA Research Institute, Chiba, Japan*

KENJI YOKOYAMA • *Research Center of Advanced Bionics, National Institute of Advanced Industrial Science and Technology (AIST), Tsukuba, Ibaraki, Japan*

MINORU YOSHIDA • *Chemical Genetics Laboratory and Chemical Genomics Research Group, RIKEN Advanced Science Institute, Saitama, Japan*

XIAOBO YU • *NMI Natural and Medical Sciences Institute at the University of Tübingen, Reutlingen, Germany*

Part I

The Importance of Fully-Characterized Genomic Resources and Informatics for Reverse Chemical Genetics

Chapter 1

ORFeome Cloning

Osamu Ohara

Summary

Reverse chemical genomic approach is expected to greatly expedite the discovery of new compounds, which modulate biological phenotypes in various ways. However, toward this end, various contents and platforms must be well prepared in the research community. In this regard, genome-wide preparation of clones for production of proteins in either a native or a fusion form, which are conventionally called ORFeome clones, would play a crucial role in realizing reverse chemical genomics as an approach of choice. In this chapter, currently available ORFeome cloning technologies are overviewed and a selection guideline for them is provided.

Key words: ORFeome cloning, Protein production, Recombination, Fusion protein

1. Introduction

Genome information provides us with various lines of biological information of a particular organism, because all the genetic information must be encoded on the genome. One of the most interesting lines of information is regarding proteins; genome information is expected to give us a complete catalog of proteins encoded by the genome, which has been long been dreamed of by biologists. In reverse chemical genomics, this protein catalog would serve as a solid basis of this approach. More clearly speaking, reagents which enable us to produce proteins of interest in vitro and/or in vivo play a pivotal role in reverse chemical genomic approaches. Thus, most researchers to date have tried to prepare these protein-expression clones by themselves. However, the research community has started to realize that these independent efforts are often redundant,

Hisashi Koga (ed.), *Reverse Chemical Genetics*, Methods in Molecular Biology, vol. 577
DOI 10.1007/978-1-60761-232-2_1, © Humana Press, a part of Springer Science+Business Media, LLC 2009

costly, time-consuming, and labor-intensive. If somebody successfully establishes a set of clones for production of proteins in a
genome-wide manner and allows the research community to
share it, reverse chemical genomic approaches must become
a method of choice for screening of modulators of protein
functions. This set would greatly accelerate the reverse
chemical genomic approach and would certainly release the
research community from an uncomfortable burden of redundant preparation of protein-production clones. This is a basic
and general motivation to initiate "ORFeome" cloning of the
genomics community (1–3).

In a strict sense, "ORFeome" is nothing but a jargon.
According to conventional terminology, we should remember
that open-reading frame (ORF) is not identical to protein-coding
sequence (CDS) that covers a region from the translation start
site to the termination site because ORF is literally defined only
as a contiguous region uninterrupted by a stop codon. However,
mainly because "ORFeome" sounds nice, the term "ORFeome"
is widely and preferentially used as an equivalent to a complement
of CDSs encoded by the genome. In this context, ORF should be
certainly read as CDS hereafter in this chapter.

ORF clones are artificially prepared by excising only
CDS from the genome or cDNA. In this regard, it should
be noted that ORFeome cloning aims to prepare expression
clones not only for production of native proteins but also for
that of fusion proteins of interest. For production of fusion
proteins, ORF clones carrying ORF without an original stop
codon must be prepared in a genome-wide manner. Although
this inevitably doubles our effort in ORFeome cloning, the
set of ORF clones which can direct the synthesis of fusion
proteins of interest is highly important; the resultant fusion
proteins can be used for versatile purposes for functional
analyses of genes. For example, genome-wide protein–protein
interaction analysis based on the yeast two-hybrid method is
a well-known example of the applications of fusion-type ORF
clones (4). A technical challenge in ORFeome cloning is thus
how to prepare many such ORF clones effectively in parallel
and this has been already reviewed (5). In this chapter, a
general guideline of selection of ORFeome cloning methods
is given for researchers who want to prepare their own ORF
clone sets. The information regarding public resources of
ORF clones is also provided because tremendous amounts of
efforts have already been made to generate such resources for
various organisms in the research community. These lines of
information must be highly useful for researchers who want to
first come to the field of reverse chemical genomics.

2. Materials

Sets of reagents for respective high-throughput cloning systems are commercially available from the following suppliers: Gateway® cloning system, Invitrogen; The Echo™ cloning system, Invitrogen; In-Fusion cloning system, Clontech; Creator cloning system, Clontech; Flexi® vector system, Promega. However, if an appropriate expression vector is not commercially available in either system, you may generate a new master ORFeome vector to fit your applications by yourself (*see* **Note 1**).

3. Methods

The ORFeome cloning system is broken down into two steps: Step 1, Generation of a master ORF clone for each gene; Step 2, transfer of the DNA insert from the master clones to other expression vectors. **Figure 1** shows a flowchart of the overall process of ORFeome cloning. To select an ORFeome cloning system most suitable for your purpose, you should seriously consider an overall design of your project at the beginning.

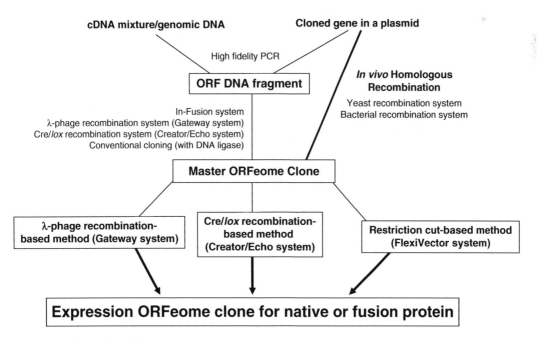

Fig. 1. A selection guide of ORF cloning methods.

Commercial availability of expression vectors fitting your purpose may serve as a key factor for the practical selection of the ORFeome cloning system. In this sense, there are three high-throughput cloning systems commercially available and suitable for step 2 in ORFeome cloning (**Fig. 1**): Gateway cloning system based on in vitro λ-phage recombination (Invitrogen), Creator cloning system or Echo cloning system based on in vitro Cre/*lox* recombination (Clontech or Invitrogen, respectively), and Flexi cloning system based on restriction digestion–ligation (Promega).

3.1. Excision of ORF Followed by Subcloning into a Master ORFeome Vector

As shown in **Fig. 1**, the first thing to do in step 1 of ORFeome cloning is excision of the ORF for each gene from the cloned gene or cDNA/gene library (*see* **Note 2**). This is usually done by polymerase chain reaction (PCR) with high-fidelity polymerase or by direct cloning based on homologous recombination *(6, 7)*. Whereas cloning based on the homologous recombination method in vivo enables us to directly generate master ORF clones from an original cDNA clone, the excised ORF region produced by PCR must next be connected to a master ORFeome vector by recombination-based (e.g., In-Fusion cloning system from Clontech; Gateway cloning system from Invitrogen) or conventional ligation-based cloning method (*see* **Note 3**). In addition, the application of in vivo Cre/*lox* recombination for this purpose was recently reported *(8)*. In the former case, the PCR products must carry homologous recombination sites at both ends; 15-bp and 25-bp for the In-Fusion and the Gateway cloning systems, respectively. On the other hand, because the Cre/*lox* recombination system requires a longer homologous recombination site, is less frequently used in this subcloning step for ORFeome cloning. Because the structure of the master ORFeome vector decides which high-throughput method for transfer of the insert ORF fragment becomes compatible, the selection of the vector of master ORF clones is highly crucial. By recombinational cloning systems such as the Creator, the Ecoh, and the Gateway systems, DNA fragments coding for ORF must shuttle between acceptor and donor vectors. Thus, a master ORF clone is usually in a format of donor plasmid and actual expression plasmids are generated after transfer of the ORF fragment to the corresponding acceptor plasmid. It is impossible to directly transfer the ORF fragment from one acceptor plasmid to another as long as we use a homologous recombination method. In contrast, a restriction cut–ligation-based cloning system enables us to directly transfer an ORF fragment from one expression plasmid to another with a different vector backbone. In other words, a master ORF clone for the restriction cut–ligation based cloning method can be used also as an expression clone, whereas this cannot be the case for a master ORF clone generated by a recombinational cloning method.

3.2. Transfer of ORF by High-Throughput Methods

Although multiple methods are available for preparation of master ORF clones as described above, a limited number of high-throughput methods for transfer of the DNA insert to other vectors are commercially available at present, as described above (**Fig. 1**): Gateway cloning system (Invitrogen), Creator cloning system or Echo cloning system (Clontech or Invitrogen, respectively), and Flexi cloning system (Promega). Each commercial system provides a set of various types of expression vectors compatible for easy transfer of the DNA insert in the master ORF clone (*see* **Note 4**). If you would plan to use these ORF clones for production of fusion proteins, availability of the expression vectors for fusion partners in each selected high-throughput cloning system may become a key issue for the selection of ORFeome cloning systems. In this regard, it is worth noting that the Flexi cloning system enables us to seamlessly apply the HaloTag technology, which provides us with a unique fusion partner for functional analyses of genes (Chaps. 3 and 10 in this volume). In the same context, the Gateway cloning system has a wide range of expression vectors and enables us to readily use the Lumio technology for functional analyses using ORF clones *(9)*. Thus, it is strongly recommended to first consider how you will use the resultant ORF clones and then decide which high-throughput cloning system will be applied. Except for downstream applications, another obvious difference among ORF clones derived from the Gateway, the Creator/Echo, and the Flexi cloning systems is in the size of the region inevitably flanked with insert ORFs in the ORF clones; the recombination sites in the Gateway and Creator/Echo systems are 25 bp and 34 bp, respectively, while the restriction site in the Flexi system is only 8 bp. Although this difference has not been reported to make any detectable difference in protein production, we recently found that a shorter flanking sequence was better for in vitro production of proteins particularly using insect lysate *(7)*.

3.3. Quality Control of ORF Clones and Public ORFeome Resources

The resultant master ORF clones should be checked by several different criteria: DNA sequence, protein productivity, and the structure of produced proteins (*see* **Note 5**). Once these master ORF clones whose quality has been well-checked become available to the research community, a wealth of time, labor, and cost will surely be saved and provide a solid basis for reverse chemical genomic approaches. In this context, many groups working on ORFeome cloning have made their ORF clones open to the research community: For human ORF clones, the ORFeome collaboration is actively working to generate a complete set of human ORF clones as an international collaboration (http://www.orfeomecollaboration.org/); *Schizosaccharomyces pombe* ORF clones are already available at the DNA bank of RIKEN

Bioresource center (http://www.brc.riken.jp/lab/dna/en/yoshidayeast_en.html). Although ORF clones publicly available are often generated by the Gateway system as in the case of these two resources, it is interesting to note that human ORF clones compatible with the Flexi cloning system are available from Kazusa DNA Research Institute (http://www.kazusa.or.jp/kop/). Those who are interested in ORF clones of a particular organism should first check the availability of ORF clones of the organism of interest through the internet. Because it is strongly recommended to share these ORF clones with the research community in the field of genomics, the chance of finding a good resource of ORF clones is high.

4. Notes

1. As for the Gateway system, a kit for the preparation of a new vector is available. However, a similar kit is not available for the Flexi system at present. This is because either system uses a trick to reduce the number of nonrecombinational background clones upon cloning by using a lethal gene. Remember that a special *Escherichia coli* strain is needed to propagate a new cloning vector for either cloning system. Because other systems (Creator/Echo systems) take advantage of antibiotic selection, they do not need any special *E. coli* strain for preparation of a new cloning vector.

2. For some model organisms, cDNA resources are already prepared and shared in the research community. Thus, when there is a need to study about functional genomics of a model organism, a search for appropriate cDNA resources open to the public should be made first. These lines of information may be found in genomic databases and/or Web sites of publicly funded genome projects. For example, human and mouse ORF clones are available from the ORFeome collaboration (http://www.orfeomecollaboration.org/html/index.shtml).

3. Even when a high fidelity polymerase for PCR is used, the full DNA sequences of the ORF clone must be confirmed after cloning, just in case. In particular, it should be kept in mind that oligonucleotides used as PCR primers sometimes have incorrect sequences, which could take place more frequently as the length of oligonucleotides increases. Because incorrect oligonucleotide sequences can cause a detrimental effect on the performance of ORFeome clones, the flanking sequences of the ORF in a master clone should also be examined as carefully as the ORF.

4. A variety of available expression vectors compatible for the Gateway, Creator, Echo, and Flexi systems can be accessed at the following URLs, respectively: http://www.invitrogen.com/content.cfm? pageid = 10287, http://www.clontech.com/products/detail.asp?product_id = 10400, https://catalog.invitrogen.com/index.cfm?fuseaction = viewCatalog.view ProductDetails&productDescription = 767https://catalog.invitrogen.com/index.cfm?fuseaction = viewCatalog.view ProductDetails&productDescription = 767, http://www.promega.com/catalog/catalogproducts.aspx?categoryname = productleaf_1636.

5. This quality check step may be the most time-consuming and labor-intensive step in the overall ORFeome cloning. However, the availability of these quality-check data is extremely important for future uses. Although examination of a DNA sequence is rather straightforward, a quality check at the gene product level is usually more tedious. The use of HaloTag technology and/or Lumio technology *(9)* in combination with the Flexi and Gateway cloning systems might make this situation much easier because of their readiness of detection of fusion proteins.

References

1. Reboul, J., et al. (2003) *C. elegans ORFeome version 1.1: experimental verification of the genome annotation and resource for proteome-scale protein expression*. Nat Genet. **34**, 35–41.

2. Rual, J.F., et al. (2004) *Toward improving Caenorhabditis elegans phenome mapping with an ORFeome-based RNAi library*. Genome Res. **14**, 2162–2168.

3. Brasch, M.A., J.L. Hartley, and Vidal, M. (2004) *ORFeome cloning and systems biology: standardized mass production of the parts from the parts-list*. Genome Res. **14**, 2001–2009.

4. Uetz, P., et al. (2004) *From ORFeomes to protein interaction maps in viruses*. Genome Res. **14**, 2029–2033.

5. Marsischky, G. and LaBaer, J. (2004) *Many paths to many clones: A comparative look at high-throughput cloning methods*. Genome Res. **14**, 2020–2028.

6. Nakajima, D., et al. (2005) *Preparation of a set of expression-ready clones of mammalian long cDNAs encoding large proteins by the ORF trap cloning method*. DNA Res. **12**, 257–267.

7. Nagase, T., et al. (2008) *Exploration of Human ORFeome: High-throughput preparation of ORF clones and efficient characterization of their protein products*. DNA Res **15**, 137–149.

8. Khalil, A.M., Julius, J.A. and Bachant, J. (2007) *One step construction of PCR mutagenized libraries for genetic analysis by recombination cloning*. Nucleic Acids Res. **35**, e104.

9. Griffin, B.A., Adams, S.R. and Tsien, R.Y. (1998) *Specific covalent labeling of recombinant protein molecules inside live cells*. Science. **281**, 269–272.

Chapter 2

Systematic Cloning of an ORFeome Using the Gateway System

Akihisa Matsuyama and Minoru Yoshida

Summary

With the completion of the genome projects, there are increasing demands on the experimental systems that enable to exploit the entire set of protein-coding open reading frames (ORFs), viz. ORFeome, en masse. Systematic proteomic studies based on cloned ORFeomes are called "reverse proteomics," and have been launched in many organisms in recent years. Cloning of an ORFeome is such an attractive way for comprehensive understanding of biological phenomena, but is a challenging and daunting task. However, recent advances in techniques for DNA cloning using site-specific recombination and for high-throughput experimental techniques have made it feasible to clone an ORFeome with the minimum of exertion. The Gateway system is one of such the approaches, employing the recombination reaction of the bacteriophage lambda. Combining traditional DNA manipulation methods with modern technique of the recombination-based cloning system, it is possible to clone an ORFeome of an organism on an individual level.

Key words: ORFeome, The Gateway system, Cloning, High-throughput, *Schizosaccharomyces pombe*

1. Introduction

As the genomes of many organisms have been sequenced, a flood of new information has been provided. A huge volume of information has brought about a great change in the way for the study toward understanding complex biological systems. Especially, thanks to the entire sequence information, classical (forward) proteomics has been greatly facilitated because it usually uses mass spectrometric techniques based on DNA sequence databases. On the other hand, completion of the genome project has set off a flood of new large-scale protein functional analyses called reverse

Hisashi Koga (ed.), *Reverse Chemical Genetics*, Methods in Molecular Biology, vol. 577
DOI 10.1007/978-1-60761-232-2_2, © Humana Press, a part of Springer Science+Business Media, LLC 2009

proteomics. Reverse proteomics is a methodology that starts from the entire set of protein-coding ORFs (ORFeome) of an organism. Therefore, one of the crucial missions at the beginning of this type of research is to construct a platform, that is, cloning of an ORFeome. Of course, cloning of an ORFeome is not anywhere near as simple as it sounds, since the number of ORFs is at least well into the thousands even in lower organisms. Therefore, the conventional cloning methods in which a DNA fragment is digested with restriction endonucleases and ligated to a vector are insufficient for ORFeomes. However, recently developed cloning techniques that employ site-specific and homologous recombination have made it feasible to manipulate thousands of ORFs en masse. The Gateway® system is one of such the recombination-based ORF cloning systems *(1, 2)*. This system consists of two recombination reactions, viz. the BP and LR reactions **(Fig. 1)**. The first step to clone an ORF is the BP reaction that transfers an ORF flanked by the *att*B sequences (*att*B1 and *att*B2) usually from PCR products to an *Escherichia coli* vector containing the *att*P sites (*att*P1 and *att*P2), called the "Donor vector." The resultant plasmid having an insert of interest is called "Entry clone." Since the recombination at these *att* sites is highly specific

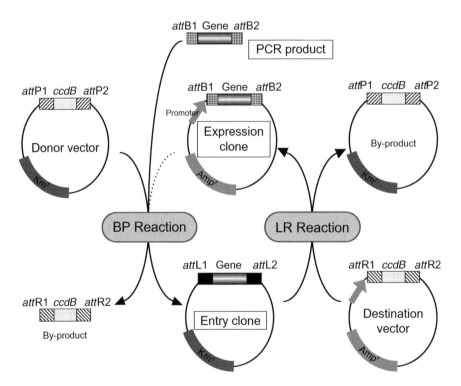

Fig. 1. Schematic representation of the Gateway system. The byproducts containing the *ccd*B cassette are generated in both BP and LR reactions. These diminish from the *E. coli* transformants, since the *ccd*B product activates DNA gyrase and kill *E. coli* cells *(7)*, thereby allowing only transformants harboring appropriate plasmids to grow.

and unique, *att*B1 reacts only with *att*P1, and *att*B2 reacts only with *att*P2. This ensures the correct orientation of the gene transferred. Once a gene is flanked by *att*L sites (*att*L1 and *att*L2) as an Entry clone, it can be transferred into any expression vectors designed for the Gateway system, called "Destination vectors" by the other recombination reaction named the LR reaction, resulting in the generation of a plasmid called "Expression clone" in which the gene is flanked again by *att*B1 and *att*B2 sites. The orientation of the gene is also maintained through the LR reaction, since *att*L1 reacts only with *att*R1, and *att*L2 reacts only with *att*R2. If required, a DNA fragment in an Expression clone can be transferred back to the Donor vector to give an Entry clone. Furthermore, both BP and LR reactions are carried out by simply mixing several reagents in a tube, allowing high-throughput manipulation. These features are extremely advantageous since it is required to manipulate a number of ORFs en masse in cloning of an ORFeome. Therefore, the Gateway system is particularly useful for construction of the whole ORF library (ORFeome), thereby being used in cloning of ORFeomes of many organisms (as reviewed by Yashiroda et al.) *(3)*.

The fission yeast *Schizosaccharomyces pombe*, which diverged from *Saccharomyces cerevisiae* several hundred million to one billion years ago and from animals about one billion years ago *(4, 5)*, shares many traits, notably cell division, with cells of higher eukaryotes, hence the information that the fission yeast proteome study provides, will be invaluable for functional and comparative studies of eukaryotic cell processes. Nonetheless, *S. pombe* has the extremely compact genome *(6)*, which is suitable as a resource for reverse proteomics. Here we describe the methodology for cloning of the fission yeast ORFeome using the Gateway system. However, it is also essentially applicable for cloning of ORFeomes of any other organisms except the preparation for the template DNA.

2. Materials

2.1. Preparation of the Fission Yeast Genomic DNA

1. *YE liquid medium.* 0.5% yeast extract, 2% glucose, 50 μg/ml adenine. To make 1 l of this medium, these materials are added to 1 l of water, dissolved well, and then autoclaved (120°C, 10–15 min). The concentration of glucose is often increased to 3%.

2. Zymolyase 100T (Seikagaku Kogyo, Tokyo, Japan) is suspended at 10 mg/ml in water and stored at less than –20°C. This enzyme is not completely dissolved at this concentration.

3. *Tris solution.* 50 mM Tris–HCl [pH 7.5], 20 mM EDTA.

4. Sorbitol solution is prepared by dissolving the following materials in water and then autoclaved: 1 M Sorbitol, 10 mM EDTA.

5. 10% (w/v) SDS. Autoclaving is not needed.

6. Potassium acetate is dissolved at 5 M in water, and then autoclaved.

7. 2-propanol and 70% (v/v) ethanol.

8. *TE buffer.* 10 mM Tris–Cl [pH 8.0], 1 mM EDTA.

9. Ribonuclease A (RNase A) is dissolved at 1 mg/ml in water, and stored at –20°C. To inactivate the possible contaminated DNase completely, RNase A solution is sometimes boiled once when prepared.

10. 3 M of Sodium acetate is dissolved in water, and then autoclaved.

11. Water-saturated phenol/chloroform is prepared in the following way. Phenol is fused by heating the bottle in hot water (55–60°C). After addition of an excess amount of water, they are mixed well and left to allow separation of water from the mixture at room temperature. After water–phenol separation, the same amount of chloroform as the water-saturated phenol is added. These are then mixed well and left again to allow separation. Use the lower layer for phenol/chloroform extraction. The upper water can be discarded if the volume is too excessive.

2.2. Amplification of ORFs by PCR

To clone a gene of interest using the Gateway technology, it should be sandwiched between two specific sequences, viz. *att*B1 and *att*B2. This is easily accomplished by attaching each sequence to primers for PCR. However, as both *att*B1 and *att*B2 are 25 bp in length, gene-specific primers would become too long to perform PCR cloning at small cost. To solve this problem, it is recommended to generate the final insert fragments by two-step PCR as described below. Firstly, an ORF is amplified by PCR with a set of gene-specific primers, each of which is fused with a part of *att*B1 or *att*B2. Second, the first PCR products are extended using universal primers that contain full sequences of *att*B1 or *att*B2. There are many kinds of software available for prediction of an optimal sequence and position for PCR primers. However, to clone full-length ORFs, it is impossible to change the position of primers. Although there are many other things that someone concerns about in designing PCR primers, we recommend simply using fixed number of bases from the initiation codon and the termination codon of an ORF. In our cases, for example, 20 bases starting from an initiation codon were attached to the universal sequence AAAAAGCAGGCTCTCAT containing a part of *att*B1 and a spacer sequence to generate a forward primer. The spacer sequence (CACAT in the above case) is not essential for use in the Gateway system. This sequence is just for adjusting the reading frame of an ORF with a tag in a vector, or for addition of a restriction enzyme recognition site. Similarly, a complementary sequence of 20 bases just upstream of the stop codon was attached to the other universal sequence AGAAAGCTGGGTA containing a part of *att*B2, resulting in the generation of a reverse primer (*see* **Note 1**). Using this simple set of primers, we have successfully cloned more than 99% of the fission yeast ORFeome without any nonspecific bands (*see* **Note 2**).

1. *Polymerase for amplification.* Pyrobest DNA Polymerase (TaKaRa BIO inc.) or PrimeSTAR DNA Polymerase (TaKaRa BIO INC.) are our recommendation. Other polymerases are also possible, but it is essential to select ones with extremely high fidelity. Buffers and dNTPs are usually supplied together with polymerases from manufactures.

2. *Universal primers for secondary PCR: attB1 adaptor primer.* 5′- GGGGACAAGTTTGTACAAAAAAGCAGGCT -3′, and attB2 adaptor primer: 5′- GGGGACCACTTTGTACAA-GAAAGCTGGGT -3′. The four guanine (G) residues at the 5′ end of these universal primers should be required to make the PCR fragment an efficient BP reaction substrate.

3. *Agarose gel for DNA electrophoresis.* Agarose is suspended in TAE buffer (40 mM Tris–acetate [pH 8.3], 1 mM EDTA) and dissolved by heating in a microwave oven. When the temperature drops to around 65°C, pour it into trays and allow for gelation.

4. Ethidium bromide solution is supplied from many manufactures (e.g., AMRESCO, Ohio, Code No. E406).

2.3. BP Reaction

1. The BP Clonases enzyme mix and buffers are supplied from Invitrogen. Although the product is provided with two different versions (premix and separate), we recommend the separate type for saving costs.

2. *Donor vector.* An *E. coli* vector containing the *ccd*B gene *(7)* flanked by *att*P sites. This vector can be purchased from Invitrogen.

3. *E. coli competent cells.* We usually use the DH5a strain, but other strains that are generally used are also possible. However, strains harboring F plasmid seem to work poorly in this system from our experiences.

4. *2 × YT liquid medium.* 1% Yeast extract, 1.6% Pepton (Becton, Dickinson and Company, cat. No. 211677), 0.5% NaCl. Adjust pH to 7.0 with 2N NaOH. Premix powder is also commercially available (e.g., Becton, Dickinson and Company, cat. No. 244020). Sterilize by autoclaving. Ampicillin or kanamycin should be added at 50 µg/ml if needed.

5. Kanamycin stock solution is prepared by dissolving at 50 mg/ ml in water, and is filter-sterilized. Stock solution should be kept at −20°C.

6. *LB (+Km) solid medium.* 1% Trypton (Becton, Dickinson and Company, cat. No. 211705), 0.5% Yeast extract, 1% NaCl, 0.2% Glucose, 1.5% Agar. Adjust pH to 7.2 with a 2N NaOH solution. Premix powder is also commercially available (e.g., Becton, Dickinson and Company, cat. No. 244520). When the temperature drops to around 65°C after autoclaving, add kanamycin at 50 µg/ml, mix immediately, and pour it into dishes. After gelation, store the plates in a cool and dark space.

2.4. Plasmid DNA Preparation in a 96-Well Format

1. *2 × YT liquid medium.* Prepared as described above. Ampicillin or kanamycin should be added at 50 µg/ml if needed.

2. *Cell resuspension solution.* 50 mM Tris–HCl [pH 7.5], 10 mM EDTA, 100 µg/ml RNase A.

3. *Cell lysis solution.* 0.2N NaOH, 1% SDS.

4. *Neutralization solution.* 7.5 M Ammonium acetate. Since ammonium acetate is highly hygroscopic, add 90 ml of deionized water per 100 g of ammonium acetate directly to the reagent bottle.

5. Plate sealer, breathseal, 80.0/140 mm (Greiner Bio-One, cat. No. 676051), or Breathe-EASIER™ (DIVERSIFIED BIO-TECH, cat. No. BERM-2000). These are air-permeable plastic films to seal 96-well plates.

6. MASTERBLOCK, 96-well, 2 ml, V-bottom (Greiner Bio-One, Cat. No. 780270). This product is a deep well plate in a 96-well format to culture *E. coli*. Other equivalent 96-well plates can be used. One should select a product that can be repeatedly used by autoclaving for saving costs.

7. 1.1 ml 96 Well Deep Well Plate (AXYGEN SCIENTIFIC, cat. No. P-DW-11-C). This product is a 96-well deep well plate with round wells. Other 96-well plates with similar features are also possible.

8. *2-notch polystyrene lid for deep well plates and assay plates (AXYGEN SCIENTIFIC, cat. No. P-LID-PS).* A rubber lid for 96-well plates. This item is suitable for repeatedly opening and covering samples. It should conform closely to the 96-well plate used for 2-propanol precipitation. This can be used repeatedly by autoclaving.

2.5. LR Reaction

1. The LR Clonases enzyme mix and buffers are also supplied from Invitrogen. There are also two types of packages, and we recommend the separate type product for saving cost. Although proteinase K solution is also supplied with the enzyme, it is not required in general use.

2. *Destination vector.* A vector for expression of a cloned ORF in an organism of interest. This vector should have the *ccd*B cassette at the position where the ORF is to be inserted, as is the case for a Donor vector (*see* **Note 3**).

3. *LB (+Amp) solid medium.* Prepare LB as in the case for LB (+Km). Just before pouring into Petri dishes, add ampicillin at 50 µg/ml. Store the plates at 4°C.

2.6. Check of Plasmid DNAs by Restriction Enzyme Digestion in a 96-Well Plate

1. Flexible plate, 96 well, U-bottom without lid (BECTON DICKINSON, cat. No. 353911). There are several 96-well plates, but this product is easily handled especially for restriction enzyme digestion of a large number of DNA samples.

3. Methods

In general, a full-length cDNA library has been used for ORF cloning of eukaryotic genes, because each cDNA clone has a real "ORF" without introns, which can be applied to heterologous expression systems such as bacterial expression lacking the splicing machinery. However, it is sometimes difficult to globally collect ORFs from cDNAs at a high coverage rate, since the successful cloning largely depends on the amounts of mRNA of target ORFs but some genes are not expressed or are expressed at very low levels under normal culture conditions. For instance, stress-inducible genes might be rarely cloned unless various culture conditions are tested. On the other hand, the genomic genes were expected to be easily collected at a high rate. In the case of *S. pombe*, unlike the budding yeast *S. cerevisiae*, it is predicted that almost half of the genes have one or more introns, although many of them are not experimentally confirmed *(6)*. Therefore, it does not seem useful to construct an ORFeome library from the genomic DNA in fission yeast. However, most proteome studies can be done with the self-expression system in fission yeast, since the proteins are likely expressed from the cloned genomic genes after correct splicing. We therefore used genomic DNA as a template based on the genome sequence database.

3.1. Preparation of the Template DNA (The Fission Yeast Genomic DNA)

1. Inoculate cells (wild-type is suitable) in YE medium and culture them at 30°C overnight.

2. Count cells using a blood cell counting chamber, and calculate the cell concentration.

3. Inoculate an appropriate amount of cells into YE medium, and culture them at 30°C for appropriate time. At 30°C, cells generally divide every 2.2–2.5 h, although the doubling time

depends on the genotype of a strain. It is of note that exponentially growing cells should be used for experiments, since saturated cells are generally somewhat resistant to many reagents. Generally, most experiments are done using cells at the density of $0.5–1.0 \times 10^7$ cells/ml. Calculate the number of cells required for the experiment in consideration of cultured time and an amount of the medium.

4. Harvest cells in a 50 ml tube by centrifugation ($2,000 \times g$, 3 min) and discard the medium.

5. Suspend cells with 5 ml of Sorbitol solution.

6. Add 200 μl of Zymolyase T100 solution and incubate at 37°C for 1 h with agitation.

7. Harvest cells by centrifugation ($1,700 \times g$, 3 min) and resuspend them in 5 ml of Tris buffer.

8. Add 500 μl of SDS solution, mix well, and incubate at 65°C for 30 min.

9. Add 2 ml of potassium acetate solution, mix well, and leave on ice for 10 min.

10. Centrifuge at $2,000 \times g$ at 4°C for 15 min.

11. Transfer the supernatant to another tube, add equal amount of 2-propanol, mix well, and leave for 5 min.

12. Centrifuge at $2,000 \times g$ at 4°C for 20 min.

13. Rinse the pellet with 70% ethanol, and dry up.

14. Dissolve the pellet with 2 ml of TE buffer.

15. Add 100 μl of RNase A solution, and then incubate at 37°C for 1 h.

16. Add equal amount of phenol/chloroform solution, mix well, and centrifuge at $17,000 \times g$ for 3 min.

17. Transfer the upper aqueous layer to another tube. If the amount of debris is so high, repeat the previous step.

18. Add 200 μl of sodium acetate solution, mix well, and then add 2 ml of 2-propanol.

19. After 5 min incubation, centrifuge at $17,000 \times g$ for 3 min, discard the aqueous solution, and rinse the pellet with 70% ethanol.

20. Dissolve the pellet with 1 ml of TE buffer.

3.2. Amplification of ORFs by PCR

1. For 96 samples, prepare 100 samples' premix. Assemble the following recipe: The fission yeast genomic DNA (0.1–1.0 μg/μl) 100 μl, 5× buffer 400 μl, dNTPs (2.5 mM each of dGTP, dATP, dTTP, and dCTP) 160 μl, deionized water 1,130 μl, PrimeSTAR DNA Polymerase (2.5 U/μl) 10 μl.

2. Dispense 18 μl of the premix solution to each well of a 96-well plate (*see* **Note 4**).

3. Mix each pair of primers in each well of a 96-well plate. Prepare 10 μM solution of each primer at first, and then mix each 1 μl of primer with the same volume of an appropriate counterpart. For quick and easy handling, primers are mixed in a 96-well plate when 10 μM solutions are prepared, and then 2 μl of each primer mix is transferred by using a multichannel pipette. Seal the plate with thermotolerant films and spin down the samples.

4. The conditions for the first PCR are as follows: 95°C for 3 min, 15 cycles of (95°C for 15 s, 52°C for 15 s, 72°C for XX s), and 72°C for 3 min, where XX is determined according to the length of an ORF (~45 s/kbp).

5. To do the second PCR, assemble a recipe as follows: 5× buffer 400 μl, dNTPs (2.5 mM each) 160 μl, attB1 adaptor primer (100 μM) 5 μl, attB2 adaptor primer (100 μM) 5 μl, deionized water 1,320 μl, PrimeSTAR DNA Polymerase (2.5 U/μl) 10 μl.

6. Dispense 19 μl of the premix solution to each well of the 96-well plate, as is the case for the first PCR.

7. Dispense 1 μl of 100-fold diluted first PCR solution to each well. Seal and spin down the plate.

8. The conditions for the second PCR are the same as the first PCR except that the number of cycles is 20.

9. Check 2 μl of the resultant solution by agarose gel electrophoresis (**Fig. 2**). If a desired DNA band is observed (*see* **Notes 5** and **6**), proceed to the next step.

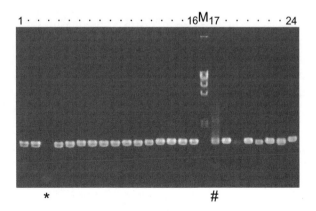

Fig. 2. Amplification of ORFs by 2-step PCR. The products of the second PCR were electrophoresised using a 1% agarose gel. There are some ORFs having the same 5′- and 3′- sequences, although the internal sequences are distinct (marked by #). This property is typical in *wtf* genes *(6)*. These ORFs were simultaneously amplified by the same set of primers and distinguished by sequencing after cloning. Primer dimers are sometimes observed when a desired ORF is not amplified (*). M: λ/HindIII marker.

3.3. BP Reaction in a 96-Well Format

The BP reaction is a recombination reaction that transfers a DNA fragment (such as a PCR product) flanked by *att*B recombination sites into an *E. coli* vector, called "Donor vector" containing *att*P sites, to produce a new plasmid, called "Entry clone." This reaction is catalyzed by the BP Clonase mix of recombination proteins. In this reaction, the *ccd*B gene is removed from the Donor vector, thereby allowing the transformants to grow.

1. For 96 samples, prepare 100 samples' premix. Assemble the following recipe: Donor vector (pDONR221: 150 ng/µl) 50 µl, BP reaction buffer (5×) 100 µl, TE buffer 150 µl, BP Clonase enzyme mix 100 µl.

2. Dispense 4 µl of the premix solution to each well of a 96-well plate using an 8- or 12-channel pipette. For quick and easy handling as is the case for PCR, transfer 48 µl of the premix solution to the first well of each lane, and then dispense 4 µl out of the solution to other wells along with each lane using an 8-channel pipette. Or, transfer 32 µl of the premix to each well of the top lane, and then dispense 4 µl using a 12-channel pipette.

3. Add 1 µl of a PCR product to each well.

4. After sealing and spin-down, incubate the plate at 25°C overnight.

5. Add 1 µl of Proteinase K solution and incubate at 37°C for 10 min.

6. Transform *E. coli* cells with 3 µl of the solution.

7. After addition of 2 × YT liquid medium followed by 37°C incubation for an hour, spread cells onto LB (+Km) plate and culture them at 37°C.

8. Check successful cloning by restriction enzyme digestion and sequencing of the plasmid DNA (*see* **Note 7**).

3.4. Plasmid DNA Preparation in a 96-Well Format

There are many protocols for alkali-method to isolate plasmid DNA from *E. coli*. The protocol described below is specialized for handling a large number of samples using a 96-well plate.

1. Culture *E. coli* transformants in 0.8–1.0 ml of 2× YT (+Km or Amp) with a 2 ml 96-well plate at 37°C overnight. Seal the plate with air-permeable plastic sheet. Shake the plate vigorously (>120 min^{-1}).

2. Harvest cells by direct centrifugation of the culture plate (2,000 × *g*, 15 min). Discard medium by inverting the plate. Wipe the opening of the container with lint-free paper.

3. Suspend cells with 100 µl of Resuspension solution and vortex vigorously until cells are well suspended.

4. Dispense 100 µl of Cell lysis solution and mix mildly until the solution becomes clear.

5. Dispense 100 μl of Neutralization solution and mix vigorously (*see* **Note 8**).

6. Centrifuge at 2,000 × *g* for 15 min.

7. Transfer the supernatants to a 1.1 ml 96-well plate prefilled with 300 μl 2-propanol. Seal the plate with a rubber lid and mix well.

8. Centrifuge at 2,000 × *g* for 20 min, then discard the supernatant by inverting the plate. Wipe the opening of the plate with lint-free paper.

9. Rinse each well with 100 μl of 70% ethanol. Centrifuge at 2,000 × *g* for 5 min and discard the supernatant. Wipe the opening of the plate with lint-free paper.

10. Dry up the plate.

11. Dissolve DNA with 50 μl of TE buffer or deionized water.

3.5. LR Reaction in a 96-Well Format

Compared with the BP reaction, the LR reaction shows extremely high activity. Therefore, the reaction requires less time and enzymes (*see* **Note 9**).

1. For 96 samples, prepare 100 samples' premix, as is the case for the BP reaction. Assemble the following recipe: Destination vector (~10 ng/μl) 25 μl, LR reaction buffer (5×) 60 μl, TE buffer 105 μl, LR Clonase enzyme mix 10 μl.

2. Dispense 2 μl of the premix solution to each well of a 96-well plate, as is the case for the BP reaction.

3. Add 1 μl of an Entry clone diluted to 1–10 ng/μl to each well (*see* **Note 10**).

4. After sealing and spin down, incubate the plate at 26°C for more than an hour.

5. Transform *E. coli* cells with the reaction mixture directly (*see* **Note 11**). Plate the cells on LB (+Amp) and incubate at 37°C overnight.

6. Pick up a colony (*see* **Note 12**) and check the plasmid by restriction enzyme digestion followed by agarose gel electrophoresis.

3.6. Restriction Enzyme Digestion of Plasmid DNAs in a 96-Well Plate

1. For 96 samples, prepare 100 samples' premix. Assemble the following recipe: 10× buffer 100 μl, deionized water 800 μl, restriction endonuclease 10 μl.

2. Dispense 9 μl of the premix solution to each well of a 96-well plate. For quick and easy handling, transfer 108 μl of the premix solution to the first well of each lane, and then dispense 9 μl out of the solution to other wells along with each lane using an 8-channel pipette. Or, transfer 72 μl of the premix to each well of the top lane, and then dispense 9 μl using a 12-channel pipette.

3. Add a DNA sample to each well using an 8- or 12-channel pipette. Mix well by pipetting.

4. Seal the plate with vinyl tape, and incubate the plate at the appropriate temperature (usually 37°C).

4. Notes

1. If the fusion of a tag is planned, it is important to consider the reading frames of an ORF and the tag so that they are properly translated in-frame. In addition, removal of the termination codon is essential for production of C-terminally tagged proteins.

2. For extremely long ORFs that exceed 10 kb in length, it is recommended to amplify the ORFs as two divided fragments at first. They are subsequently connected by the in vivo standard method using restriction endonucleases and a DNA ligase, or by the in vivo recombinational cloning method (8). In the latter case, two fragments are generated as partially overlapping fragments, each of which contain one or other of the attB sequences. These fragments are simultaneously reacted with a donor vector in the BP reaction, resulting in the generation of full-length ORFs by transformation of E. coli with the reaction mixture.

3. Many destination vectors are commercially available. However, it is also possible to construct a destination vector that is suitable for individual experiments. To construct such vectors, one should insert the ccdB-containing cassette (commercially available from Invitrogen) into the appropriate locus of a Gateway-incompatible vector. The resultant plasmids can be amplified only in the DB3.1 strain, due to the toxic ccdB gene (7).

4. For quickly dispensing without using an autodispenser, transfer 216 µl of the premix solution to the endmost well of each lane, and then dispense 18 µl out of the solution to other wells along with each lane using an 8-channel pipette. Similarly, if a 12-channel pipette is used, transfer 144 µl of the premix solution to the top wells of a 96-well PCR plate at first, and then dispense 18 µl of the premix in sequence (**Fig. 3**).

5. There is little possibility that unknown bands are amplified in the PCR. However, when an extra band(s) is observed in the electrophoretic analysis, the correct band should be gel-extracted using a standard protocol, purified and then subjected to the BP reaction. Especially, since long (>2 kb) fragments are relatively less effective for the BP reaction, elimination of

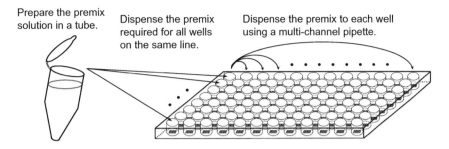

Fig. 3. Quick dispensation of samples. An appropriate amount of premix solutions is taken into the endmost well of each line. An aliquot is then dispensed from these into each well in the same line using a multi-channel pipette.

the extra band(s) is often essential. As for primer dimers that are sometimes observed, one can remove them using the 30% PEG/MgCl$_2$ solution (supplied together with the BP Clonase Enzyme Mix) according to the manufacture's instructions.

6. When no band is observed, there are some tips for enhancement of effectiveness of PCR. The simplest way to get better results is just to increase the amount of a polymerase. Increase of the template DNA may also result in an increase of PCR products. Use of another polymerase may give better results in some cases. For example, by using PrimeSTAR DNA Polymerase, we obtained some PCR products that were not amplified when Pyrobest DNA Polymerase was used. On the contrary, some ORFs were amplified only when Pyrobest DNA Polymerase was used. Thus, polymerases have some preference in sequence. Therefore, it is worth testing another polymerase to expand the coverage of cloned ORFs.

7. The specificity and accuracy is very high in the BP reaction. Therefore, most of the *E. coli* colony has correct plasmids. However, to ensure the cloning, we recommend to check at least two colonies. In addition, we recommend confirming the correct ORF cloning by sequencing. To alleviate some of this economic burden by the full-length sequencing, we recommend sequencing of at least both ends of the inserts. In cloning of the fission yeast ORFeome, we detected many apparent base-exchanges by sequencing *(9)*. Of course, these may be a sum of errors in PCR or sequence analyses, and due to substantial differences in strains used in the genome project and our study. However, the errors tended to be enriched within regions synthesized as primers. Therefore, it is suggested that a considerable number of errors occur in the synthesis of oligo DNAs.

8. It is also possible to use 5 M sodium acetate [pH 4.8] in place of ammonium acetate in this step. However, the debris resulted from the addition of ammonium acetate would become highly compact so that the transfer of the supernatant becomes easier.

9. The activity of the LR Clonase enzymes is so high that considerable degree of dilution of the enzymes is possible. At least, we have succeeded in obtaining proper expression plasmids using 1/40-diluted enzymes (data not shown).

10. The concentration of an Entry clone plasmid should be kept at a low level (1–10 ng/μl) in the LR reaction. A high amount of an Entry clone proved to be adverse, contrary to our expectations. Similarly, the concentration of the destination vector should be kept low. In contrast to the LR reaction, it would be better to use the insert DNA (PCR products) at a high concentration in the BP reaction.

11. Although the manufacture's instructions directs that the LR reaction should be terminated by addition of the Proteinase K solution as is the case for the BP reaction, this step can be skipped from our experiences.

12. The specificity and accuracy of the LR reaction seem higher than those of the BP reaction. In addition, there is almost no possibility that some errors (such as mutation and deletion) occur unlike PCR followed by the BP reaction. Therefore, most of the *E. coli* colony has correct plasmids. However, we recommend to check at least two colonies per expression plasmid to ensure acquisition of proper plasmids.

Acknowledgments

This work was supported by CREST Research Project, Japan Science and Technology Agency.

References

1. Hartley JL, Temple GF, Brasch MA. (2000) DNA cloning using in vitro site-specific recombination. *Genome Res* 10, 1788–1795.

2. Walhout AJ, Temple GF, Brasch MA, et al. (2000) GATEWAY recombinational cloning: application to the cloning of large numbers of open reading frames or ORFeomes. *Methods Enzymol* 328, 575–592.

3. Yashiroda Y, Matsuyama A, Yoshida M. (2008) New insights into chemical biology from ORFeome libraries. *Curr Opin Chem Biol* 12, 55–59.

4. Sipiczki M. (2000) Where does fission yeast sit on the tree of life? *Genome Biol* 1, REVIEWS1011.

5. Heckman DS, Geiser DM, Eidell BR, Stauffer RL, Kardos NL, Hedges SB. (2001) Molecular evidence for the early colonization of land by fungi and plants. *Science* 293, 1129–1133.

6. Wood V, Gwilliam R, Rajandream MA, et al. (2002) The genome sequence of *Schizosaccharomyces pombe*. *Nature* 415, 871–880.

7. Bernard P, Couturier M. (1992) Cell killing by the F plasmid CcdB protein involves poisoning of DNA-topoisomerase II complexes. *J Mol Biol* 226, 735–745.

8. Oliner JD, Kinzler KW, Vogelstein B. (1993) In vivo cloning of PCR products in *E. coli*. *Nucleic Acids Res* 21, 5192–5197.

9. Matsuyama A, Arai R, Yashiroda Y, et al. (2006) ORFeome cloning and global analysis of protein localization in the fission yeast *Schizosaccharomyces pombe*. *Nat Biotechnol* 24, 841–847.

Chapter 3

High-Throughput Construction of ORF Clones for Production of the Recombinant Proteins

Hisashi Yamakawa

Summary

Expression-ready cDNA clones, where the open reading frame (ORF) of the gene of interest is placed under the control of an appropriate promoter, are critical for functional characterization of the gene products. To create a resource of human gene products, we attempted to systematically convert original cDNA clones to expression-ready forms for recombinant proteins. For this purpose, we adopted a rare-cutting restriction enzyme-based system, the Flexi® cloning system, to construct ORF clones. Taking advantage of the fully sequenced cDNA clones we accumulated to date, a number of sets of Flexi® ORF clones in a 96-well format have been prepared. In this section, two methods for the preparation of Flexi® ORF clones in a 96-well format are described. A protocol for transferring ORFs between Flexi® vectors in a 96-well format is also described. We believe that the resultant clone set could be successfully used as a versatile reagent for functional characterization of human proteins.

Key words: cDNA, KIAA, Proteomics, ORFeome, Protein expression, Flexi® cloning

1. Introduction

A protein-coding region on a eukaryotic genome is typically divided into pieces of exons by introns. After transcribing the nucleotide sequence of this region to mRNA, these introns are removed and the remaining exons are concatenated. This maturated mRNA is eventually used as a template of protein synthesis in vivo, and thus suitable for investigation of structural and functional analyses of proteins. Actually, cDNA, an artificial copy of mRNA, is used for such experiments because manipulation of cDNA is convenient for the construction of expression vectors and alteration of nucleotide sequences. Thus cDNA should be a

Hisashi Koga (ed.), *Reverse Chemical Genetics*, Methods in Molecular Biology, vol. 577
DOI 10.1007/978-1-60761-232-2_3, © Humana Press, a part of Springer Science + Business Media, LLC 2009

significant material for protein synthesis in vivo and in vitro and has become a major focus of molecular biologists.

In this context, we have started a sequencing project focused on human large cDNAs at the Kazusa DNA Research Institute since 1994 to accumulate information of the predicted amino acid sequences encoded on the cDNAs for newly identified genes *(1)*. These newly identified genes were designated as "KIAA" plus a four-digit number and comprehensively characterized by expression profiling and computer prediction *(2, 3)*. In recent years, cDNA clones for mouse homologs of human KIAA genes (mKIAA genes) *(4, 5)* and polyclonal antibodies against mKIAA proteins *(6, 7)* have also been accumulated at the Kazusa DNA Research Institute to investigate the function of KIAA gene products using an animal model in vivo *(8–10)*.

Recently, whole genome sequences from various species, including human and mouse, have been determined, and the worldwide trends in molecular biology are shifting from the discovery of novel genes to the comprehensive analysis of structure and function of the gene products (mRNAs and proteins). In this context, many efforts have been made to prepare sets of ORF clones for protein expression that contain protein coding sequences of cDNA without a 5′/3′-untranslated region (UTR) by a process called ORFeome cloning *(11–13)*. We have also begun to prepare such ORFeome clones, taking advantage of the thousands of fully sequenced human cDNA clones already accumulated through the project *(14)*.

The aim of ORFeome cloning is to prepare clones that can be used for comprehensive analysis of structure and function of protein products. Nevertheless, it will be necessary to reconstruct expression vectors to produce differently tagged proteins according to the purpose of use. The HaloTag® is a highly versatile protein tag that was developed to solve this problem *(15–18)*. This system is flexibly adaptive to the imaging (in vivo and in vitro) and capture of tagged proteins through the exchange of appropriate HaloTag® ligands suitable for specific purposes *(16)*. This HaloTag® technology is seamlessly integrated into the Flexi® cloning system *(19)*, which is one of the rare-cutting restriction enzyme-based directional cloning systems. Once ORFs are incorporated into this system, they can be easily transferred to any Flexi® vectors, including HaloTag®-fused forms. Therefore, we decided to use the Flexi® cloning system for preparation of ORF clones to apply HaloTag® technology in proteomic explorations. We have prepared nearly 3,500 Flexi®-format human ORF clones so far *(20)*, and the number continues to grow. The information on our ORF clones is available through our database (Kazusa ORFeome Project, http://www.kazusa.or.jp/kop/).

Here we present the protocols for cloning of ORFs from cDNA clones into the Flexi® system by a PCR method and an ORF trap method and transferring them to expression vectors in a 96-well format.

2. Materials

2.1. Enzymes

1. *Sgf*I.
2. *Pme*I.
3. DNA Ligation Kit Ver.2 (BioDynamics Laboratory Inc., Bunkyo-ku, Tokyo, Japan).
4. PrimeSTAR® HS DNA Polymerase (Takara Bio Inc., Ohtsu, Shiga, Japan).
5. Illustra TempliPhi™ DNA Amplification Kit (GE Healthcare Bio-Sciences Corp., Piscataway, NJ, USA).

2.2. Buffers

1. *Flexi® Digest Buffer (10×)*. 100 mM Tris–HCl, pH 7.9, 100 mM MgCl$_2$, 500 mM NaCl, 10 mM DTT and 1 mg/mL acetylated BSA.
2. *TE buffer*. 10 mM Tris–HCl, pH 8.0 and 0.1 mM EDTA.
3. *Cell Stock Buffer*. 50% glycerol.

2.3. E. coli Culture

1. *E. coli* strain JC8679 (*recB21, recC22, sbcA23, thr-1, leuB6, phi-1, lacY1, galK2, ara-14, xyl-5, mtl-1, proA2, his-4, argE3, rpsL31, tsx-33, supE44, his-328*) *(21)* from the Health Science Research Resources Bank (HSRRB) of the Japan Health Sciences Foundation.
2. High efficiency JM109 competent cells for CaCl$_2$ method (over 10^8 cfu/µg).
3. Materials for media (Bacto™ Tryptone, Bacto™ Yeast Extract and Difco™ SOB Medium, agar powder and NaCl) and antibiotics (ampicillin sodium and kanamycin sulfate).
4. Sterile No.2 square dish (10 cm × 14 cm × 1.5 cm) for square agar plates.
5. 96-well deep well culture plate.
6. Air-permeable plate sealer.

2.4. Kits for DNA Purification

1. Wizard® SV 96 Plasmid DNA Purification System (Promega Corp., Madison, WI, USA).
2. Wizard® SV 96 PCR Clean-Up System (Promega).

3. Wizard® SV Gel and PCR Clean-Up System (Promega).

4. CloneChecker™ System (Invitrogen Corp., Carlsbad, CA , USA).

2.5. Other Materials

1. pF1K T7 Flexi® Vector (Promega).

2. Oligonucleotides for cloning of ORFs and for the sequencing of pF1K T7 clones (cf. **Fig. 1**).

3. 96-well plate for PCR.

4. PCR apparatus compatible with 96-well plate reactions.

5. Plate sealer.

6. *E. coli* Pulser™ (Bio-Rad Laboratories, Inc., Hercules, CA, USA).

7. Gene Pulser®/MicroPulser™ Cuvettes, 0.1 cm gap (Bio-Rad Laboratories).

3. Methods

To construct Flexi® ORF clones from cDNA plasmids in a 96-well plate format, we routinely use two types of ORF-cloning methods, a PCR method **(Fig. 1a)** and an ORF trap method **(Fig. 1b)** *(14)*. The ORF trap method is a cloning technique based on a homologous recombination in *E coli*. By using PCR, specific cloning vectors tagged with the gene-specific sequences corresponding to both the ends of the ORF, called a trap vector, are prepared. *E. coli* strain JC8679, which shows high homologous recombination activity, is transformed with the gene-specific trap vector and the corresponding cDNA plasmid that encodes the target ORF sequence to be cloned. Then homologous recombination occurs in *E. coli* and the ORF region is transferred into the trap vector.

It is necessary to certify the nucleotide sequences of the fragments cloned by the PCR method, because the use of thermophilous DNA polymerase frequently results in unintended nucleotide substitutions. If the ORF length is smaller than 1.2 kb, single-pass sequencings from both the ends are sufficient for confirmation of the entirety of the ORF sequence, whereas in the case of a relatively large ORF, it often fails to obtain an intact clone without any mutations and is accompanied by tremendous task for the sequencing. On the other hand, ORF sequence cloned by the ORF trap method does not easily involve mutations because the cloned sequence is amplified in *E. coli* by the endogenous replication enzymes, though PCR primers for trap vector preparation are relatively long (about 60-mer each) (*see* **Note 1**). Thus the choice of a method depends on an ORF length.

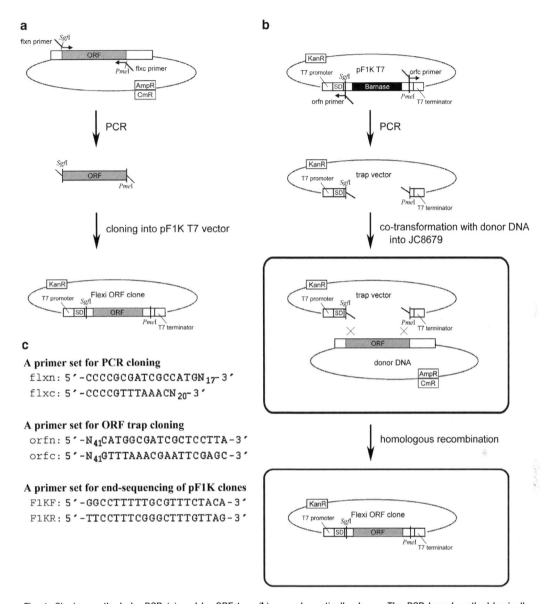

Fig. 1. Cloning methods by PCR (**a**) and by ORF trap (**b**) are schematically shown. The PCR-based method basically follows the instructions of the Promega. For ORF trap method, a cloning vector is tagged with the both the ends of the ORF sequence by using PCR. The *E.coli* strain JC8679 is transformed with this vector called trap vector and the cDNA plasmid encoding the target ORF sequence. Then homologous recombination occurs in *E. coli* and the ORF sequence is transferred into the trap vector. (**c**) The basic primer structure for PCR cloning and ORF trap cloning, and the primer sequences for the sequencing of pF1K T7 clones are shown. In "A primer set for PCR cloning," N_{17} in flxn indicates a 17nt-sense sequence after the start codon of ORF and N_{20} in flxc indicates a 20nt-antisense sequence before the stop codon of ORF. Similarly, in "A primer set for ORF trap cloning," N_{41} in orfn indicates a 41nt-antisense sequence after the start codon of ORF, and N_{41} in orfc indicates a 41nt-sense sequence before the stop codon of ORF. Note that the ORF region is amplified in PCR cloning while a vector is amplified in ORF trap cloning. Thus the directions of the corresponding nucleotide sequences in ORF (flxn – orfn, flxc – orfc) are opposite.

ORFs compatible with the Flexi® cloning system can be easily transferred between expression vectors with different antibiotics (ampicillin-resistant and kanamycin-resistant vectors) (*see* **Note 2**) using a restriction enzyme-based protocol. Though this is a basic manipulation in the recombinant DNA technology, several optimizations are needed when using a 96-well format. Our routine protocol is described at the end of this section.

Basic reagents are prepared by a standard protocol for molecular biological experiments. The SOB medium used here contains 20 mM of magnesium.

3.1. Cloning of PCR Fragments into pF1K T7 Vectors in a 96-Well Plate Format

1. The PCR-based ORF cloning is basically done according to the instructions provided by Promega. The sequences of the basic primers used for the PCR are shown in **Fig. 1c**. PCR products of 20 µL in a 96-well plate format are purified by using the Wizard® SV 96 PCR Clean-Up System. As a result, purified PCR products in 100 µL of H_2O are prepared.

2. An aliquot of the purified PCR products (typically 7.5 µL) is treated with 2.5 U of *Sgf*I and 2.5 U of *Pme*I in a 10 µL-reaction volume containing 1× Flexi® Digest Buffer at 37°C for 90 min in a 96-well plate, and then the enzymes are inactivated by incubating the reaction mixture at 65°C for 20 min.

3. For preparation of a cloning vector, 2.5 µg of pF1K T7 vector is treated with 30 U of *Sgf*I and 30 U of *Pme*I in a 100 µL-reaction volume (equivalent amount of 96 constructions) containing 1× Flexi® Digest Buffer at 37°C for 90 min, and then the enzymes are inactivated by incubating the reaction mixture at 65°C for 20 min.

4. Two microliters of the *Sgf*I/*Pme*I-treated PCR products and 1 µL of the *Sgf*I/*Pme*I-treated pF1K T7 vector are mixed and placed in a 96-well plate. Three microliters of 2× Ligation Buffer and 0.3 µL of the Ligase Mixture from a DNA Ligation Kit Ver.2 are blended in advance and added to the DNA mixture. After pipetting them twice using an 8-channel autopipetter, this ligation reaction mixture set is incubated at 16°C for 30 min.

5. Fifteen microliters of JM109 competent cells and 1.5 µL of the ligation reaction mixture are mixed in a 96-well plate followed by sealing with plate sealers, and the mixture is left on ice for 30 min. Then heat-shock is applied to the cells by placing the 96-well plate at 42°C for 45 s. The plate is then immediately placed on ice for 2 min (*see* **Note 3**), and then each transformation reaction mixture is transferred into 150 µL of SOC medium in a 96-well deep well culture plate. The plate is sealed with an air-permeable sheet and incubated at 37°C for 90 min with gentle shaking.

6. One hundred microliters of the culture is spotted onto a square LB agar plate containing 50 µg/mL of kanamycin. Several spots and one streak are formed on the LB agar plate for each

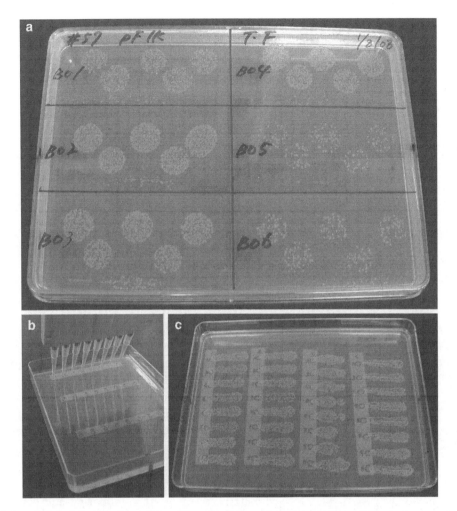

Fig. 2. In order to isolate clones from a 96-well format culture, we have to spread the cultures one by one onto an agar plate with appropriate antibiotics. (a) In order to isolate clones for the PCR cloning method, 100 μL of culture is placed onto a square LB agar plate with 50 μg/mL of kanamycin. Several spots and one streak are formed on the LB agar plate for each transformation reaction. A culture streak can be used if the spotted colonies are too dense for analysis. An example of a square plate incubated at 37°C overnight is shown. Relatively dense colonies are formed in the samples B01 to B04, and single colonies are recovered from the streak area. In the samples B05 and B06, colonies are sparsely formed and single colonies are recovered from the spotted area. (b) When transferring a plasmid set from JC8679 into JM109, single colony isolation is needed after the transformation process by streaks of cell suspensions onto a square LB agar plate with appropriate antibiotic. In that case, it is functional to use an 8-channel autopipetter for streak. (c) The suspensions of 32 samples (8 samples × 4 rows) are placed onto a square LB agar plate by using an 8-channel autopipetter and incubated at 37°C overnight. Three to several colonies for each sample are recovered from each streak area and inoculated for 96-well plasmid preparation.

transformation reaction (**Fig. 2a**), and the plate is kept at 37°C overnight (*see* **Note 4**). The remaining transformation reaction mixtures (about 50 μL each) are used for glycerol stock solution; these reaction mixtures are transferred into 25 μL of Cell Stock Buffer in each well of a 96-well plate.

7. Two colonies per transformation reaction are separately inoculated in 600 µL of LB medium containing 50 µg/mL of kanamycin in a pair of 96-well culture plates and cultured at 37°C overnight. Consequently two sets of cultures are prepared. For glycerol stock, 50 µL of culture is added to 25 µL of Cell Stock Buffer in a 96-well plate. *E. coli* cells in the remaining suspensions are harvested by centrifugation and the pellets are preserved by freezing. Then plasmids are prepared from one set of the harvested cells (*see* **Note 5**) using the Wizard® SV 96 Plasmid DNA Purification System (*see* **Note 6**).

8. One microliter of the plasmids thus prepared is treated with *Sgf*I/*Pme*I and analyzed by agarose gel electrophoresis (*see* **Note 7**). Clones with an appropriate insert size are applied to sequencing analysis. Sequencing samples are prepared from the purified plasmids using an illustra TempliPhi™ DNA Amplification Kit, because the yields of plasmid in a 96-well format preparation are sometimes insufficient for sequencing.

3.2. ORF Trap Cloning of Long ORFs into pF1K T7 Vectors in a 96-Well Plate Format

1. For preparation of donor DNAs, 2 µg of the cDNA clones carrying the desired ORF are linearized by a restriction enzyme that can cleave the vector sequence but not ORF (*see* **Note 8**). Prepared cDNAs are digested in 50 µL of a reaction mixture with 20 U of the restriction enzyme at the appropriate temperature for the enzyme for 1 h in a 96-well format, and the enzyme is inactivated by heating the reaction mixture whose condition is suitable for the enzyme.

2. For ethanol precipitation, 5 µL of 3 M sodium acetate and a 125 µL of 100% ethanol are added and mixed by gentle shaking. The 96-well plate is covered with a rubber lid and placed on ice for 10 min.

3. The plate is centrifuged at 2,380 g at 4°C for 30 min using EX-126 with a TS-40 rotor (Tomy Seiko Co., Ltd., Nerima-ku, Tokyo, Japan), and then the supernatants are discarded by reversing the plate. Then the plate is put onto sheets of paper towel upside down and the residual liquids are completely removed from the plate by spin down at 2,380 g at 4°C for 1 s.

4. Eighty microliters of 70% ethanol is added to each well. The plate is centrifuged at 2,380 g at 4°C for 30 min, and the supernatants are discarded by reversing the plate. Immediately, the residual liquids are completely removed from the plate as described above. The samples are dried by keeping them at room temperature for 10 min and dissolved into 10 µL of H_2O. These are the "donor DNA solutions."

5. Trap vectors are prepared (*see* **Note 9**). For each gene, the set of trap vector primers described in **Fig. 1c** is designed. Thus 96 pairs of primers are needed for 96 samples. Corresponding

primer sets (orfn:orfc) are blended to create an H_2O solution of 10 pmol/μL each in a 96-well format. This primer mix set is used for the Trap vector preparation.

6. The pF1K T7 vector is used as a template for the PCR. Reaction volume, 50 μL; pF1K T7 vector, 2 μL (1 ng/μL); primer mix, 1 μL; dNTP, 0.2 mM; 5× PrimeSTAR Buffer, 10 μL. The reaction conditions are as follows: preincubation at 98°C for 30 s, followed by 30 cycles at 98°C for 10 s, at 55°C for 5 s and at 72°C for 3 min, and postincubation at 72°C for 5 min. Amplification of the trap vector is confirmed by agarose gel electrophoresis, and concentrated by ethanol precipitation as well as donor DNA preparation followed by dissolution in 20 μL of H_2O. These are the "trap vector solutions."

7. Three microliters of the donor DNA solution and 1 μL of the trap vector solution are blended with a 20 μL of competent JC8679 cells for electroporation (*see* **Note 10**), and the mixture is transferred into an electroporation cuvette with a 0.1 cm electrode gap. After an electric pulse of 1.67 kV is applied, 1 mL of SOC medium is added to the suspension, and incubated at 37°C for 3 h with vigorous shaking. This process is applied to each gene one by one.

8. Thirty microliters of the suspension is spread on one quarter of a square LB agar plate containing 50 μg/mL of kanamycin and incubated at 37°C overnight. Thus four kinds of samples are on one plate and 24 plates are needed per a 96-sample set. In addition, glycerol stocks are prepared by blending 100 μL of the cell suspension with 50 μL of Cell Stock Buffer in a 96-well format.

9. Colonies are examined with the CloneChecker™ System. Plasmid sizes are analyzed by cutting with *Pme*I according to the supplier's recommendations. Clones with a plasmid of an appropriate size are selected, and the corresponding suspensions that are prepared for analysis with the CloneChecker™ System are respectively inoculated to 600 μL of LB medium containing 50 μg/mL of kanamycin in a 96-well format and cultured at 37°C overnight.

10. For glycerol stock, 50 μL of the culture is added to 25 μL of Cell Stock Buffer in a 96-well plate. The remaining suspensions are applied to plasmid preparation using the Wizard® SV 96 Plasmid DNA Purification System (*see* **Note 6**). One microliter of resultant plasmid solution is applied to agarose gel electrophoresis to examine the yields of plasmids.

11. The end-sequences of these plasmids are examined by DNA sequencing (*see* **Note 11**). Sequencing samples are prepared from the purified plasmids using an illustra TempliPhi™

DNA Amplification Kit as well as the PCR cloning check. The plasmids with appropriate end-sequences are selected (one clone for one gene) and re-arrayed to their primary positions in a 96-well format.

12. These plasmids are transformed into JM109 (*see* **Note 12**). One microliter of plasmid solution is added to a 10 μL of JM109 competent cells, and is left on ice for 30 min in a 96-well plate. Then heat-shock is applied to the cells by placing the 96-well plate at 42°C for 45 s using a heat block incubator such as a PCR apparatus. The plate is immediately placed on ice for 2 min, and then each transformation reaction mixture is transferred into 100 μL of SOC medium in a 96-well culture plate. The plate is sealed with an air-permeable sheet and incubated at 37°C for 1 h with gentle shaking. A 10 μL of the suspension is placed onto a square LB agar plate containing 50 μg/mL of kanamycin using an 8-channel autopipetter (32 samples per plate, see **Fig. 2b, c**) and kept at 37°C overnight.

13. Three to several colonies for each sample are inoculated into the same 600 μL of LB medium containing 50 μg/mL of kanamycin and cultured at 37°C overnight. For glycerol stock, 50 μL of the culture is added to 25 μL of Cell Stock Buffer in a 96-well plate. The remaining suspensions are applied to the plasmid preparation with the Wizard® SV 96 Plasmid DNA Purification System (*see* **Note 6**). One microliter of the resultant plasmid solution is directly applied to agarose gel electrophoresis for estimation of the size of plasmid in a form of covalently closed circular. Similarly, another 1 μL of the plasmid solution is treated with *Sgf*I/*Pme*I and analyzed by agarose gel electrophoresis for an insert size check. This plasmid solution set is the final product and is reserved in a freezer.

3.3. Transfer Flexi® ORF to Flexi Expression Vectors

1. Five micrograms of an expression vector solution (an ampicillin-resistant vector is used here because pF1K T7 is kanamycin-resistant) is treated with 50 U of *Sgf*I and 50 U of *Pme*I (expression vector for no-tagged or N-terminal tagged protein) or *Eco*ICRI (expression vector for C-terminal tagged protein) in a 500 μL of reaction volume containing 1× Flexi® Digest Buffer at 37°C for 60 min, and then the enzymes are inactivated by incubating the reaction at 65°C for 20 min. The vector is about 50% digested under this condition.

2. The digested vector is purified by using the Wizard® SV Gel and PCR Clean-Up System. The plasmid concentration of the resultant solution is measured by UV absorbance, and adjusted to 25 ng/μL.

3. Two microliters of pF1K-ORF plasmid solutions prepared with the Wizard® SV 96 Plasmid DNA Purification System are treated with 5 U of *SgfI* and 5 U of *PmeI* in a 10 μL reaction volume containing 1× Flexi® Digest Buffer at 37°C for 60 min, and then the enzymes are inactivated by incubating at 65°C for 20 min.

4. Three microliters of this solution and 1 μL of the vector solution are mixed in a 96-well plate. Four microliters of 2× Ligation Buffer and 0.4 μL of Ligase Mixture from a DNA Ligation Kit Ver.2 is blended and added to the DNA mixture. After pipetting twice using an 8-channel autopipetter, this ligation reaction mixture set is incubated at 16°C for 30 min.

5. One microliter of this ligation mixture is added to 10 μL of JM109 competent cells, and is left on ice for 30 min in a 96-well plate. Then heat-shock is applied to the cells by placing the 96-well plate at 42°C for 45 s using a heat block incubator such as a PCR apparatus. The plate is then immediately placed on ice for 2 min, after which each transformation reaction mixture is transferred into 100 μL of SOC medium in a 96-well culture plate. The plate is sealed with an air-permeable sheet and incubated at 37°C for 60 min with gentle shaking.

6. The cultures are thoroughly spread onto one-sixth of a square LB agar plate containing 100 μg/mL of ampicillin and left at 37°C overnight. Thus six kinds of samples are on one plate and 16 plates are needed per 96-sample set. Two of the obtained colonies are suspended into 6 μL of LB medium, and 1 μL of each suspension is spotted onto two kinds of LB agar plates (one containing 100 μg/mL of ampicillin and one containing 50 μg/mL of kanamycin) and placed at 37°C overnight.

7. Clones with ampicillin resistance but without kanamycin resistance are examined with the CloneChecker™ System. By this antibiotic selection, the undesired vector heterodimer is removed. If both of the clones are false, additional clones are analyzed using the same protocol. When appropriate clones are obtained for almost all of the genes, they are inoculated from the ampicillin plates to prepare plasmids in a 96-well format by using the Wizard® SV 96 Plasmid DNA Purification System (*see* **Note 6**).

8. Prepared plasmids are examined by a restriction enzyme digestion and an agarose gel electrophoresis. Insert sizes are examined and plasmids with an insert of an appropriate size are used for the next experiment.

4. Notes

1. Because the oligonucleotides primers are not free from mutations originating from synthesis errors, sequence confirmation around the oligomers (i.e., the N-terminus and C-terminus of the ORF) is indispensable. It is also important to use high-quality oligonucleotides.

2. In the case of vectors for expression of the C-terminal-tagged protein, the *Pme*I site is disrupted by fusion with *Eco*ICRI to remove the termination codon. Thus the ORF in this type of vector is no longer removable by *Sgf* I and *Pme* I digestion.

3. The reaction mixtures are cooled by placing the 96-well PCR plate on top of a 96-well aluminum block chilled on ice. Heat-shock of 42°C is accomplished by placing the plate in a water bath. Recooling on ice is done first by placing the plate in an ice-water bath and then by placing the plate on top of a 96-well aluminum block chilled on ice.

4. Typically, several colonies appear in a single spot, but some-times the number of colonies is too high for analysis. In such cases, isolated colonies are available from the streak.

5. The cloning efficiency of the present method is sufficient to obtain positive clones from a single culture set, although arti-ficial alterations of nucleotide sequences originating from the PCR process are inevitable.

6. The plasmid preparation using the Wizard® SV 96 Plasmid DNA Purification System follows the protocol from Promega, except that TE buffer instead of H_2O is used for the final plas-mid elution buffer. This alteration is applied to all the plasmid preparation processes in this chapter.

7. Image analyzing software is very useful for efficient verification of the insert sizes of a 96-well format sample set. We routinely digitize electrophoretic images using a BioDoc-It™ Imaging system (BM Equipment Co., Ltd., Bunkyo-ku, Tokyo, Japan) and insert sizes are estimated by MultiGauge (Fujifilm Corp., Minato-ku, Tokyo, Japan).

8. Because our cDNA libraries are mostly cloned after digestion by *Not*I, the restriction enzyme for linearization is typically *Not*I. To raise the cloning efficiency of the homologous recombination reaction, the insert fragment including the ORF should be purified by agarose gel electrophoresis. In that case, *Bss*HII is available because the backbone of our libraries is pBluescript® II or pBC, unless the ORF involves the *Bss*HII site(s).

9. Homologous recombination happens elsewhere than in a target region if the region has an unexpected homologous sequence. If a donor DNA clone and a trap vector have the same replication origin and the origin is in the same direction relative to the ORF, recombination often occurs at the origin instead of the additional region for recombination, and a part of the ORF is eliminated. This is not a problem, of course, when the fragment encoding the ORF is excised from the cDNA plasmid and purified before use. We prepare in advance a modified pF1K T7 vector in which the replication origin is inversed, and choose two types of vectors according to the direction of origin of the donor DNA clones.

10. Because JC8679 competent cells for electroporation are not commercially available, we had to produce our own. We routinely prepare competent cells following the protocol reported previously *(14)*. Although JC8679 competent cells for electroporation of 10^8–10^9 cfu/μg pUC19 are routinely prepared, the apparent transformation efficiency for the ORF trap is much lower (typically 50–100 colonies per 30 μL of transformation culture).

11. Because a trap vector is prepared by PCR, a mutation within a vector region sometimes occurs. This is not a problem in most cases because we are interested only in an insert fragment, but in some cases, such a mutation happens to influence the vector function (multimerization, reduction of transformation efficiency, *etc.*). This situation can be avoided by selecting another clone or transferring the insert to another intact vector.

12. JC8679 is *End*A⁺, which codes for endonuclease I, and plasmids from this strain are often unstable over long-term storage. In addition, prepared plasmids are in a multimer form. Therefore, we immediately transfer the plasmid from JC8679 to JM109, and prepare it from JM109 for stable storage and for dissolution of the multimer form.

Acknowledgments

I would like to thank T. Watanabe, M. Tamura, K. Yamada, E. Suzuki, C. Mori, and H. Kinoshita for their technical assistance. The Kazusa ORFeome Project of which this report is a part is organized by Dr. O. Ohara and Dr. T. Nagase (Kazusa DNA

Research Institute). This work is supported in part by a grant from the Promega Corporation and by a special grant from the Chiba Prefectural Government for acceleration of the practical application of biotechnology.

References

1. Nomura N, Miyajima N, Sazuka T, et al. (1994) Prediction of the coding sequences of unidentified human genes. I. The coding sequences of 40 new genes (KIAA0001-KIAA0040) deduced by analysis of randomly sampled cDNA clones from human immature myeloid cell line KG-1 *DNA Res* **1**, 27–35.

2. Nagase T, Ishikawa K, Nakajima D, et al. (1997) Prediction of the coding sequences of unidentified human genes. VII. The complete sequences of 100 new cDNA clones from brain which can code for large proteins in vitro *DNA Res* **4**, 141–150.

3. Nagase T, Ishikawa K, Suyama M, et al. (1998) Prediction of the coding sequences of unidentified human genes. XI. The complete sequences of 100 new cDNA clones from brain which code for large proteins in vitro *DNA Res* **5**, 277–286.

4. Okazaki N, Kikuno R, Ohara R, et al. (2002) Prediction of the coding sequences of mouse homologues of KIAA gene: I. The complete nucleotide sequences of 100 mouse KIAA-homologous cDNAs identified by screening of terminal sequences of cDNA clones randomly sampled from size-fractionated libraries *DNA Res* **9**, 179–188.

5. Okazaki N, Kikuno R, Ohara R, et al. (2004) Prediction of the coding sequences of mouse homologues of KIAA gene: IV. The complete nucleotide sequences of 500 mouse KIAA-homologous cDNAs identified by screening of terminal sequences of cDNA clones randomly sampled from size-fractionated libraries *DNA Res* **11**, 205–218.

6. Hara Y, Shimada K, Kohga H, Ohara O, Koga H. (2003) High-throughput production of recombinant antigens for mouse KIAA proteins in Escherichia coli: computational allocation of possible antigenic regions, and construction of expression plasmids of glutathione-S-transferase-fused antigens by an in vitro recombination-assisted method *DNA Res* **10**, 129–136.

7. Koga H, Shimada K, Hara Y, et al. (2004) A comprehensive approach for establishment of the platform to analyze functions of KIAA proteins: generation and evaluation of anti-mKIAA antibodies *Proteomics* **4**, 1412–1416.

8. Kikuno R, Nagase T, Nakayama M, et al. (2004) HUGE: a database for human KIAA proteins, a 2004 update integrating HUGEppi and ROUGE *Nucleic Acids Res* **32 Database issue**, D502–D504.

9. Koga H, Yuasa S, Nagase T, et al. (2004) A comprehensive approach for establishment of the platform to analyze functions of KIAA proteins II: public release of inaugural version of InGaP database containing gene/protein expression profiles for 127 mouse KIAA genes/proteins *DNA Res* **11**, 293–304.

10. Murakami M, Shimada K, Kawai M, Koga H. (2005) InCeP: intracellular pathway based on mKIAA protein-protein interactions *DNA Res* **12**, 379–387.

11. Brizuela L, Richardson A, Marsischky G, Labaer J. (2002) The FLEXGene repository: exploiting the fruits of the genome projects by creating a needed resource to face the challenges of the post-genomic era *Arch Med Res* **33**, 318–324.

12. Rual JF, Hill DE, Vidal M. (2004) ORFeome projects: gateway between genomics and omics *Curr Opin Chem Biol* **8**, 20–25.

13. Temple G, Lamesch P, Milstein S, et al. (2006) From genome to proteome: developing expression clone resources for the human genome *Hum Mol Genet* **15 Spec No 1**, R31–R43.

14. Nakajima D, Saito K, Yamakawa H, et al. (2005) Preparation of a Set of Expression-Ready Clones of Mammalian Long cDNAs Encoding Large Proteins by the ORF Trap Cloning Method *DNA Res* **12**, 257–267.

15. Lang C, Schulze J, Mendel RR, Hansch R. (2006) HaloTag: a new versatile reporter gene system in plant cells *J Exp Bot* **57**, 2985–2992.

16. Los GV, Wood K. (2007) The HaloTag: a novel technology for cell imaging and protein analysis *Methods Mol Biol* **356**, 195–208.

17. Zhang Y, So MK, Loening AM, Yao H, Gambhir SS, Rao J. (2006) HaloTag protein-mediated site-specific conjugation of bioluminescent proteins to quantum dots *Angew Chem Int Ed Engl* **45**, 4936–4940.

18. Hata T, Nakayama M. (2007) Rapid single-tube method for small-scale affinity purification

of polyclonal antibodies using HaloTag Technology *J Biochem Biophys Methods* **70**, 679–682.

19. Blommel PG, Martin PA, Wrobel RL, Steffen E, Fox BG. (2006) High efficiency single step production of expression plasmids from cDNA clones using the Flexi Vector cloning system *Protein Expr Purif* **47**, 562–570.

20. Nagase T, Yamakawa H, Tadokoro S, et al. (2008) Exploration of Human ORFeome: High-Throughput Preparation of ORF Clones and Efficient Characterization of Their Protein Products *DNA Res* **15**, 137–149.

21. Gillen JR, Willis DK, Clark AJ. (1981) Genetic analysis of the RecE pathway of genetic recombination in Escherichia coli K-12 *J Bacteriol* **145**, 521–532.

Chapter 4

Computational Overview of GPCR Gene Universe to Support Reverse Chemical Genomics Study

Makiko Suwa and Yukiteru Ono

Summary

In order to support high-throughput screening for ligands of G-protein coupled receptors (GPCRs) by using bioinformatics technology, we introduce a database (SEVENS) with genome-scale annotation and software (GRIFFIN) that can simulate GPCR function. SEVENS (http://sevens.cbrc.jp/) is an integrated database that includes GPCR genes that are identified with high accuracy (99.4% sensitivity and 96.6% specificity) from various types of genomes, by a pipeline that integrates such software as a gene finder, a sequence alignment tool, a motif and domain assignment tool, and a transmembrane helix (TMH) predictor. SEVENS provides the user a genome-scale overview of the "GPCR universe" with detailed information of chromosomal mapping, phylogenetic tree, protein sequence and structure, and experimental evidence, all of which are accessible via a user-friendly interface. GRIFFIN (http://griffin.cbrc.jp/) can predict GPCR and G-protein coupling selectivity induced by ligand binding with high sensitivity and specificity (more than 87% on average), based on the support vector machine (SVM) and hidden Markov Model (HMM). SEVENS and GRIFFIN are expected to contribute to revealing the function of orphan and unknown GPCRs.

Key words: Reverse chemical genomics, G-protein coupled receptor, Eukaryote genome, Gene finding, Comparative genome analysis, Orphan receptor, Chemical compound

---

1. Introduction

The rapid influx of biological information in the postgenomics era has paved the way to establishing the field of "chemical genomics" as infrastructure for drug screening. Chemical genomics is often compared with "chemical biology," the latter being categorized into two types: "forward" and "reverse." Analogous to these two types, "forward chemical genomics" aims to identify genes (proteins) and their function hidden under some phenotypes that

Hisashi Koga (ed.), *Reverse Chemical Genetics*, Methods in Molecular Biology, vol. 577
DOI 10.1007/978-1-60761-232-2_4, © Humana Press, a part of Springer Science+Business Media, LLC 2009

are induced by some specific chemical compounds. This process does not require prior information of target proteins. In contrast, "reverse chemical genomics" starts from specific protein information; by adding ligands to these protein groups, the behavior of the protein and the phenotype are directory linked. Although both types are indispensable to the screening for ligands that have potential use as a drug, reverse chemical genomics is more suitable for high-throughput screening for ligands based on a massive number of protein sequence information.

In this context, we focus on G-protein coupled receptors (GPCRs) with seven transmembrane helices (TMHs) that act as the gateway for signal transduction at the cell surface membrane. An external ligand stimulus applied to GPCR induces coupling with G-proteins ($G_{i/o}$, $G_{q/11}$, G_s, and $G_{12/13}$, etc.), followed by different types of signal transduction (**Fig. 1**). Since approximately half *(1)* of all drugs distributed throughout the world are designed to control these mechanisms, GPCRs are important targets for the development of effective drugs.

From the viewpoint of drug design, it is of utmost importance to construct a screening system for ligand molecules that can effectively control specific GPCRs and G-proteins, by monitoring their activation. If this is accomplished, high-throughput screening for ligand molecules that activate orphan receptors having yet-unknown ligands will be possible. Furthermore, the system can assist in the experimental design of a cell system suitable for target GPCR expression.

Although these are the most important requirements, it is extremely difficult to construct a high-throughput and comprehensive biochemical experimental system because it requires

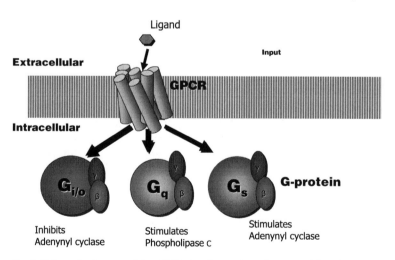

Fig. 1. Schematic diagram of the GPCR signaling system. An external ligand stimulus applied to GPCR induces coupling with G-proteins followed by different types of signal transduction, such as the inhibition and stimulation of adenynyl cyclase and the stimulation of phospholipase C.

enormous cost and much time. To solve these problems, we use bioinformatics methodology. First, we created a database that contains a comprehensive collection of GPCR genes identified from genome sequences. Then, we developed software that can predict the behavior of GPCRs, particularly that of orphan receptors, by conducting many ligand-binding trials. The database provides an overview of the "GPCR universe" that will allow us to list novel or orphan receptors. The software is important especially for sequences that show no sequence similarity to other known GPCRs. In other words, it is necessary to formulate an algorithm to predict G-protein coupling selectivity when the user inputs various kinds of ligand information. In this chapter, we introduce SEVENS *(2)*, a database containing a comprehensive collection of GPCR genes, and GRIFFIN *(3)*, a software for predicting GPCR behavior.

2. Materials

1. *Genome sequence ftp sites.* NCBI (http://www.ncbi.nlm.nih.gov/), UCSC (http://genome.ucsu.edu), IRGSP (http://rgp.dna.affrc.go.jp/IRGSP/), SilkDB (http://silkworm.genomics.org.cn/) and dictybase (http://dictybase.org/).

2. *Reference sequences.* GPCRDB (http://www.gpcr.org/7tm/) and NCBI (http://www.ncbi.nlm.nih.gov/), SwissProt/TrEMBL (http://www.expasy.org/sprot/).

3. *Motif and domain databases.* PROSITE (http://www.expasy.org/cgi-bin/nicesite) and PFAM (http://www.sanger.ac.uk/cgi-bin/Pfam/getacc).

4. *Sequence databases.* UniGene sequences and their expression profiles (http://www. ncbi. nlm. nih. gov/sites/entrez? db = unigene).

5. *Gene expression information.* (http://www. ncbi. nlm. nih. gov/sites/entrez? db = unigene).

3. Methods

3.1. SEVENS: A Comprehensive GPCR Database

From the viewpoint of comprehensive collection of GPCR gene sequences, currently available are such useful integrated GPCR databases as GPCRDB *(4)*, GPCR-PD™ *(5)*, and ORDB *(6)*. GPCRDB is the most popular and includes known GPCR sequences from Swiss-prot, TrEMBL, and GENBANK.

GPCR-PD™, a database for commercial purposes, accumulates literature information as well as sequences. ORDB focuses on the olfactory receptor, a GPCR subfamily. All of them are based on only GPCR genes that have been expressed and well characterized. However, to gain an overview of the GPCR universe, it is necessary to treat a large data space that includes not only expressed sequences but also newly identified sequences that cannot be detected by in vivo experiments, although they definitely exist on the genome sequence and are just waiting for the opportunity to express their functions. For this purpose, we introduce SEVENS database (http://sevens.cbrc.jp/) that summarizes GPCR genes that are comprehensively identified from genome sequences.

3.2. GPCR Sequence Collection

1. Genome sequences are downloaded from database (*see* **Subheading 2**, **item 1**).

2. Genomic regions where at least partial regions of known GPCR gene sequences (*see* **Subheading 2**, **item 2**) show hits with a significant score of TBLASTN are listed.

3. Around the hit regions, the full gene structure is reconstructed using the ALN program *(7)*. This program expands the alignment regions of a GPCR gene sequence along the upper and lower regions of genomic sequences by taking exon/intron boundary consensus into consideration.

4. When a stop codon is found at the exon region or a frame shift occurs by insertion or deletion, the gene is defined as a pseudogene (*see* **Note 1**).

5. Redundancies, which are overlaps at the same genomic position, were adjusted with the clustering method, in which sequences were merged together only when they showed hits for more than 50 amino acids with higher than 99% identity.

6. The identified amino acid sequences are subjected to an analyzing filter using items (*see* **Subheading 2**, **item 3**) of BLAST *(8)* for similarity search, HMMER for PFAM domain assignment *(9)*, an in-house program for PROSITE *(10)* pattern assignment, SOSUI *(11)*, and our original tool for predicting TMH regions, and DISOPRED2 *(12)* for predicting disorder regions. The threshold of each tools first assessed to evaluate sensitivity and specificity for the reference dataset (GPCRs and non-GPCRs in Swiss-prot/TrEMBL, *see* **Subheading 2**, **item 2**).

7. By combining these thresholds, we generate datasets of various qualities (Levels A, B, C, and D. *see* http://sevens.cbrc.jp/for details). The most accurate dataset (Level A, *see* **Note 4**) is obtained by "AND" combination of the threshold of sequence similarity search (E value $<10^{-80}$) and PFAM domain assignments (E value $< 10^{-10}$), and has 99.4% sensitivity and 96.6% specificity for known GPCR datasets.

8. We classify these sequences according to the score of significant hits (E value $< 10^{-30}$) to each subfamily of Swiss-Prot classification.

9. We also classify the sequences as known products when they show hits with known sequences with 96% similarity for more than 100 residues of the alignment regions. For sequences that do not satisfy this condition, we define them as novel ones (*see* **Note 1**).

10. For selected GPCR gene sequences the phylogenetic trees were constructed by using ClustalW *(13)* and TreeView *(14)* programs.

11. Expression information for genes was obtained by assigning them to the known information in Unigene (*see* **Subheading 2, item 5**).

12. Finally, GPCR gene sequences are summarized with the following annotations (a) novel judgment, (b) family information, (c) data level, (d) chromosome number, (e) genomic coordinate information, (f) exon number, (g) sequence length, (h) DNA sequence and protein sequence, (i) sequence search information, (j) TMH, motifs, and domain information, and (k) phylogenetic tree, (l) gene expression information.

13. Now, it compiles 34,250 (Level A) to 53,331 (Level D) GPCR genes from 34 eukaryote genomes (*see* **Note 3**). The total GPCR number is 1,000–2,000 in mammals (~50 subfamilies), several hundreds in fishes and birds (~50 subfamilies), approximately 300–400 in insects (~20 subfamilies) etc. **Table 1** lists the GPCR distribution in mammalian genomes, as an example.

3.3. Usage of SEVENS

1. SEVENS database is available for free at http://sevens.cbrc.jp/.

2. On the top page (**Fig. 2a**), selection of a representative genome navigates the user to the next page for search (the human genome is shown as an example).

3. At the upper part of the search page, the chromosomal viewer, the phylogenetic map button, and the content search area are shown. As an initial value, all GPCR genes of Level A are displayed at chromosomal map.

4. Clicking the phylogenetic map button links the user to the phylogenetic tree viewer of all GPCR genes of Level A. The branch color can be selected according to subfamily or chromosomal number.

5. By clicking "submit" bottun, after the "AND" combinations of several conditions, the content search area retrieve the selected GPCR genes that again appear on the chromosomal viewer, the phylogenetic tree viewer, and the lower scroll list page.

Table 1
Computationally identified GPCRs in mammal genomes

	hsap	ptro	rmac	etel	mmus	rnor	cpor	cfam	fcat	btau	lafr	dnov	oana	ggal	acar	xtro	drer	tnig	frub	olat	gacu
Odorant/olfactory and gustatory receptor	759	726	551	921	1272	1557	1022	1018	612	2058	3119	1812	467	321	133	1074	121	42	53	60	115
Chemokines and chemotactic factors receptor	34	31	32	24	36	38	23	27	24	27	18	17	23	18	21	33	54	23	26	38	35
Pheromone receptors	33	27	16	18	521	325	155	21	20	67	65	154	829	0	70	634	3	1	1	3	1
Family T1R receptors (taste receptors)	31	35	23	20	43	40	34	19	14	32	21	9	6	3	37	7	0	0	0	0	0
Adenosine and adenine nucleotide receptor	23	20	20	15	19	19	15	20	17	19	12	12	19	23	28	34	53	20	34	56	45
Serotonin receptor	14	13	14	7	12	12	8	12	9	15	9	5	9	13	12	14	24	16	15	16	16
Lysolipids receptor	11	9	13	8	11	10	6	11	10	12	8	5	7	9	12	13	16	13	16	14	16
Opsin	10	8	8	5	8	8	3	8	7	7	4	2	8	14	25	21	41	31	32	32	32
Adrenergic receptor	9	9	8	7	9	8	3	9	5	9	5	3	5	9	9	8	19	15	16	17	15
Prostanoids receptor	8	7	8	5	8	11	6	7	6	11	3	6	5	3	6	8	12	10	10	12	11
Trace amine receptor	8	8	7	19	16	19	27	4	8	42	14	8	4	4	3	6	125	35	21	34	61
Dopamine receptor	7	6	5	5	5	5	5	5	5	3	4	3	3	8	7	5	12	12	12	11	9
Somatostatin and urotensin receptor	6	6	6	3	6	6	6	5	4	5	5	1	5	9	9	10	16	11	13	12	11
Acetylcholine (muscarinic) receptor	5	5	5	4	5	5	4	5	4	5	2	4	3	4	4	5	5	10	8	8	8
Melanocortins receptor	5	5	5	4	5	5	3	5	4	6	3	2	5	4	4	5	6	4	4	4	4
Neuropeptide Y receptor	5	5	4	4	5	5	4	5	4	6	6	6	6	7	6	8	6	5	6	4	
Other receptor	5	5	5	0	6	6	1	5	2	4	0	3	2	9	10	9	13	8	7	9	10
Relaxin receptor	5	5	5	2	4	4	3	3	1	5	4	3	3	3	5	11	10	10	9	9	
Releasing hormones receptor	5	4	5	4	4	4	3	5	5	9	4	1	5	6	6	9	13	12	12	11	11
Histamine receptors	4	4	4	2	5	4	4	4	3	6	2	2	4	2	5	13	6	5	5	5	5
Opioid peptides receptor	4	3	4	3	4	4	2	4	4	4	3	3	4	4	4	4	6	6	6	4	6
Proteinase-activated receptor	4	4	4	3	4	3	1	4	3	4	2	3	3	5	5	3	7	16	8	7	6
Vasopressin / oxytocin receptor	4	3	4	3	4	4	1	4	4	3	3	3	4	5	5	8	7	7	7	7	
Bombesin receptor	3	3	3	0	3	3	2	3	2	3	1	1	3	3	3	3	2	2	3	4	3
Cysteinyl leukotriene receptor	3	3	3	2	3	3	3	2	3	3	1	2	3	3	2	3	7	3	3	5	4
Free fatty acid receptor	3	4	2	3	3	3	3	4	4	4	2	2	2	21	5	6	7	4	5	6	2
Glycoprotein hormone receptor	3	3	3	3	3	3	2	3	3	4	4	3	2	3	3	3	3	3	4	4	
Melanotonin receptor	3	3	3	0	3	3	2	3	2	5	1	1	3	3	4	6	7	4	4	4	4
Tachykinin receptor	3	3	3	0	3	2	1	3	1	3	2	0	0	3	3	2	6	5	5	6	4
Angiotensin receptor	2	2	2	1	3	3	0	2	2	2	2	1	2	2	4	3	2	2	3	2	
Bradykinin receptor	2	2	2	0	2	2	1	2	2	2	1	0	2	2	1	1	3	2	2	5	3
Cannabinoids receptor	2	2	2	2	2	2	0	2	2	1	1	2	2	2	2	2	3	3	3	3	3
Cholecystokinin / gastrin receptor	2	2	2	3	2	1	1	2	2	2	1	0	0	2	2	1	3	3	3	3	3
Endothelin receptor	2	2	2	0	2	1	0	2	2	2	1	2	3	3	3	4	5	5	5	5	
Krebs cycle intermediates receptor	2	2	2	0	2	2	0	2	2	2	1	2	3	3	5	4	2	2	4	2	
Melanin-concentrating hormone receptor	2	2	2	1	1	1	0	2	1	2	2	1	2	4	4	2	3	2	2		
Neuromedin U receptor	2	2	1	2	2	2	2	2	1	2	2	0	2	2	2	3	3	3	3	3	
Neuropeptide FF receptor	2	2	2	1	2	3	1	2	2	2	2	2	1	2	3	2	9	3	4	4	3
Neuropeptides B/W receptor	2	2	2	1	2	1	1	2	1	2	1	1	0	3	2	2	2	1	1	1	1
Neurotensin receptor	2	2	2	0	2	1	0	2	0	2	1	0	1	0	1	2	1	1	1	1	
Nicotinic acid receptor	2	2	1	2	1	1	1	1	1	1	1	0	0	2	4	5	7	5			
Orexins receptor	2	2	2	0	2	2	2	2	1	2	1	1	2	2	2	0	1	1	2		
Prokineticin receptor	2	2	2	2	2	2	1	2	2	2	1	1	1	2	2	1	2	3	2		
Adrenomedullin receptor	1	1	1	0	1	1	1	1	1	1	1	0	1	1	1	1	1	1			
Apelin receptor	1	1	1	2	1	1	1	1	0	1	1	1	2	2	1	3	3	3	3	3	
Arachidonyl glycine receptor	1	1	1	1	1	1	1	1	0	1	1	2	1	1	1	1	1	1	1		
Bile acid receptor	1	1	1	1	1	1	0	1	0	1	1	0	0	1	1	2	1	1	1	1	
Eicosanoid receptor	1	1	1	0	0	0	2	2	0	0	0	0	0	1	0	0	0	0			
Estrogen receptor	1	1	1	1	1	1	1	1	1	1	0	1	1	1	1	2	2	2	2		
Family OA	1	1	1	0	1	1	1	0	1	0	0	1	0	1	2	0	1	1			
Insect chemosensory receptor	1	0	0	0	0	0	0	0	0	1	0	0	0	0	0	0	0	0	0	0	
Kisspeptins receptor	1	1	1	0	1	1	0	1	0	1	0	0	2	1	3	2	1	1	2	1	
Neuropeptide S receptor	1	1	1	0	0	1	0	1	0	1	0	0	1	0	0	0	0	0			
Platelet-activating factor receptor	1	1	1	1	1	1	0	1	0	1	1	0	2	1	2	2	2	4	2		
Family 2 (B) receptor	62	58	54	26	55	48	21	59	33	58	28	19	39	41	39	55	86	55	63	71	67
Family 3 (C) receptor (metabotropic glutamate)	26	25	23	26	23	22	17	22	24	26	18	15	23	17	25	151	97	50	64	65	67
Family fz/smo receptor	11	11	11	8	11	10	6	11	7	16	9	6	10	12	10	11	15	15	14	14	14
UNKNOWN	27	23	17	7	57	23	19	14	6	17	16	19	185	4	33	100	84	60	60	62	49
Novel by Our definition	24	89	87	936	229	102	696	345	686	264	1691	1147	362								
Pseudo gene	386	372	260	281	304	416	725	209	162	810	1755	1024	536								
Total	1265	1203	1000	1232	2320	2334	1466	1438	931	2606	3470	2191	1777								

hsap Human, *ptro* Chimpanzee, *rmac* Rhesus, *etel* Lesser hedgehog tenrec
mmus Mouse, *rnor* Rat, *cpor* Guinea pig, *cfam* Dog, *fcat* Cat, *btau* Cow, *lafr* Elephant,
dnov Armadillo, *oana* Platypus.

6. Selection of a query gene from these regions (the chromosomal viewer or the phylogenetic tree vewer or the lower
list page) navigates the user to the page for gene annotation
information.

7. At the upper part of this page (**Fig. 2b**) is a chromosomal
viewer that provides gene coordinate information of a selected

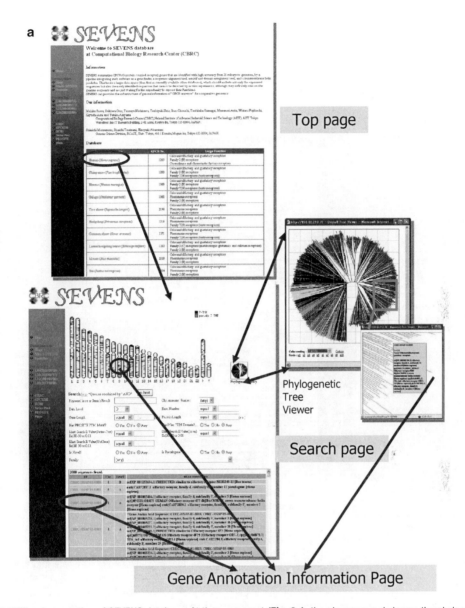

Fig. 2. WEB representation of SEVENS database. At the upper part **(Fig. 2a)**, the chromosomal viewer, the phylogenetic map button, and the content search boxes are shown. Using the "AND" combinations of several conditions, the content search boxes retrieve GPCR genes. Selection of a query gene from these viewers or the list table navigates the user to the gene annotation information page.

gene indicated with other GPCR genes on the board where background color changes according to the GC content of the genome sequence.

8. The lower part shows information of selected protein sequence. The small table shows the results of sequence search against UNIPROT(Swiss-prot/TrEMBL), nr.aa, and UniGene database (*see* **Subheading 2**, **items 2** and **4**) using BLAST.

b

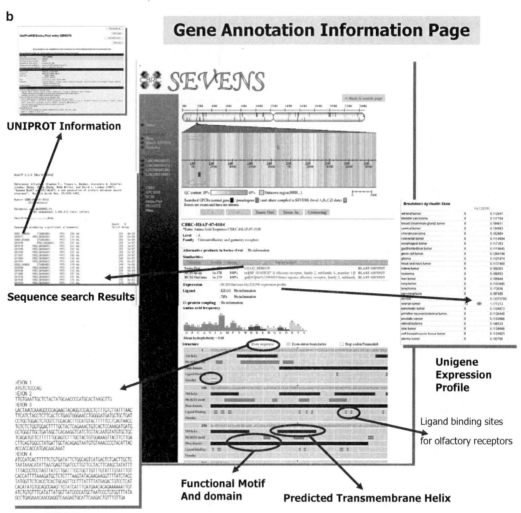

UNIPROT Information

Sequence search Results

DNA Sequence

Functional Motif And domain

Predicted Transmembrane Helix

Unigene Expression Profile

Ligand binding sites

for olfactory receptors

Predicted Disorder regions

Fig. 2. (continued) On this page **(Fig. 2b)** is a chromosomal viewer that provides gene coordinate information of a selected gene (*red*) indicated with other GPCR genes. The middle part indicates sequence similarity of genes and experimental information, such as alternative products, gene expression profiles, binding ligands, and G-proteins. The lower "Structure" part shows the results of structural analysis. Along the protein sequence, exon/intron boundaries, stop codon/frame shift positions (for pseudogenes), and structural features: TMH (*red*), PROSITE motif pattern (*green*), PFAM domain (*blue*), and predicted disorder regions (*gray*) are indicated. When the sequence is an odorant receptor, ligand-binding sites (*sky blue*) are also displayed.

9. We can observe experimental evidence of alternative products, profiles, binding ligands, and G-proteins.

10. The description in Expression category links to experimental evidence of gene expression in the NCBI Unigene expression profile (*see* **Subheading 2, item 5**).

11. Amino acid frequency of the selected receptor is shown as the graph.

12. The lower "Structure" part shows the results of structural analysis. Along the protein sequence, exon/intron boundaries (yellow squares), stop codon/frame shift positions (for pseudogenes), and structural features: TMH (red), PROSITE motif (green), PFAM domain (blue), and predicted disorder regions (gray), are indicated. Furthermore, ligand-binding sites (sky blue) are displayed if odorant receptors are selected.

13. Each exon appears as a DNA sequence when the *"Exon Sequence"* button is clicked.

14. Each piece of colored bars is directly linked to tools (*see* **Subheading 2**, **item 2**) or related databases (*see* **Subheading 2, item 3**)

3.4. GRIFFIN: Software for Predicting GPCR Behavior

For in-silico functional prediction, the established way involves classifying protein sequences into functional groups whose members are linked by sequence similarity, by using a conventional sequence search method. However, in the case of GPCR, the "function-similarity" relationship is unclear. For example, (a) homologous GPCR pairs that have the same ligands sometimes bind to different G-proteins; (b) GPCR pairs that bind the same G-protein sometimes have different ligands; and (c) GPCR pairs sometimes bind the same ligand and the same G-protein, although those pairs show less than 25% sequence similarity *(15)*. Given this situation, various computational methods have been developed by using not simple sequence search but more powerful methods, such as the Hidden Markov Model (HMM), the machine learning classifier (support vector machine (SVM)), and other statistical analyses. These methods are divided into two main branches: classification of GPCRs by ligand type *(16–21)* and that by G-protein type *(22–24)*. We have developed a unique program called GRIFFIN *(3)* to predict GPCR–G-protein coupling specificity from ligand information as well as the GPCR sequence. The main part of GRIFFIN includes a hierarchical combination of SVM classifier with feature vectors obtained from the physical properties of ligand, GPCR, and G-protein. This part is useful for the classification of Family 1(A) (Class A), the major family. While, for opsin and olfactory subfamilies of Class A and other minor families (Family 2(B), Family 3(C), fz/smo receptors), binding G-protein kind is predicted with high accuracy by HMM. Applying this system to known GPCR sequences, each binding G-protein is predicted with high sensitivity and specificity (more than 87% on average). We believe that GRIFFIN will contribute immensely to the research of functional assignment of orphan GPCRs and to the design of experimental systems for drug screening.

3.5. Usage of GRIFFIN

1. GRIFFIN is available for free at http://griffin.cbrc.jp/ (**Fig. 3a**).

2. Input the sequence and it's name into the first two boxes.

3. Three small text boxes that appear at the bottom of the page are for the user to enter the range of ligand molecular weight (onset, termination, and differential values) in a left-to-right fashion.

4. Of course, the user can also predict the type of G-protein by entering only one value of ligand molecular weight.

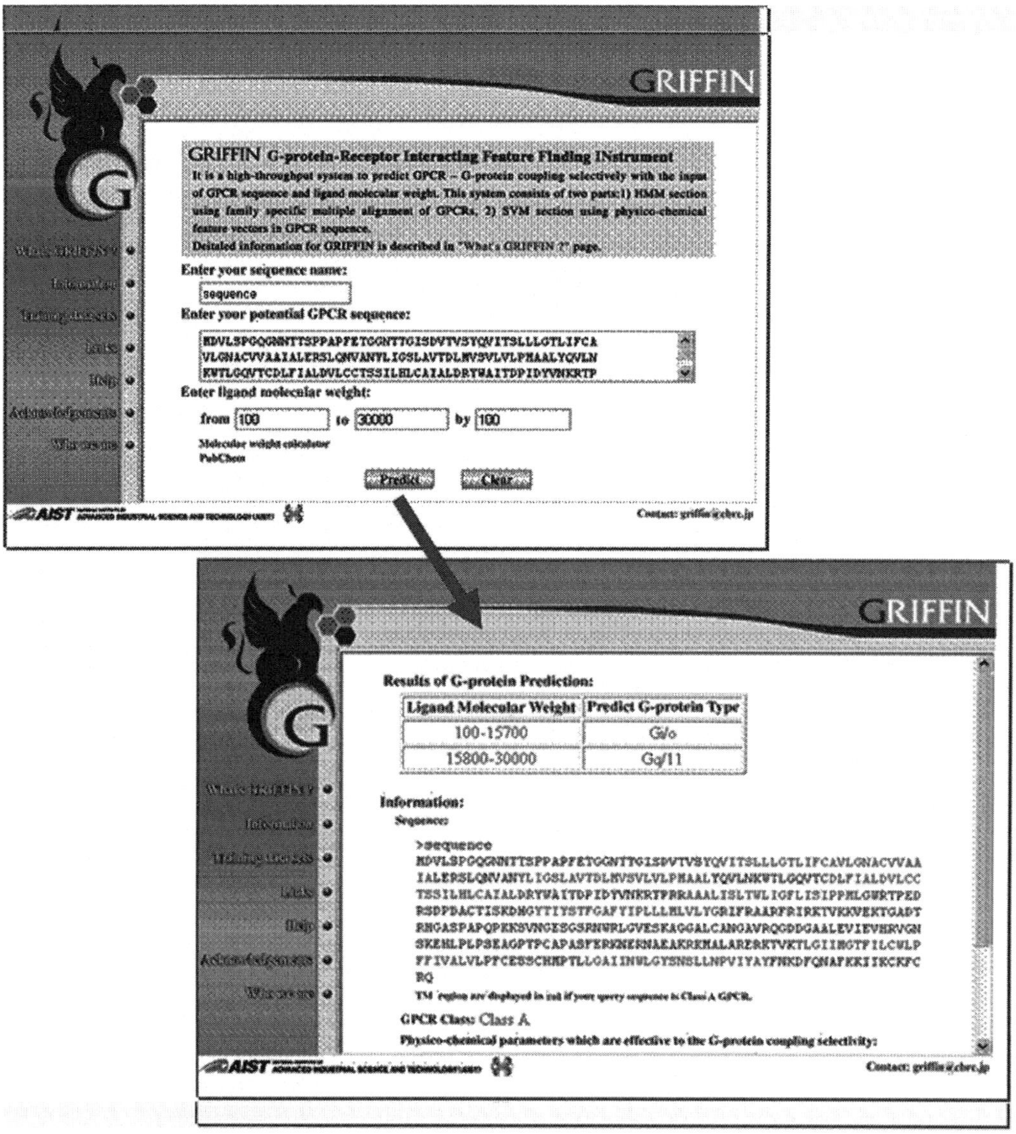

Fig. 3. WEB representation of GRIFFIN, which allows the user to predict G-protein binding selectivity by entering GPCR sequence and ligand molecular weight.

5. The molecular weight calculater bottun or PubChem bottun shows the information of specific ligands.

6. By changing the range of ligand molecular weight, the user can perform computational experiments to monitor G-protein binding of orphan receptors whose ligands are still unknown (*see* **Note 8**). For example, **Fig. 3** shows the result when a wide molecular weight range (from 100 to 30,000 by 100 MW) is entered; this query sequence changes between coupling G-proteins $G_{i/o}$ and $G_{q/11}$.

7. At the result page, the query sequence is displayed with TMH regions in red, when the query GPCR belongs to Class A family.

8. In addition, feature vector elements and their scores, which are calculated in the prediction process, are displayed in a table.

3.6. Application of SEVENS and GRIFFIN to Reverse Chemical Genomics

Figure 4 shows the flow of GPCR gene analysis for the purpose of supporting the reverse chemical genomics approach.

1. GPCR genes were collected from SEVENS database, in which genes are classified into the 57 known GPCR subfamilies, or into orphan or unknown receptor families. **Table 1** shows the example case of family distribution in mammal GPCRs.

2. Since GRIFFIN requires sequence and ligand size as input information, we apply this program to all GPCR sequences

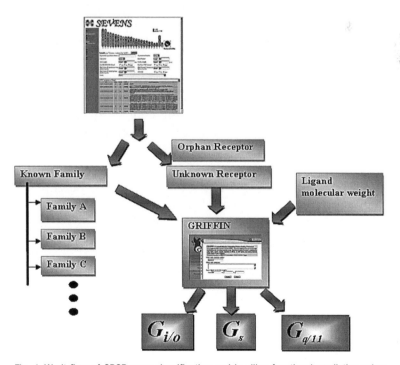

Fig. 4. Work flow of GPCR gene classification and in-silico functional prediction using SEVENS and GRIFFIN, to support reverse chemical genomics.

and monitor G-protein binding type by changing ligand size from small (molecular weight of several hundreds order) to large (molecular weight of 10,000 order).

3. In the case of human, 1,265 GPCR genes (879 normal genes and 386 pseudogenes) are compiled in Level A datasets (*see* **Note 3**). Of the 879 normal GPCR genes, there are 83 orphan receptors and 27 unknown receptors.

4. The distribution of predicted binding G-proteins by GRIF-FIN, when ligand molecular weight is fixed to several hundred order), is 66.6% G_s, 21% $G_{q/11}$, 6.7% $G_{i/o}$, and 5.5% other types, such as fz/smo family. The 110 genes (27 unknown receptors + 83 orphan receptors) are classified and it is predicted that 60 belong to G_s protein binding type, 38 to $G_{q/11}$ binding type, and 12 to $G_{i/o}$ binding type.

5. For GPCR gene sequences predicted to be the $G_{q/11}$ binding type, we choose them as candidates for experimental analysis, because this type controls intracellular calcium content, enabling us to monitor GPCR activity more easily.

4. Notes

1. In the case of computational gene identification, the pseudogenes is judged from only information of stop codon and frame shift on the protein coding regions. Therefore, we cannot identify such pseudogenes that are caused with abnormal regulatory region.

2. In the case of computational gene identification, the criteria of novel sequence is based on analysis of recent reference databases. However it is required to redefine the criteria with every update opportunity of reference datasets.

3. As regards the comprehensive GPCR gene analysis of individual genomes, many publications, including those of insect, plant, human, and mouse, are available. It seems that the GPCR gene number collected by our pipeline is somewhat larger than previous studies.

4. Our data must be sufficiently accurate because our pipeline can predict GPCR genes from known sequences with 99.4% sensitivity and 96.6% selectivity. Because these dataset is the most accurate one (Level A), the statistical description in this chapter is based on this dataset.

5. Therefore, using SEVENS database, it is possible to cover the GPCR universe by including a larger number of accurate GPCR genes than that of previous studies.

6. Currently, additional information (tertiary structure, gene regulatory regions, etc.) is required for SEVENS database.

7. Since the amount of genome sequence is rapidly increasing, such additional information will be included in the database with every update opportunity of increasing species of genome sequences.

8. For all GPCRs compiled in SEVENS database, we are planning to create G-protein selectivity profiles according to information of various number of ligands (>several million).

9. In current GRIFFIN, only molecular weight is used as a descriptor of ligands. However, in order to increase prediction accuracy, it is required to describe ligand by using larger numbers of physical properties. To accomplish this, we intend to modify GRIFFIN in the near feature.

Acknowledgment

This work was supported by a Grant-in-Aid for special projects in genome science from the Ministry of Education Culture, Sports, Science, and Technology of Japan. We would like to thank Dr. Wataru Fujibuchi, Dr. Takatsugu Hirokawa, Mr. Yukimitsu Yabuki, and Mr. Tatsuya Nishizawa for helpful discussion in the course of SEVENS and GRIFFIN development.

References

1. Drews, J. (1996) Genomic sciences and the medicine of tomorrow. *Nat Biotechnol* **14**, 1516–1518.

2. Ono, Y., Fujibuchi, W. and Suwa, M. (2005) Automatic gene collection system for Genome-Scale overview of G-protein coupled receptors in Eukaryotes. *Gene* **364**, 63–73.

3. Yabuki, Y., Muramatsu, T., Hirokawa, T., Mukai, H. and Suwa, M. (2005) GRIFFIN: a system for predicting GPCR–G-protein coupling selectivity using support vector machines and a hidden Markov model. *Nucleic Acid Res* **33**, W 148–W153.

4. Horn, F., Vriend, G. and Cohen, F. E. (2001) Collecting and harvesting biological data: the GPCRDB and Nuclear DB information systems. *Nucleic Acids Res* **29**, 346–349.

5. Hodges, P. E., et al. (2002) Annotating the human proteome: the Human Proteome Survey Database (HumanPSD™) and an in-depth target database for G protein-coupled receptors

(GPCR-PD) from Incyte Genomics. *Nucl Acids Res* **30**, 137–141.

6. Crasto, C. et al. (2002) Olfactory Receptor Database: a metadata-driven automated population from sources of gene and protein sequences. *Nucl Acids Res* **30**, 354–360.

7. Gotoh, O. (2000) Homology-based gene structure prediction: simplified matching algorithm using a translated codon (tron) and improved accuracy by allowing for long gaps. *Bioinformatics* **16**, 190–202.

8. Altschul, S. F., et al. (1997). Gapped BLAST and PSI-BLAST: a new generation of protein database search programs. *Nucleic Acids Res* **25**, 3389–3402.

9. Bateman, A., Birney, E., Durbin, R., Eddy, S. R., Howe, K. L. and Sonnhammer, E. L. (2000) The Pfam protein families' database. *Nucleic Acids Res* **28**, 263–266.

10. Hulo, N., Bairoch, A., Bulliard, V., Cerutti, L., Cuche, B. A., de Castro, E., Lachaize, C.,

Langendijk-Genevaux, P. S. and Sigrist, C. J. (2008) The 20 years of PROSITE. *Nucleic Acids Res* **36**, D245–9.

11. Hirokawa, T., Boon-Chieng, S. and Mitaku, S. (1998) SOSUI: classification and secondary structure prediction system for membrane proteins. *Bioinformatics* **14**, 378–379.

12. Ward JJ, Sodhi JS, McGuffin LJ, Buxton BF and Jones DT (2004) Prediction and functional analysis of native disorder in proteins from the three kingdoms of life *J Mol Biol* **337**, 635–645.

13. Larkin MA, Blackshields G, Brown NP, Chenna R, McGettigan PA, McWilliam H, Valentin F, Wallace IM, Wilm A, Lopez R (2007) Clustal W and Clustal X version 2.0. *Bioinformatics* **23**, 2947–2948.

14. Page, RD, (1996) TREEVIEW: An application to display phylogenetic trees on personal computers. *Comput Appl Biosci* **12**, 357–358.

15. Gaulton, A. and Attwood, T. K. (2003) Bioinformatics approaches for the classification of G-protein-coupled receptors. *Curr Opin Pharmacol* **3**, 114–120.

16. Karchin, R., Karplus, K. and Haussler, D. (2002) Classifying G-protein coupled receptors with support vector machines. *Bioinformatics* **18**, 147–159.

17. Bhasin, M. and Raghava, G.P. S. (2004) GPCRpred: an SVM-based method for prediction of families and subfamilies of G-protein coupled receptors. *Nucleic Acid Res* **32**, 383–389.

18. Lapnish, M., Gutcaits, A., Prusis, P., Post, C., Lundstedt, T. and Wikberg, J. E. S. (2002) Classification of G-protein coupled receptors by alignment-independent extraction of principle chemical properties of primary amino acid sequences. *Protein Sci* **11**, 795–805.

19. Huang, Y., Cai, J., Ji, L. and Li, Y. (2004) Classifying G-protein coupled receptors with bagging classification tree. *Comput. Biol. Chem* **28**, 275–280.

20. Qian, B., Soyer, O. S., Neubig, R. R. and Goldstein, R. A. (2003) Depicting a protein's two faces: GPCR classification by phylogenetic tree-based HMMs. *FEBS Lett* **554**, 95–99.

21. Attwood, T. K., Croning, M. D. R. and Gaulton, A. (2001) Deriving structural and functional insights from a ligand-based hierarchical classification of G protein-coupled receptors. *Protein Eng* **15**, 7–12.

22. Cao, J., Panetta, R., Yue, S., Steyaert, A., Young-Bellido, M. and Ahmad, S. (2003) A naive Bayes model to predict coupling between seven transmembrane domain receptors and G-proteins. *Bioinformatics* **19**, 234–240.

23. Möller, S., Vilo, J. and Croning, M. D. R. (2001) Prediction of the coupling specificity of G protein coupled receptors to their G proteins. *Bioinformatics* **17**, 174–181.

24. Sreekumar, K. R., Huang, Y., Pausch, M. H. and Gulukota, K. (2004) Predicting GPCR–G-protein coupling using hidden Markov models. *Bioinformatics* **20**, 3490–3499.

Chapter 5

High-Performance Gene Expression Module Analysis Tool and Its Application to Chemical Toxicity Data

Wataru Fujibuchi, Hyeryung Kim, Yoshifumi Okada, Takeaki Taniguchi, and Hideko Sone

Summary

Gene clustering is one of the main themes of data mining approaches in bioinformatics. Although it has the power to analyze gene function, interpretation of the results becomes increasingly difficult when the number of experiments (samples) exceeds hundreds or more. A new type of clustering called "biclustering," where genes and experiments are coclustered in a large-scale of gene expression data, has been extensively studied in the last decade. We have developed "SAMURAI," an original program that detects all the biclusters or "gene modules" whose genes have similar expression patterns to query profile using the ultrafast data mining algorithm called Linear-time Closed itemset Miner (LCM). Using chemical toxicity dataset from J&J rat liver experiments, we compiled an exhaustive dictionary of gene modules by searching datasets of gene modules with each chemical exposure experiment as query. Through the module analysis, we found that our program can detect up/down-regulated gene sets that significantly represent particular GO functions or KEGG pathways, thereby unraveling reactions and mechanisms common to different toxicochemical treatments of hepatocytes.

Key words: Gene expression module, Biclustering, Chemical toxicity, Data mining, Linear time common itemset miner, Common reaction and mechanism

1. Introduction

Microarrays or other high-throughput gene expression analysis systems provide extensive information on gene expression differences under various experimental conditions, such as cell type, developmental stage, and reaction to stimulus. Recent easy access to such experimental techniques has promoted the accumulation of gene expression data in public gene expression data

Hisashi Koga (ed.), *Reverse Chemical Genetics*, Methods in Molecular Biology, vol. 577
DOI 10.1007/978-1-60761-232-2_5, © Humana Press, a part of Springer Science+Business Media, LLC 2009

repositories, such as GEO and ArrayExpress *(1, 2)*. Among available tools to analyze such large-scale data, a promising method called "biclustering" *(3)* has emerged and has been widely studied *(4–9)* for its ability to mine datasets containing hundreds of experiments. Biclustering detects common gene expression patterns or "gene expression motifs" that are represented in any combination of experiments. A subset of genes that contain a common expression pattern in a subset of experiments is called a "gene module."

We have developed a high-performance biclustering method that has high calculation speed and high biological evaluation accuracy. Our biclustering system called "SAMURAI (System for Assembling Modules by Ultra Rapid Algorithm on Itemsets)" *(10)* can search thousands of microarray data for gene modules in several seconds in most cases. In addition, the detected gene modules show surprisingly high accuracy of matching to known gene function groups in the study of 2,988 disease microarray data provided by the Critical Assessment of Microarray Data Analysis meeting *(11)*. Here we applied this system to a chemical toxicity dataset obtained from J&J rat liver experiments and compiled an exhaustive dictionary of gene modules by searching the dataset with each chemical exposure experiment as query. From the resultant gene modules, we found that there are a total of 92,100 modules of which 10,805 (11.7%) represent known functions (GO or KEGG) at a high significance threshold ($p < 1e – 5.5$ and $p < 1e – 4$, respectively).

2. Materials and Methods

To obtain and analyze gene modules from large-scale gene expression data, we first normalize and convert them into a unified file format. After obtaining formatted data, we discretize them to certain degrees of expression to find common expression patterns in a limited search space. Then, to reduce search space effectively and to detect gene modules in real time, we perform "query-and-database" search. In this approach, given query gene expression data by a user, all of the discretized values not common to the query in the database are erased, thus reducing database size extensively. This process is critical to the calculation of the following module detection process, giving exhaustive (not partial) results.

After fully reducing search space by discretizing and erasing data unrelated to query, we perform rapid data mining where common gene expression patterns that are preserved in all combinations of (maximum) experiments are exhaustively retrieved.

However, the gene modules retrieved in this step have rigid patterns with no relaxation (i.e., noise), which contrasts to real data containing noise and biological flexibility. Thus, in the next step, these "core modules" are compared with each other and merged into bigger modules containing noise. As the final output, we obtain each module consisting of a subset of genes and a subset of experiments. By scrutinizing both gene functions and experimental relationships in each module, we can formulate new and interesting hypotheses on gene functions and experimental groups.

2.1. Rat Chemical Exposure Dataset and Normalization

1. Download gene expression data of chemical effects on rat liver by J & J from the Web site: http://cebs.niehs.nih.gov/. To retrieve the data, select the subject "J&J Hepatotoxicant Library" in the "Display All Studies" page or limit data by the organization name "Johnson and Johnson" in the "Study Characteristics" page. There are 133 toxicochemical groups containing 964 microarray experiments. Go to "View Selected Microarray Data by Studies/Experiments" from the bottom of page, select the dataset, and go to "View Details about Selected Experiment(s)." Then, download microarray data files after entering "Click to Download" page. As the file size is 117.3 MB, downloading will take 5 min to hours depending on the user's network conditions.

2. Unzip downloaded files and select files to analyze. In this study, we select only experiments that have both chemical exposure done and control data collected on the same day. The number of such experiments is 298. Among 9,215 probes in the dataset, we delete low-abundance genes that show no expression in all of the 298 experiments and select only 7,614 probes. Every pair of gene expression values is transformed into log-fold-change abundance by subtracting control values from the chemical exposure after taking $\log_2$ and subtracting the median value in each array (*see* **Note 1**). Finally, the log-fold-change values are normalized to Z-score by $(x - \text{mean})/\text{SD}$.

3. To perform gene functional analysis in later process, check if each probe has a link to UniGene database. Only 5,832 probes have links to UniGene database. Then, to remove probe redundancies, take the average if multiple probes correspond to the same UniGene ID. As a result, we obtain 2,497 averaged probes that have links to UniGene database for 298 chemical exposure experiments.

2.2. Formatting Database by Discretization

1. Convert normalized dataset into rank-ordered discrete data within each experiment. To do this, select one experiment and sort genes by expression value. Then, put all the genes into 10,000 bins of the same size and assign every gene a rank value equal to the number of bins (1st–10,000th from low to high) that it belongs to.

2. Select one gene and make a distribution of rank values for all the 298 experiments. Then, set a discretization parameter and thresholds. In this study, we set the degree of discretization at 3 (±1, 0) and the thresholds at 3% or 5% from each side of top and bottom (i.e., 6% or 10% in total) in rank value distribution. Using these parameters, we assign discrete values to rank values.

2.3. Query Data and Database Compression

1. Given query gene expression data, discretize gene expression values using the same procedure as that employed in the above database formatting process. Use the same degree and thresholds to discretize query data as that used in the database discretization.

2. Compare discretized query to discretized database at the gene level. Then, delete all discrete values that differ from the query in the database. In addition, delete all zero values in the database. This procedure compresses the database to an extremely small size (*see* **Note 2**).

2.4. LCM for Data Mining of Core Gene Modules

1. LCM *(12, 13)* is an ultrafast algorithm for data mining that has been used to retrieve maximum common itemsets from a large list of itemsets called a transaction database (*see* **Note 3**). To apply this algorithm, assign item names to all the existing combinations of gene names and discrete values in the gene expression database. For example, we give item names "a – 1" and "a – 2" to the case that gene "a" has values of both "–1" and "–2" in the database. This procedure converts each gene expression experiment datum into an itemset list that symbolizes gene expression status consisting of gene names and their discrete values.

2. Write itemset list to a file in the format of one experiment in one line. Then, download the LCM program from the Web site: http://research.nii.ac.jp/~uno/codes.htm. Run the LCM program with the itemset list file with parameters of minimum size of gene modules to extract: *m* genes × *n* experiments. For example, the input command to run LCM on a Linux machine is: % lcm CqI –l *m* [input_file] *n* [output_file] (*see* **Note 3**).

2.5. Merging Redundant Modules

1. Raw gene modules (core modules) extracted by LCM are expected to be highly redundant. To reduce almost the same or quite similar gene modules in output data, merge them if they meet conditions specified by the following procedure. First, sort gene modules by size. Then, select the largest module and merge it with other modules one by one from large to small ones. Suppose we are merging modules A and B. If A and B share genes g1 and g2 and experiments e1 and e2 but A has another gene g3 and B has another experiment e3, the merged module will have genes g1, g2, and g3 and experiments e1, e2,

and e3 by adding missing gene (g3) and experiment (e3) to B and A, respectively. However, if any gene or experiment of the merged module contains inconsistent values, such as missing or different discrete values, the percentages of inconsistencies in each line and row of the merged module should be checked. If the inconsistency in every line and row is less than the threshold (in this study, 0.4 and 0.5 are adopted), execute the merge and replace the larger module with it. (Delete the smaller one.) Repeat this "check and merge" process for this larger module until it reaches the smallest one.

2. Repeat the above "check and merge" process from the next largest module to the smallest module. Once the smallest module is reached, sort the modules by size again and perform "check and merge" from the largest module to the smallest one for a new list of modules.

3. Repeat the above "sort, check, and merge" until no merge happens. Then, output the final (merged) modules to a file (*see* **Note 4**). The whole process from formatting data to merging modules is illustrated in **Fig. 1**. Here an example of two degrees (high and low expressions, or +1 and −1) of discretization is shown.

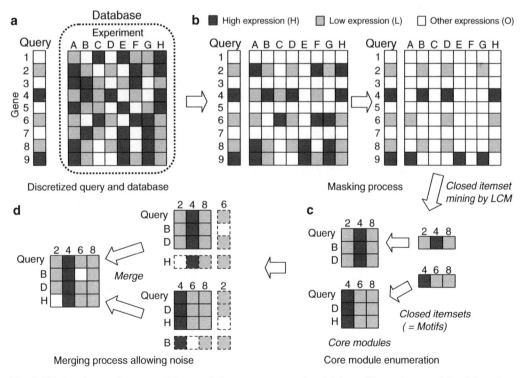

Fig. 1. Whole scheme of gene module search from gene expression database. The system consists of four steps (**a**) discretization of query and database, (**b**) database masking, (**c**) enumeration of core modules, and (**d**) module merging. In this example, the query and the database are discretized into only three degrees "High (+1)," "Low (−1)," and "Other expressions (O)".

2.6. Evaluation by GO and KEGG

Once the final set of modules is obtained, it is necessary to check the biological validities of those modules to verify if the selected parameters (discretization degree, noise threshold, module size, etc.) work properly. To approach this, compare each gene module with known biological functions or pathways to investigate if genes in a single module are statistically "enriched" for a particular category of functions. Here we describe the method of performing categorical enrichment analysis based on Gene Ontology (GO) functions and KEGG biological pathways.

1. Download necessary files from two FTP sites (a) gene2unigene and gene2go.gz files from ftp://ftp.ncbi.nlm.nih.gov/gene/DATA/ for gene name conversion and GO term information, respectively; and (b) gene_map.tab for KEGG pathway map index information and rno_gene_map.tab files for rat specific pathway gene list from ftp://ftp.genome.ad.jp/pub/kegg/pathway/.

2. Take one gene expression module. Convert UniGene IDs into EntrezGene IDs via the cross-reference list in gene2unigene file (*see* **Note 5**).

3. Assign GO function terms to the converted (Entrez-) genes. Obtain four parameters (a) U, the number of EntrezGenes found in the input gene expression data (2,497 UniGenes); (b) M, the number of EntrezGenes assigned to each GO term; (c) k, the number of EntrezGenes in each gene module; and (d) m, the number of EntrezGenes in each GO term found in each module.

4. Assign KEGG pathway map names to the converted (Entrez-) genes. Obtain the four parameters for each pathway map in the same way as the GO terms.

5. Evaluate each GO term and KEGG pathway map names for each gene module with standard hypergeometric distribution statistics by giving m as positives out of k samples and M known positives among the total population of U. To critically assess p value threshold, shuffle gene names (UniGene IDs) in the input dataset and do the same statistical analysis for each module, and use them as a null-distribution model.

6. The numbers of extracted modules for 298 query chemicals under two different discretization thresholds (3% and 5%) are summarized in **Table 1**. Two different noise ratios in the module merging process are also tested in both data.

2.7. Analysis of Common Reactions Among Chemicals by Gene Modules

The main objective in gene module analysis of reverse chemical genomics is to find new functional relationships between different chemicals. Once a set of gene modules annotated by GO and KEGG is obtained, check the common function names for every combination of query chemicals with a significant p value threshold.

Table 1
Numbers of obtained modules under various parameter conditions

Discretization	Noise ratio	
	0.4	0.5
3%	2,859	2,088
5%	92,100	61,852

1. First, assign p values to each gene module by GO and KEGG categorical enrichment analysis as described in **2.6**. Choose the most significant (the smallest) p value among various functional candidates for a single gene module. Then, plot each module by its (–log) p value, as shown in **Fig. 2a**.

2. Plot the same module in which gene IDs are shuffled by its p value, as shown in **Fig. 2b**. Compare the two plots. Set the p value threshold at the critical point where raw modules are still observed but gene-shuffled modules disappear. Here, we arbitrarily choose 1e – 5.5 and 1e – 4 as the thresholds for GO and KEGG, respectively, for the modules extracted by the parameters of 5% discretization and 0.4 of noise ratio.

3. Take every pair of query chemicals and check if they share common function or pathway names at the above threshold. Store the results.

4. Find biological hypotheses that can explain the obtained relationships among two or more chemicals. For example, in our data, some modules obtained from a query of Benzbromarone are found to affect the pathway of "Biosynthesis of unsaturated fatty acids." This pathway was also found with queries of Fenbufen, Clofibrate, and Dichloroacetate. Three genes are involved in the obtained modules: acyl-CoA thioesterase 3 (Rn.11326), acyl-CoA thioesterase 7 (Rn.6024), and acyl-Coenzyme A oxidase 1, palmitoyl (Rn.31796), all of which are important in unsaturated fatty acid metabolism. This result and information from literature suggest that these chemicals could affect the rat liver in a similar manner that is related to carcinogenesis via PPARα-derived oxidative reaction. **Figure 3b** is an example of the graphical output of these modules produced by the web-based GUI version of the SAMURAI system.

2.8. Usage of SAMURAI System

To enhance the above analysis in a coordinated way, we have developed a gene module extraction and evaluation system called SAMURAI. The free trial version of the program coded in java/ C++/Perl is available from http://samurai.cbrc.jp/download/ SAMURAI-Progressive/ (*see* **Note 6**). Here we describe briefly the usage of the system.

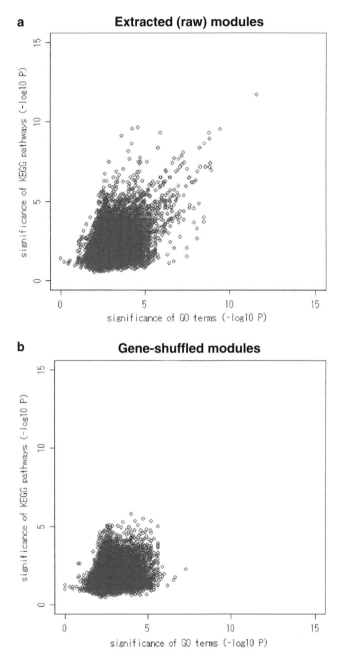

Fig. 2. Analysis of significant gene modules by GO and KEGG function groups. Each gene module (with 5% discretization threshold and 0.4 noise ratio) is evaluated with GO terms and KEGG pathway maps based on hypergeometric distribution statistics and plotted by the most significant *p* values. A total of 92,100 obtained gene modules are plotted in (**a**), and the same gene modules in which their gene ids are shuffled are plotted in (**b**). *p* values are dramatically increased due to randomness in (**b**). There is a significant correlation between *p* values of GO and KEGG in only (**a**). We arbitrarily choose $1e-5.5$ and $1e-4$ as the threshold for GO and KEGG, respectively.

1. Download SAMURAI program from the above site. Select SAMURAI-P program. Uncompress and untar the frozen file on your Linux machine. Go to the expanded directory and type "make compile" to compile all the programs in the system.

2. Transform your gene expression dataset into the "CellMontage" format *(14)* where a gene expression profile consists of a single description line, starting with ">," followed by one or more data lines. The data consist of elements separated by a space or a new line. Each element consists of a UniGene identifier and an expression value separated by a colon. See **Fig. 3a** for example data.

a

An example of partial profile in CellMontage format, where only three genes and their expression values are shown.

```
>Clofibrate_600mg_HybGrpOA2
Rn.98209:0.26226233    Rn.53257:0.550381825
Rn.94195:-0.285033381
```

A gene expression profile consists of a single description line, starting with ">", followed by one or more data lines. The data consist of elements, separated by a space or a new line. Each element consists of a UniGene identifier and an expression value separated by a colon.

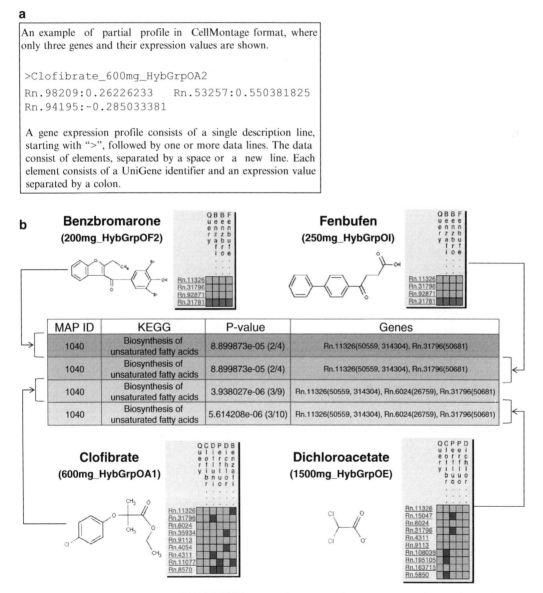

Fig. 3. Examples of input and output of SAMURAI-GUI system. An example of analysis with queries tnts (**a**) the CellMontage format as input and (**b**) graphical output of modules that share common biological function. Four example modules are searched by Benzbromarone, Fenbufen, Clofibrate, and Dichloroacetate. KEGG pathway functions for each module with the first and the second most significant *p* values are only shown.

3. Format data as described in **2.2** "Formatting Database by Discretization." Use the "formatdb" command. To discretize your data with the thresholds, as exemplified in **2.2**, type "%formatdb dataset_file 0.03 (or 0.05)." This command takes a while and creates both the discretized data "dataset_file.db" and its gene index file "dataset_file.idx."

4. Run the LCM algorithm to extract core modules and merge them by typing: "% java –Xmx2000m xSamurai –M –i dataset_file.idx –d dataset_file.db –q query_file –n noise_threshold –s minimum_module –r result_dir."

    The query_file must also be written in the CellMontage format. The "noise_threshold" must be in the range of [0,1]. The "minimum_module" parameter sets the minimum size of gene modules to output. The "result_dir" parameter indicates the directory to write the results of final gene modules.

5. To perform module evaluations with GO and KEGG, execute the command: "%EA = GO_KEGG_test GO_KEGG_test/ assignKEGG.pl dataset_file.idx P result_dir/*."

    The "GO_KEGG_test" is the directory for GO/KEGG evaluation package (*see* **Note** 7).

6. The GUI-based web version for multi-CPU calculation and module visualization in color is also available from a commercial site. To view free test results, visit: http://samurai.cbrc.jp/ and try the "Module search from a large-scale database" Web page (*again, see* **Note 6**).

---

3. Notes

1. Actually, the purpose of subtracting median values and *Z*-transformation in each data is only to improve visualization; they do not change the results as the following discretization process is based on rank values.

2. With an average query that represents only 10% of its discrete values are active (up- or down-regulated) genes, it is estimated that the database will be reduced to $(0.05 \times 0.05 \times 2 =)$ 0.5% of its original size.

3. LCM program usually takes several seconds to finish, but sometimes takes several minutes. A faster program is currently available from the developers' Web site.

4. Many versions of merging processes are available. For example, implementing merge after finishing all the "checks" of module pairs is an option. Take the best approach depending on the situation (computational resource, purpose, etc.).

5. The conversion of genes from UniGene into EntrezGenes generates often more than single (one-to-one) correspondences.

6. The full license and web-enhanced server versions are available from HPC Solutions Inc. (http://www.hpc-sol.co.jp/).

7. Before running GO/KEGG evaluation script, do not forget to download necessary data files, including gene2unigene, gene2go.gz, and KEGG pathway maps. To do this, add your species code to "getKEGGmaps.pl" script in the "GO_KEGG_test" directory and then type "make compile" at the top directory.

Acknowledgments

We would like to thank Dr. Takeaki Uno at National Institute of Informatics for advice and kindly providing the LCM program for free use.

References

1. Barrett, T., Suzek, T.O., Troup, D.B., Wilhite, S.E., Ngau, W.C., Ledoux, P., Rudnev, D., Lash, A.E., Fujibuchi, W., and Edgar, R. (2005) NCBI GEO: mining millions of expression profiles – database and tools. *Nucleic Acids Res.* **33** (Database issue), D562–D566.

2. Brazma, A., Parkinson, H., Sarkans, U., Shojatalab, M., Vilo, J., Abeygunawardena, N., Holloway, E., Kapushesky, M., Kemmeren, P., Lara, G.G., Oezcimen, A., Rocca-Serra, P., and Sansone, S.A. (2003) ArrayExpress – a public repository for microarray gene expression data at the EBI. *Nucleic Acids Res.* **31**, 68–71.

3. Cheng, Y., and Church, G. (2000) Biclustering of expression data. *Proc. Int. Conf. Intell. Syst. Mol. Biol.*, 93–103.

4. Tanay, A., Sharan, R., and Shamir, R. (2002) Discovering statistically significant biclusters in gene expression data. *Bioinformatics* **18**, S136–S144.

5. Ben-Dor, A., Chor, B., Karp, R., and Yakhini, Z. (2002) Discovering local structure in gene expression data: the order-preserving submatrix problem. *Proceedings of the 6th Annual International Conference on Computational Biology, ACM Press, New York, NY, USA*, 49–57.

6. Murali, T.M., and Kasif, S. (2003) Extracting conserved gene expression motifs from gene expression data. *Pac. Symp. Biocomput.* **8**, 77–88.

7. Ihmels, J., Bergmann, S., and Brkai, N. (2004) Defining transcription modules using large-scale gene expression data. *Bioinformatics* **20**, 1993–2003.

8. Wu, C.J., and Kasif, S. (2005) GEMS: a web server for biclustering analysis of expression data. *Nucleic Acids Res.* **33**, W596–W599.

9. Prelic, A. et al. (2006) A systematic comparison and evaluation of biclustering methods for gene expression data. *Bioinformatics* **22**, 1122–1129.

10. Okada, Y., and Fujibuchi, W. (2007) Mining a Large-scale Microarray Database for Similar Gene Expression Modules to Find Distant Relationships between Down Syndrome and Huntington's Disease. *Proceedings of Critical Assessment of Microarray Data Analysis 07, Valencia, Spain.*

11. http://camda.bioinfo.cipf.es/camda07/

12. Uno, T., Asai, T., Uchida, Y., and Arimura, H, (2004) An efficient algorithm for enumerating closed patterns in transaction databases, *Lecture Notes in Artificial Intelligence* **3245**, 16–31.

13. Uno, T., Kiyomi, M., and Arimura, H, (2002) LCM ver.2: Efficient Mining Algorithms for Frequent/Closed/Maximal Itemsets, *IEEE ICDM'04 Workshop FIMI'04* **126**.

14. Fujibuchi, W., Kiseleva, L., Taniguchi, T., Harada, H. and Horton, P. (2007) CellMontage: Similar Expression Profile Search Server, *Bioinformatics* **23**, 3103–3104.

Chapter 6

Human Protein Reference Database and Human Proteinpedia as Discovery Tools for Systems Biology

T.S. Keshava Prasad, Kumaran Kandasamy, and Akhilesh Pandey

Summary

Although high-throughput technologies used in biology have resulted in the accumulation of vast amounts of data in the literature, it is becoming difficult for individual investigators to directly benefit from this data because they are not easily accessible. Databases have assumed a crucial role in assimilating and storing information that could enable future discoveries. To this end, our group has developed two resources – Human Protein Reference Database (HPRD) and Human Proteinpedia – that provide integrated information pertaining to human proteins. These databases contain information on a number of features of proteins that have been discovered using various experimental methods. Human Proteinpedia was developed as a portal for community participation to annotate and share proteomic data using HPRD as the scaffold. It allows proteomic investigators to even share unpublished data and provides an effective medium for data sharing. As proteomic information reflects a direct view of cellular systems, proteomics is expected to complement other areas of biology such as genomics, transcriptomics, classical genetics, and chemical genetics in understanding the relationships among genome, gene functions, and living systems.

Key words: Bioinformatics, Biomarker, Clinical proteomics, Proteotypic peptides, Signal transduction, Signaling pathways, Protein–protein interaction, Post translation modification

1. Introduction

The genome of an organism provides a blue print for its structural and functional attributes. Genome functions through the synthesis, regulation, and activity of proteins. A dynamic and well balanced network of DNA–protein, RNA–protein, and protein–protein interactions (PPIs) maintain the cellular system as a complex but cohesive unit *(1)*. Proteomics serves as a medium to unravel protein functions and ultimately to understand a living system or a disease condition *(2–5)*. Over the years, classical genetic

Hisashi Koga (ed.), *Reverse Chemical Genetics*, Methods in Molecular Biology, vol. 577
DOI 10.1007/978-1-60761-232-2_6, © Humana Press, a part of Springer Science+Business Media, LLC 2009

methodologies including both forward and reverse genetics have been popular in studying gene functions. These approaches are carried out either by introducing mutations in genes and studying their phenotypes or by studying certain phenotypes to uncover the underlying genetic mutations. In recent times, chemical genetics has emerged as a complementary approach to understand gene function. Chemical genetics makes use of small molecules to perturb protein function in lieu of mutations or RNA interference that are used in classical genetic approaches *(6)*. These small molecules can often be highly specific in their action to the extent that they can differentiate between protein isoforms or even between protein domains of a multidomain protein *(7, 8)*. This high specificity combined with the ease in handling and reversibility is a major advantage of chemical genetics over classical genetics. Small molecule screening built on the concept of forward chemical genetics has become an invaluable segment of drug discovery industry *(9, 10)*. In contrast, reverse chemical genetics has been used to investigate the function of proteins by perturbing a known protein and then studying the phenotype *(6)*. Prior knowledge of target protein is very important for this approach *(11)* and perhaps it is in this area that proteomics meets reverse chemical genetics. Protein features such as PPIs, post-translational modifications (PTMs), subcellular localization, and availability of antibodies and their tested efficiencies are important in the development of high-throughput screening platforms in reverse chemical genetics. In addition, expression patterns of proteins of interest in normal or pathological conditions and role of these proteins in diverse signaling pathways are also very useful in establishing relationships among genes and altered phenotype in order to determine probable gene function.

A large number of individual systematic and low-throughput experiments aimed at studying proteins of interest have enriched our knowledge in the area of proteomics. Successful sequencing of human and other mammalian genomes has provided the basic scaffold needed to study proteins. Development of computational infrastructure and its applications to manage biological data has also increased the efficiency and speed of proteomic studies. In the last decade, high-throughput technologies such as the yeast two-hybrid, mass spectrometry (MS), protein/peptide arrays and fluorescence microscopy have become popular in experimental proteomics and resulted in accumulation of proteomics data. Such a rapid escalation of biological data poses a challenge for biologists *(12, 13)*. Biomedical community will be benefited if data on diverse features of proteins are arranged in data repositories, wherein information is regularly updated, exchanged, and analyzed to decipher greater biological implications *(14)*. Here, we will discuss the utility of Human Protein

Reference Database (HPRD) and Human Proteinpedia for systems biology approaches.

2. Human Protein Reference Database as a Centralized Repository for Proteomic Data Annotation

HPRD (http://hprd.org) was developed in response to a growing need of centralized resource for protein data (15–18). HPRD serves scientific community with curated protein data pertaining to the human proteome, which are updated regularly (18). HPRD is a rich source of protein data for over 25,650 human proteins including 6,360 isoforms for which curated sequences are reported so far in RefSeq database (19). Proteomic data in HPRD is comprised of over 38,167 unique PPIs, 16,972 PTMs, 19,670 subcellular localization, and 65,536 tissue expression (Table 1). More than ten PPIs are annotated for 10% of proteins in HPRD and 50% of molecules have at least one PPI. HPRD is richer in various aspects of PPI data evaluated as compared to several other publicly available databases (20). These databases include MINT (http://mint.bio.uniroma2.it/mint) (21), IntAct (http://www.ebi.ac.uk/intact) (22) BIND (23), DIP (http://dip.doe-mbi.ucla.edu) (24), MIPS (http://mips.gsf.de/proj/ppi) (25), and PDZBase (http://icb.med.cornell.edu/services/pdz) (26). HPRD is unique in that it assimilates diverse protein features such as PPIs, PTMs, subcellular localization, tissue expression, biological motifs, and domains derived from a variety of experimental platforms (Fig. 1). Thus HPRD can be used to perform complex queries involving multiple features of proteins.

Table 1
Proteomic data annotation by HPRD team and scientific community

Protein feature type	Total number of annotations added to HPRD (From 2003 to 2008)	Total number of annotations contributed by Human Proteinpedia (in 2008)
Protein–protein interactions	>38,000	>34,500
Post-translational modifications	>16,500	>17,000
Sites of subcellular localization	>19,600	>2,900
Sites of tissue expression	>65,500	>150,300

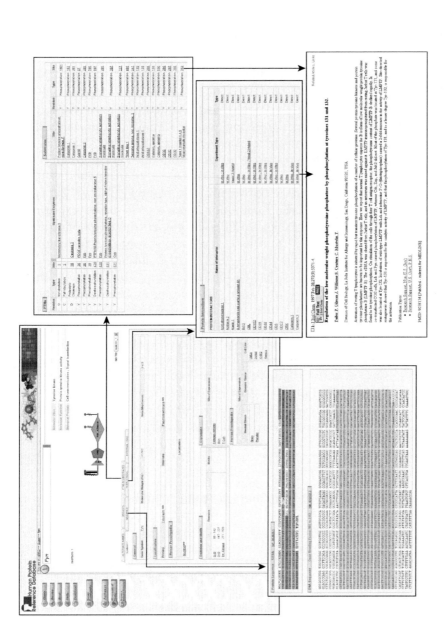

Fig. 1. Display of a HPRD pages providing a composite view of the protein tyrosine kinase, Fyn. The screenshots show molecule page of Fyn, which is a tyrosine kinase involved in several cancer and immune signaling pathways. The summary page of the molecule displays the essential details of the protein, its molecular function and biological process along with subcellular localization, tissue expression and biological motifs, and domains. The "Sequence" page contains RefSeq identifiers along with cDNA and protein sequences. The "PTMs and Substrates" page provides a list of PTMs of Fyn and its substrates. Information pertaining to the modified site from the literature is mapped to the sequences provided in HPRD. The substrates include those proteins whose PTMs are directly brought about by Fyn without any intermediate molecules. The site of each PTM is linked to PubMed citation of the article in which the experiment is described. Information on diseases, alternate names, and external links are also provided in separate pages. If available, data annotated by Human Proteinpedia is also listed in separate tables for PPIs, PTMs, and substrates, subcellular localization and expression.

3. Manual Curation and Controlled Vocabularies

There are no standard protocols or a centralized authority for the nomenclature of proteins, which has resulted in common names for different proteins. Unfortunately, this is one of the impediments faced in the use of text mining algorithms for the curation of proteomic data. Manual curation of the scientific articles in HPRD serves to alleviate such confusion to certain extent. Remapping of site and residue of PTM information derived from literature to a standard sequence in the database is also a very crucial outcome of manual annotation. It is important to note that controlled vocabularies are being established to describe certain protein features which include Proteomics Standard Initiative-Molecular Interaction (PSI-MI) *(27)*, Proteomics Standard Initiative-Mass Spectrometry (PSI-MS), RESID *(28)* Gene Ontology *(29)* and eVOC *(30)*, among others. Although these standard vocabularies are becoming increasingly popular, it will be a herculean task to accommodate these principles in various proteomic databases. HPRD has implemented Gene Ontology vocabularies to describe molecular function, biological process and subcellular localization. PPI data in HPRD is also available in PSI-MI format. PTM information in HPRD is being modified to comply with RESID standards.

4. Human Protein Reference Database as a Platform for Systems Biology Approaches

Proteomic information curated in HPRD is freely available for academic community in XML and tab delimited file formats. On an average, around 10,000 unique users visit the database per month. HPRD received over 8,000 gene comments or help requests till date. Proteomic data from HPRD has been utilized in various functional analyses such as networks and interactomes, development of databases and software utilities. HPRD has been cited by over 340 scientific articles published in peer-reviewed journals. PPI data from HPRD has been used in the analysis of human interactomes *(31, 32)* and the yeast two hybrid based human PPI network studies *(33, 34)*. This data has also been used in the network modeling to study the relationship between breast cancer susceptibility and centrosome function *(35)*. Proteomic data has been used in the development of various software utilities used in the analyses of genomic and proteomic data. PPI data from HPRD has been used in several interactome-based biological network visualization tools such as ConsensusPathDB *(36)*, VisANT *(37)*, Genes2Networks *(38)*, Cerebral *(39, 40)*, BioNet-Builder *(40)*, COXPRESdb *(41)*, STRING 8 *(42)* and UniHI *(43)*. Proteomic information from HPRD has been utilized in the functional analysis of an integrin adhesome network *(44)*. Pathway gene sets curated from HPRD has been used in Gene Set Enrichment Analysis in the differential gene expression data *(45)*. Sequence analysis tools which used HPRD data include CompariMotif *(46)* and SLiMFinder *(47)*. Phosphorylation-based databases including PhosphoPOINT *(48)* and PepCyber:P~PEP *(49)* have used phosphorylation data from HPRD. GPS 2.0 is a new kinase prediction tool which uses PPIs from HPRD in its database *(50)*. Resource of Asian Primary Immunodeficiency Diseases (RAPID) *(51)*, CentrosomeDB, a database of human centrosomal proteins *(52)*, MoKCa database, a database designed to predict consequences of mutations of kinases in cancers *(53)*, CutDB, database of proteolytic events *(54)*, PepBank – a database of peptides and associated biological information *(55)*, OKCAM, a knowledgebase for cell adhesion molecules *(56)*, and T1Dbase, a database for type 1 diabetes research *(57)* have obtained curated proteomic data from HPRD. Proteomic data in HPRD is linked to a compendium of signaling pathways known as Net-Path (http://netpath.org/) *(18)* and phosphorylation-based motifs curated from literature known as PhosphoMotif Finder (http://www.hprd.org/PhosphoMotif_finder) *(58)*. NetPath allows HPRD users to visualize the role of a protein in diverse human signaling pathways. The PhosphoMotif Finder provides a platform to visualize the presence of over 320 experimentally proven phosphorylation-based motifs in a protein of interest.

5. Human Proteinpedia as a Community Portal for Proteomic Data Annotation

Human Proteinpedia *(59, 60)* is a proteomic database with a public distribution annotation system wherein proteomic investigators can share experimental data with biomedical community by submitting the information into a centralized repository. Human Proteinpedia utilizes HPRD as a scaffold wherein proteomic information submitted through the former is mapped to corresponding protein feature in the latter and is reflected in a separate table in protein pages of HPRD **(Fig. 2)**. Human Proteinpedia

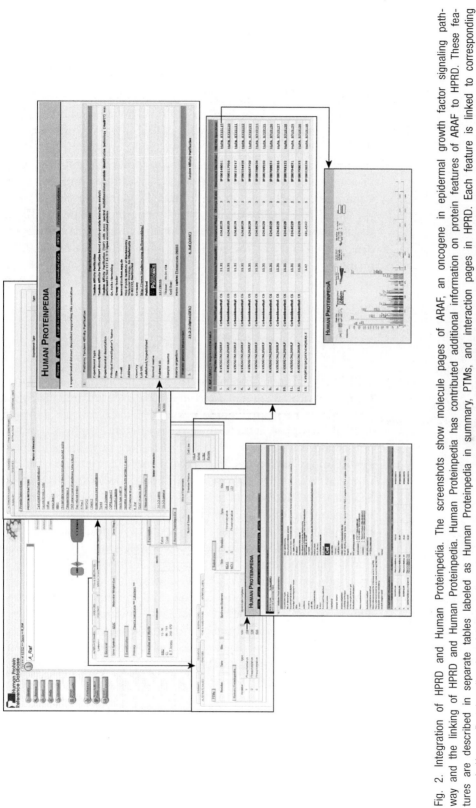

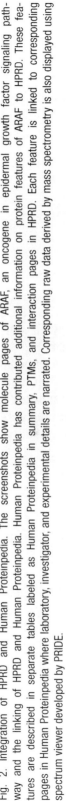

Fig. 2. Integration of HPRD and Human Proteinpedia. The screenshots show molecule pages of ARAF, an oncogene in epidermal growth factor signaling pathway and the linking of HPRD and Human Proteinpedia. Human Proteinpedia has contributed additional information on protein features of ARAF to HPRD. These features are described in separate tables labeled as Human Proteinpedia in summary, PTMs, and interaction pages in HPRD. Each feature is linked to corresponding pages in Human Proteinpedia where laboratory, investigator, and experimental details are narrated. Corresponding raw data derived by mass spectrometry is also displayed using spectrum viewer developed by PRIDE.

has certain features that distinguish it from HPRD itself. Proteomic investigators directly participate in the annotation of data in Human Proteinpedia whereas trained biologists read and interpret published information in HPRD. Both published and unpublished data can be submitted to Human Proteinpedia, which increases the speed of data dissemination. Proteomic information in Human Proteinpedia is always linked to the investigator and the laboratory along with digital images, which support the experimental findings, which makes the annotated data more comprehensive. Human Proteinpedia allows the annotation of protein expression data from disease conditions and cell lines. Community participation in Human Proteinpedia also ensures the speed and quality of data enrichment and update in HPRD which is shown by the fact that Human Proteinpedia has already doubled quantity of the proteomic information in HPRD in a relatively short period (**Table 1**) *(18)*.

6. HPRD and Human Proteinpedia as Reference Resources for Biomedical Community

HPRD and Human Proteinpedia gather information on various features of proteins obtained from diverse experimental platforms and provide them in a single resource. This offers a composite view of each protein and can serve as reference resource for scientists and students alike with regard to their proteins of interest. For example, antibodies are essential tools to study protein features. Efficiency of newly raised antibodies needs to be validated against the target protein in various tissues and cell lines. Protein expression data annotated in HPRD and Human Proteinpedia will help investigators to choose appropriate biological systems to test the specificity or sensitivity of antibodies. Human Proteinpedia documents information about primary antibodies used against a protein in various assays such as coimmunoprecipitation, Western blotting, ELISA, immunoblotting, and immunohistochemistry. This information will be invaluable for experimentalists to select a right antibody or antibodies in their investigations.

Human Proteinpedia provides a list of phosphopeptides identified in mass spectrometry-based phosphoproteomic studies. In addition, phosphorylation and dephosphorylation data curated from the literature are mapped to corresponding site and residue of sequences provided in HPRD. Using PhosphoMotif Finder one can analyze the presence of phosphorylation-based motifs, which are derived from the literature, in any protein of interest. This is a valuable data for biomedical investigators in the development of phospho-specific antibodies and peptide arrays. Availability of many raw MS datasets deposited in Human Proteinpedia can be used for further data mining. These datasets can be used to catalog various PTMs, if the original effort was done only to characterize the proteome of a particular tissue, disease condition, or cell line. Raw MS datasets obtained from different mass spectrometers, ionization methods, and separation technologies can be used to analyze the efficiency of various technologies. This analysis may also guide researchers to determine a combination of technologies to be used to maximize the discovery in proteomics. It is also possible to determine a list of highly observable peptides for most proteins by comparing available MS datasets from diverse sources. These peptides can be used as references for future differential proteomic studies.

Only a small proportion of PPIs or PTMs reported for a molecule are studied in the context of signaling pathways. Additional PPIs and PTMs listed for a protein, which is considered as an important component of a signaling pathway can be tested for their role in signaling. This may reveal novel molecules involved in signaling or responsible for crosstalk between signaling pathways. All experimental data in Human Proteinpedia is linked to the contributing laboratory and investigator. This is helpful for proteomic investigators to locate the research groups or laboratories with similar research interests, which can be complementary to their research goals. Thus, Human Proteinpedia can also lead to initiation of collaborations between various laboratories to accelerate biomedical research.

7. Proteotypic Peptides for Use in Directed Proteomics Experiments

Proteotypic peptides are experimentally derived peptides, which can serve as a unique identifier of a given protein or isoform in tandem mass spectrometry experiments *(61, 62)*. For biomarker analysis, it not sufficient to do a qualitative analysis, but also to perform a targeted quantitative proteomics across multiple samples derived from various physiological and pathological states. One of the recent developments in the field of quantitative proteomics is the use of multiple reaction monitoring or MRM *(63, 64)* on instruments such as triple quadrupole mass spectrometers where multiple precursor ions and their corresponding fragment ions can be selected and analyzed in a high-throughput and automated fashion. Though MRM has been broadly used on various biological applications such as quantification of DNA adducts *(65)* and detection of drugs in biological fluids such as blood and urine *(66–69)*; it is now increasingly being tried for biomarker analysis *(70)*. While choosing the peptide ions for MRM analysis, proteotypic peptides are of crucial importance. With Human

Proteinpedia containing over 4.8 million MS/MS spectra and ~2 million peptides, it has already become an important resource for cataloging proteotypic peptides which can be used for biomarker analysis using MRM.

8. Conclusions

HPRD and Human Proteinpedia together function as a compendium of proteomic information pertaining to humans derived from various experimental platforms. Perhaps these databases will serve as a framework in future for the unification of important proteomic resources. This will allow researchers to perform complex queries in order to retrieve candidate proteins for their study in certain biological context. Large amount of proteomic data available in these resources will also help in designing experiments and interpretation of findings in other complementary fields, namely classical genetics and chemical genetics. Proteomic data is a prerequisite for reverse chemical genetics. Investigators, in these areas of science, will be likely to increasingly depend on HPRD and Human Proteinpedia for planning purposes. Human Proteinpedia, like Wikipedia, acts as a central repository wherein researchers can annotate both published and unpublished proteomic data regardless of size of the data. This will accelerate and simplify data sharing. Data from diverse sources can be accessible in a single format, which will minimize resources spent in handling the data. *Nature Biotechnology (71)* and *Nature Methods (72)*, in their editorial, have proposed that proteomics investigators should be encouraged to submit their data into public databases before publishing in peer-reviewed journals. Human Proteinpedia and HPRD can provide such a platform by serving as discovery tools for systems biology.

References

1. Yu, H., Braun, P., Yildirim, M.A., Lemmens, I., Venkatesan, K., Sahalie, J., Hirozane-Kishikawa, T., Gebreab, F., Li, N., Simonis, N., et al, (2008) High-Quality Binary Protein Interaction Map of the Yeast Interactome Network. *Science*, **322**, 104–110.

2. Chaerkady, R. and Pandey, A. (2008) Applications of Proteomics to Lab Diagnosis. *Annu Rev Pathol: Mech Dis*, **3**, 485–498.

3. Chaerkady, R., Harsha, H.C., Nalli, A., Gucek, M., Vivekanandan, P., Akhtar, J., Cole, R.N., Simmers, J., Schulick, R.D., Singh, S., et al, (2008) A Quantitative Proteomic Approach for Identification of Potential Biomarkers in Hepatocellular Carcinoma. *J Proteome Res*, 7, 4289–4298.

4. Gronborg, M., Kristiansen, T.Z., Iwahori, A., Chang, R., Reddy, R., Sato, N., Molina, H., Jensen, O.N., Hruban, R.H., Goggins, M.G., et al, (2006) Biomarker Discovery from Pancreatic Cancer Secretome Using a Differential Proteomic Approach. *Mol Cell Proteomics*, **5**, 157–171.

5. Vermeulen, M., Hubner, N.C. and Mann, M. (2008) High Confidence Determination of Specific Protein–Protein Interactions Using

Quantitative Mass Spectrometry. *Curr Opin Biotechnol*, **19**, 331.

6. Kawasumi, M. and Nghiem, P. Chemical Genetics: Elucidating Biological Systems with Small-Molecule Compounds. *J Invest Dermatol*, **127**, 1577.

7. Knight, Z.A., Gonzalez, B., Feldman, M.E., Zunder, E.R., Goldenberg, D.D., Williams, O., Loewith, R., Stokoe, D., Balla, A., Toth, B., et al, (2006) A Pharmacological Map of the PI3-K Family Defines a Role for p110[alpha] in Insulin Signaling. *Cell*, **125**, 733.

8. Haggarty, S.J., Koeller, K.M., Wong, J.C., Grozinger, C.M. and Schreiber, S.L. (2003) Domain-Selective Small-Molecule Inhibitor of Histone Deacetylase 6 (HDAC6)-Mediated Tubulin Deacetylation. *Proc Natl Acad Sci U S A*, **100**, 4389–4394.

9. Shim, J.S. and Kwon, H.J. (2004) Chemical Genetics for Therapeutic Target Mining. *Expert Opin Ther Targets*, **8**, 653–661.

10. Dupre, A., Boyer-Chatenet, L., Sattler, R.M., Modi, A.P., Lee, J.-H., Nicolette, M.L., Kopelovich, L., Jasin, M., Baer, R., Paull, T.T., et al, (2008) A Forward Chemical Genetic Screen Reveals an Inhibitor of the Mre11-Rad50-Nbs1 Complex. *Nat Chem Biol*, **4**, 119.

11. Koga, H. (2006) Establishment of the Platform for Reverse Chemical Genetics Targeting Novel Protein–Protein Interactions. *Mol BioSyst*, **2**, 159–164.

12. Orchard, S., Hermjakob, H. and Apweiler, R. (2005) Annotating the Human Proteome. *Mol Cell Proteomics*, **4**, 435–440.

13. Mueller, M., Martens, L. and Apweiler, R. (2007) Annotating the Human Proteome: Beyond Establishing a Parts List. *Biochim Biophys Acta (BBA) – Proteins Proteomics*, **1774**, 175.

14. Orchard, S. and Hermjakob, H. (2008) The HUPO Proteomics Standards Initiative – Easing Communication and Minimizing Data Loss in a Changing World. *Brief Bioinform*, **9**, 166–173.

15. Peri, S., Navarro, J.D., Amanchy, R., Kristiansen, T.Z., Jonnalagadda, C.K., Surendranath, V., Niranjan, V., Muthusamy, B., Gandhi, T.K., Gronborg, M., et al, (2003) Development of Human Protein Reference Database as an Initial Platform for Approaching Systems Biology in Humans. *Genome Res*, **13**, 2363–2371.

16. Peri, S., Navarro, J.D., Kristiansen, T.Z., Amanchy, R., Surendranath, V., Muthusamy, B., Gandhi, T.K., Chandrika, K.N., Deshpande, N., Suresh, S., et al, (2004) Human Protein Reference Database as a Discovery Resource for Proteomics. *Nucleic Acids Res*, **32**, D497–501.

17. Mishra, G.R., Suresh, M., Kumaran, K., Kannabiran, N., Suresh, S., Bala, P., Shivakumar, K., Anuradha, N., Reddy, R., Raghavan, T.M., et al, (2006) Human Protein Reference Database – 2006 Update. *Nucl Acids Res*, **34**, D411–D414.

18. Prasad, T.S.K., Goel, R., Kandasamy, K., Keerthikumar, S., Kumar, S., Mathivanan, S., Telikicherla, D., Raju, R., Shafreen, B., Venugopal, A., et al, (2009) Human Protein Reference Database – 2009 Update. *Nucl Acids Res*, **37**, D767–D772.

19. Wheeler, D.L., Barrett, T., Benson, D.A., Bryant, S.H., Canese, K., Chetvernin, V., Church, D.M., Dicuccio, M., Edgar, R., Federhen, S., et al, (2008) Database Resources of the National Center for Biotechnology Information. *Nucleic Acids Res*, **36**, D13–D21.

20. Mathivanan, S., Periaswamy, B., Gandhi, T.K., Kandasamy, K., Suresh, S., Mohmood, R., Ramachandra, Y.L. and Pandey, A. (2006) An Evaluation of Human Protein–Protein Interaction Data in the Public Domain. *BMC Bioinform*, 7 Suppl 5, S19.

21. Chatr-aryamontri, A., Ceol, A., Palazzi, L.M., Nardelli, G., Schneider, M.V., Castagnoli, L. and Cesareni, G. (2007) MINT: The Molecular INTeraction Database. *Nucl Acids Res*, **35**, D572–D574.

22. Kerrien, S., Alam-Faruque, Y., Aranda, B., Bancarz, I., Bridge, A., Derow, C., Dimmer, E., Feuermann, M., Friedrichsen, A., Huntley, R., et al, (2007) IntAct – Open Source Resource for Molecular Interaction Data. *Nucl Acids Res*, **35**, D561–D565.

23. Alfarano, C., Andrade, C.E., Anthony, K., Bahroos, N., Bajec, M., Bantoft, K., Betel, D., Bobechko, B., Boutilier, K., Burgess, E., et al, (2005) The Biomolecular Interaction Network Database and Related Tools 2005 Update. *Nucl Acids Res*, **33**, D418–424.

24. Salwinski, L., Miller, C.S., Smith, A.J., Pettit, F.K., Bowie, J.U. and Eisenberg, D. (2004) The Database of Interacting Proteins: 2004 Update. *Nucl Acids Res*, **32**, D449–451.

25. Pagel, P., Kovac, S., Oesterheld, M., Brauner, B., Dunger-Kaltenbach, I., Frishman, G., Montrone, C., Mark, P., Stumpflen, V., Mewes, H.-W., et al, (2005) The MIPS Mammalian Protein–Protein Interaction Database. *Bioinformatics*, **21**, 832–834.

26. Beuming, T., Skrabanek, L., Niv, M.Y., Mukherjee, P. and Weinstein, H. (2005) PDZBase: A Protein–Protein Interaction Database for PDZ-Domains. *Bioinformatics*, **21**, 827–828.

27. Hermjakob, H., Montecchi-Palazzi, L., Bader, G., Wojcik, J., Salwinski, L., Ceol, A., Moore, S.,

Orchard, S., Sarkans, U., von Mering, C., et al, (2004) The HUPO PSI's Molecular Interaction Format[mdash]a Community Standard for the Representation of Protein Interaction Data. *Nat Biotech*, **22**, 177.

28. John, S.G. (2004) The RESID Database of Protein Modifications as a resource and annotation tool. *PROTEOMICS*, **4**, 1527–1533.

29. Ashburner, M., Ball, C.A., Blake, J.A., Botstein, D., Butler, H., Cherry, J.M., Davis, A.P., Dolinski, K., Dwight, S.S., Eppig, J.T., et al, (2000) Gene Ontology: Tool for the Unification of Biology. *Nat Genet*, **25**, 25.

30. Kelso, J., Visagie, J., Theiler, G., Christoffels, A., Bardien, S., Smedley, D., Otgaar, D., Greyling, G., Jongeneel, C.V., McCarthy, M.I., et al, (2003) eVOC: A Controlled Vocabulary for Unifying Gene Expression Data. *Genome Res*, **13**, 1222–1230.

31. Gandhi, T.K., Zhong, J., Mathivanan, S., Karthick, L., Chandrika, K.N., Mohan, S.S., Sharma, S., Pinkert, S., Nagaraju, S., Periaswamy, B., et al, (2006) Analysis of the Human Protein Interactome and Comparison with Yeast, Worm and Fly Interaction Datasets. *Nat Genet*, **38**, 285–293.

32. Rhodes, D.R., Tomlins, S.A., Varambally, S., Mahavisno, V., Barrette, T., Kalyana-Sundaram, S., Ghosh, D., Pandey, A. and Chinnaiyan, A.M. (2005) Probabilistic Model of the Human Protein–Protein Interaction Network. *Nat Biotechnol*, **23**, 951–959.

33. Rual, J.F., Venkatesan, K., Hao, T., Hirozane-Kishikawa, T., Dricot, A., Li, N., Berriz, G.F., Gibbons, F.D., Dreze, M., Ayivi-Guedehoussou, N., et al, (2005) Towards a Proteome-Scale Map of the Human Protein–Protein Interaction Network. *Nature*, **437**, 1173–1178.

34. Stelzl, U., Worm, U., Lalowski, M., Haenig, C., Brembeck, F.H., Goehler, H., Stroedicke, M., Zenkner, M., Schoenherr, A., Koeppen, S., et al, (2005) A Human Protein–Protein Interaction Network: A Resource for Annotating the Proteome. *Cell*, **122**, 957–968.

35. Pujana, M.A., Han, J.D., Starita, L.M., Stevens, K.N., Tewari, M., Ahn, J.S., Rennert, G., Moreno, V., Kirchhoff, T., Gold, B., et al, (2007) Network Modeling Links Breast Cancer Susceptibility and Centrosome Dysfunction. *Nat Genet*, **39**, 1338–1349.

36. Kamburov, A., Wierling, C., Lehrach, H. and Herwig, R. (2008) ConsensusPathDB – A Database for Integrating Human Functional Interaction Networks. *Nucl Acids Res*, gkn698.

37. Hu, Z., Snitkin, E.S. and DeLisi, C. (2008) VisANT: An Integrative Framework for Networks in Systems Biology. *Brief Bioinform*, **9**, 317–325.

38. Berger, S.I., Posner, J.M. and Ma'ayan, A. (2007) Genes2Networks: Connecting Lists of Gene Symbols Using Mammalian Protein Interactions Databases. *BMC Bioinform*, **8**, 372.

39. Barsky, A., Gardy, J.L., Hancock, R.E. and Munzner, T. (2007) Cerebral: A Cytoscape Plugin for Layout of and Interaction with Biological Networks Using Subcellular Localization Annotation. *Bioinformatics*, **23**, 1040–1042.

40. Avila-Campillo, I., Drew, K., Lin, J., Reiss, D.J. and Bonneau, R. (2007) BioNetBuilder: Automatic Integration of Biological Networks. *Bioinformatics*, **23**, 392–393.

41. Obayashi, T., Hayashi, S., Shibaoka, M., Saeki, M., Ohta, H. and Kinoshita, K. (2008) COXPRESdb: A Database of Coexpressed Gene Networks in Mammals. *Nucleic Acids Res*, **36**, D77–82.

42. Jensen, L.J., Kuhn, M., Stark, M., Chaffron, S., Creevey, C., Muller, J., Doerks, T., Julien, P., Roth, A., Simonovic, M., et al. (2009) STRING 8 – A Global View on Proteins and Their Functional Interactions in 630 Organisms. *Nucl Acids Res*, **37**, D412–D416.

43. Chaurasia, G., Iqbal, Y., Hanig, C., Herzel, H., Wanker, E.E. and Futschik, M.E. (2007) UniHI: An Entry Gate to the Human Protein Interactome. *Nucleic Acids Res*, **35**, D590–594.

44. Zaidel-Bar, R., Itzkovitz, S., Ma'ayan, A., Iyengar, R. and Geiger, B. (2007) Functional Atlas of the Integrin Adhesome. *Nat Cell Biol*, **9**, 858–867.

45. Subramanian, A., Tamayo, P., Mootha, V.K., Mukherjee, S., Ebert, B.L., Gillette, M.A., Paulovich, A., Pomeroy, S.L., Golub, T.R., Lander, E.S., et al, (2005) Gene Set Enrichment Analysis: A Knowledge-Based Approach for Interpreting Genome-Wide Expression Profiles. *Proc Natl Acad Sci USA*, **102**, 15545–15550.

46. Edwards, R.J., Davey, N.E. and Shields, D.C. (2008) CompariMotif: Quick and Easy Comparisons of Sequence Motifs. *Bioinformatics*, **24**, 1307–1309.

47. Edwards, R.J., Davey, N.E. and Shields, D.C. (2007) SLiMFinder: A Probabilistic Method for Identifying Over-Represented, Convergently Evolved, Short Linear Motifs in Proteins. *PLoS ONE*, **2**, e967.

48. Yang, C.Y., Chang, C.H., Yu, Y.L., Lin, T.C., Lee, S.A., Yen, C.C., Yang, J.M., Lai, J.M., Hong, Y.R., Tseng, T.L., et al. (2008) PhosphoPOINT: A Comprehensive Human Kinase Interactome and Phospho-Protein Database. *Bioinformatics*, **24**, i14–20.

49. Gong, W., Zhou, D., Ren, Y., Wang, Y., Zuo, Z., Shen, Y., Xiao, F., Zhu, Q., Hong, A.,

Zhou, X., et al, (2008) PepCyber:P~PEP: A Database of Human Protein Protein Interactions Mediated by Phosphoprotein-Binding Domains. *Nucleic Acids Res*, **36**, D679–683.

50. Xue, Y., Ren, J., Gao, X., Jin, C., Wen, L. and Yao, X. (2008) GPS 2.0, a Tool to Predict Kinase-specific Phosphorylation Sites in Hierarchy. *Mol Cell Proteomics*, **7**, 1598–1608.

51. Keerthikumar, S., Raju, R., Kandasamy, K., Hijikata, A., Ramabadran, S., Balakrishnan, L., Ahmed, M., Rani, S., Selvan, L.D.N., Somanathan, D.S., et al, (2008) RAPID: Resource of Asian Primary Immunodeficiency Diseases. *Nucl Acids Res*, **37**, D863–D867.

52. Nogales-Cadenas, R., Abascal, F., Diez-Perez, J., Carazo, J.M. and Pascual-Montano, A. (2008) CentrosomeDB: A Human Centrosomal Proteins Database. *Nucl Acids Res*, **37**, D175–D180.

53. Richardson, C.J., Gao, Q., Mitsopoulous, C., Zvelebil, M., Pearl, L.H. and Pearl, F.M.G. (2009) MoKCa Database – Mutations of Kinases in Cancer. *Nucl Acids Res*, **37**, D824–D831.

54. Igarashi, Y., Eroshkin, A., Gramatikova, S., Gramatikoff, K., Zhang, Y., Smith, J.W., Osterman, A.L. and Godzik, A. (2007) CutDB: A Proteolytic Event Database. *Nucl Acids Res*, **35**, D546–549.

55. Shtatland, T., Guettler, D., Kossodo, M., Pivovarov, M. and Weissleder, R. (2007) PepBank – A Database of Peptides Based on Sequence Text Mining and Public Peptide Data Sources. *BMC Bioinform*, **8**, 280.

56. Li, C.-Y., Liu, Q.-R., Zhang, P.-W., Li, X.-M., Wei, L. and Uhl, G.R. (2008) OKCAM: An Ontology-Based, Human-Centered Knowledgebase for Cell Adhesion Molecules. *Nucl Acids Res*, **37**, D251–D260.

57. Hulbert, E.M., Smink, L.J., Adlem, E.C., Allen, J.E., Burdick, D.B., Burren, O.S., Cassen, V.M., Cavnor, C.C., Dolman, G.E., Flamez, D., et al, (2007) T1DBase: Integration and Presentation of Complex Data for Type 1 Diabetes Research. *Nucl Acids Res*, **35**, D742–D746.

58. Amanchy, R., Periaswamy, B., Mathivanan, S., Reddy, R., Tattikota, S.G. and Pandey, A. (2007) A Curated Compendium of Phosphorylation Motifs. *Nat Biotechnol*, **25**, 285–286.

59. Mathivanan, S., Ahmed, M., Ahn, N.G., Alexandre, H., Amanchy, R., Andrews, P.C., Bader, J.S., Balgley, B.M., Bantscheff, M., Bennett, K.L., et al, (2008) Human Proteinpedia Enables Sharing of Human Protein Data. *Nat Biotechnol*, **26**, 164–167.

60. Kandasamy, K., Keerthikumar, S., Goel, R., Mathivanan, S., Patankar, N., Shafreen, B., Renuse, S., Pawar, H., Ramachandra, Y.L.,

61. Acharya, P.K., et al, (2009) Human Proteinpedia: A Unified Discovery Resource for Proteomics Research. *Nucl Acids Res*, **37**, D773–781.

61. Kuster, B., Schirle, M., Mallick, P. and Aebersold, R. (2005) Scoring Proteomes with Proteotypic Peptide Probes. *Nat Rev Mol Cell Biol*, **6**, 577.

62. Robertson Craig, J.P.C.R.C.B. (2005) The Use of Proteotypic Peptide Libraries for Protein Identification. *Rapid Commun Mass Spectrom*, **19**, 1844–1850.

63. Wolf-Yadlin, A., Hautaniemi, S., Lauffenburger, D.A. and White, F.M. (2007) Multiple Reaction Monitoring for Robust Quantitative Proteomic Analysis of Cellular Signaling Networks. *Proc Natl Acad Sci*, **104**, 5860–5865.

64. Anderson, L. and Hunter, C.L. (2006) Quantitative Mass Spectrometric Multiple Reaction Monitoring Assays for Major Plasma Proteins. *Mol Cell Proteomics*, **5**, 573–588.

65. Koc, H. and Swenberg, J.A. (2002) Applications of Mass Spectrometry for Quantitation of DNA Adducts. *J Chromatogr B*, **778**, 323.

66. Mario Thevis, G.O.W.S. (2001) High Speed Determination of Beta-Receptor Blocking Agents in Human Urine by Liquid Chromatography/Tandem Mass Spectrometry. *Biomed Chromatogr*, **15**, 393–402.

67. Ho, E.N.M., Leung, D.K.K., Wan, T.S.M. and Yu, N.H. (2006) Comprehensive Screening of Anabolic Steroids, Corticosteroids, and Acidic Drugs in Horse Urine by Solid-Phase Extraction and Liquid Chromatography-Mass Spectrometry. *J Chromatogr A*, **1120**, 38.

68. Herrin, G., McCurdy, H.H.H. and Wall, W.H. (2005) Investigation of an LCMSMS (QTrap) Method for the Rapid Screening and Identification of Drugs in Postmortem Toxicology Whole Blood Samples. *J Anal Toxicol*, **29**, 599.

69. Guan, F., Uboh, C.E., Soma, L.R., Luo, Y., Rudy, J. and Tobin, T. (2005) Detection, Quantification and Confirmation of Anabolic Steroids in Equine Plasma by Liquid Chromatography and Tandem Mass Spectrometry. *J Chromatogr B*, **829**, 56.

70. Liao, H., Wu, J., Kuhn, E., Chin, W., Chang, B., Jones, M.D., O'Neil, S., Clauser, K.R., Karl, J., Hasler, F., Roubenoff, R., Zolg, W. and Guild, B.C. (2004) Use of Mass Spectrometry to Identify Protein Biomarkers of Disease Severity in the Synovial Fluid and Serum of Patients with Rheumatoid Arthritis. *Arthritis Rheum*, **50**, 3792–3803.

71. Editorial. (2007) Democratizing Proteomics Data. *Nat Biotech*, **25**, 262.

72. Editorial. (2008) Thou shalt Share your Data. *Nat Meth*, **5**, 209.

Part II

Modification of cDNA Resources Utilized for Reverse Chemical Genetics

Chapter 7

High-Throughput Production of the Recombinant Proteins Expressed in *Escherichia coli* Utilizing cDNA Resources

Kiyo Shimada and Hisashi Koga

Summary

Conventionally, expression plasmids in *Escherichia coli* have generally been constructed using ligation reaction-assisted cloning followed by the generation of inserts. In such cases, the insert was generated by polymerase chain reaction (PCR), digestion using restriction enzymes, or oligonucleotide synthesis. To overcome the restrictions of these conventional methods, we improved them by utilizing an in vitro site-specific recombination reaction, based on the integrase–excisionase system of bacteriophage λ to insert DNA fragments. This method enabled us to insert tens of fragments into expression vectors in parallel. We applied these methods to produce glutathione S-transferase (GST)-fused or maltose-binding protein (MBP)-fused proteins in *Escherichia coli*. As a result, we successfully produced and purified more than 3,000 recombinant proteins for further study of reverse chemical genetics.

Key words: In vitro recombination, PCR, cDNA library, High throughput, GST, MBP

1. Introduction

Chemical genetics is an emerging research field that can be classified into two categories "forward" and "reverse" chemical genetics, similar to conventional genetics *(1)*. Reverse chemical genetics, corresponding to "reverse genetics," enable us to establish a phenotype-based screening based on the affinity of small molecules to a specific target protein. Such screening assays could be established not only in vivo (e.g., phenotypes of model animals) but also in vitro (e.g., biochemical assays). Especially in vitro, novel protein–protein interactions are thought to be a key to identifying small active compounds. Taking this importance into consideration, we have accumulated human cDNA resources

Hisashi Koga (ed.), *Reverse Chemical Genetics*, Methods in Molecular Biology, vol. 577
DOI 10.1007/978-1-60761-232-2_7, © Humana Press, a part of Springer Science+Business Media, LLC 2009

and established expression-ready cDNA clones *(2)*. In a parallel effort, we have also established a system for recombinant protein expression in *Escherichia coli* in a high-throughput manner *(3–5)*. Although we can now exploit several different technologies for recombinant protein expression (e.g., baculovirus and cell-free systems; see other chapters in this book), the *Escherichia coli* system is the most conventional method. To begin with the introduction of these expression systems, we present our *Escherichia coli* system in which high-throughput production is achieved by an in vitro recombination-assisted method.

2. Materials

2.1. Construction of Expression Plasmids

1. Insert DNA. 50 ng/µL PCR products (*see* **Subheading 3.1, step 10** and **Note 1**): Store at room temperature.
2. Vector DNA: pDONR207™ (Invitrogen, Carlsbad, CA, USA): Store at –20°C.
3. BP Clonase™ Enzyme Mix (Invitrogen): Store at –80°C.
4. LR Clonase™ Enzyme Mix (Invitrogen): Store at –80°C.
5. Vector DNA: 150 ng/µL pGEX–6PDES A⁺destination vector: Store at –20°C.
6. 0.75 M NaCl: Store at room temperature.
7. Proteinase K (Invitrogen): Store at –80°C.
8. Competent *Escherichia coli* DH5α cells (Toyobo, Osaka, Japan): Store at –80°C.
9. SOC medium (Invitrogen): Store at room temperature.
10. Ampicillin sodium salt (Nacalai Tesque, Kyoto, Japan): Store at room temperature.
11. LB Broth Powder Growth Media, pH 7 (Mo Bio Laboratories, Carlsbad, CA, USA): Store at room temperature.
12. LB Agar Powder Growth Media, pH 7 (Mo Bio Laboratories): Store at room temperature.
13. LA PCR™ Kit (Takara Bio, Shiga, Japan): Store at –20°C.
14. Primers for insert check **(Fig. 2a)**: Store at –20°C.pGEX 5′ primer(5′-GGGCTGGCAAGCCACGTTTGGTG).pGEX3′ primer (5′-CCGGGAGGCTGCATGTGTCAGAGG-3′).
15. Agarose S (Nippon Gene, Tokyo, Japan): Store at room temperature.
16. Tris–Acetate–EDTA buffer (50×) [TAE Buffer] pH 8.3 (Nacalai Tesque): Store at room temperature.

17. Smart Ladder (Nippon Gene, Tokyo, Japan): Store at −20°C.

18. Ethidium bromide (Sigma-Aldrich, St. Louis, MO, USA): Store at 4°C.

19. Exonuclease I (*E. coli*) (New England Biolabs, Ipswich, MA, USA): Store at −20°C.

20. Shrimp Alkaline Phosphatase (USB, Cleveland, OH, USA): Store at −20°C.

21. BigDye Terminator v3.1 Cycle Sequencing Kit (Applied Biosystems, Warrington, UK): Store at −20°C.

22. Plusgrow (Nacalai Tesque): Store at room temperature.

23. MAGNIA plasmid preparation robot: MagExtractor MFX9600 (Toyobo).

24. SpeedVac SPD1010 (ThermoQuest Scientific Equipment Group, Hants, UK).

2.2. Small-Scale Production of Recombinant Proteins

1. *E. coli* Rosetta (DE3) pLysS cells (EMD Biosciences, Novagen brand, Madison, WI, USA), a BL21 derivative designed to enhance the expression of eukaryotic proteins containing codons rarely used in *E. coli (6)*: Store at −80°C.

2. Chloramphenicol (Nacalai): Store at room temperature.

3. Isopropyl β-d-thiogalactoside (IPTG; Nacalai): Store at −20°C.

4. 3× SDS sample buffer: 150 mM Tris–HCl, pH 6.8, 6% SDS, 3% β-ME, and 0.06% BPB: Store at room temperature.

5. Bioruptor (UCW-201; Cosmo Bio, Tokyo, Japan).

6. 10× running buffer: 250 mM Tris, 1.92 M glycine, 1% SDS: Store at room temperature.

7. Stain solution: 0.25% Coomassie Brilliant Blue R250 (Wako Pure Chemical Industries, Osaka, Japan) in 25% ethanol and 7.5% acetic acid: Store at room temperature.

8. Precast gel: Real Gel Plate (Bio Craft, Tokyo, Japan): Store at 4°C.

9. PreScission plus blue standard (Bio-Rad Laboratories, Hercules, CA, USA): Store at −20°C.

2.3. Rapid Solubility Assay

1. CelLytic B II (Sigma-Aldrich): Store at room temperature.

2. Tris-buffered saline (TBS): 25 mM Tris–HCl, pH 8.0, 0.15 M NaCl: Store at room temperature.

3. Tris-buffered saline with Tween (TBST): 25 mM Tris–HCl, pH 8.0, 0.15 M NaCl, 0.02% Tween-20: Store at room temperature.

4. Immobilized glutathione on a 96-well plate (Reacti-bind glutathione coated clear strip plate; Pierce Biotechnology, Rockford, IL, USA): Store at 4°C.

5. Peroxidase-conjugated anti-GST antibody (GE Healthcare Bio-Sciences, Chalfont St. Giles, US): Store at 4°C.

6. 2,2′-azinobis (3-ethylbenzthiazoline-6-sulfonic acid) (ABTS; KPL, Gaithersburg, MD, USA): Store at 4°C.

7. Spectra MAX microplate reader (Molecular Devices, Sunnyvale, CA, USA).

2.4. Purification of Soluble Recombinant Proteins

1. Sonication buffer: TBS buffer containing 0.02% Tween 20, 5 mM EDTA, 0.2% β-ME, 1 mM PMSF, 5 μg/mL antipain, 5 μg/mL leupeptin, and 5 μg /mL pepstatin A: Store at 4°C.

2. TBS-1E: TBS containing 1 mM EDTA: Store at 4°C.

3. TBST-1E: TBST containing 1 mM EDTA: Store at 4°C.

4. Multi-beads shocker (MB501PU; Yasui Kikai, Osaka, Japan).

5. Glutathione Sepharose 4B (GE Healthcare Bio-Sciences): Store at 4°C.

6. Glutathione buffer: containing 10 mM glutathione, 0.1 M Tris (pH 8.0), and 0.2 M NaCl: Store at 4°C.

7. PreScission protease (GE Healthcare Bio-Sciences): Store at −20°C.

8. Digestion buffer: 50 mM Tris–HCl, pH 7.0, 0.15 M NaCl, 1 mM EDTA: Store at 4°C.

2.5. Purification of Insoluble Recombinant Proteins

1. Bug Buster (EMD Biosciences): Store at room temperature.

2. 2% TX wash buffer: 25 mM Tris–HCl, pH 8.0, 0.15 M NaCl, 2% TX-100, 0.02% Tween 20, 1 mM EDTA: Store at 4°C.

3. Copper negative staining (Copper Stain; Bio-Rad Laboratories): Store at 4°C.

4. Electroeluter Model 422 (Bio-Rad Laboratories).

3. Methods

We provide an outline of methods that the readers can use in their own laboratories to generate expression plasmids for GST-fused recombinant proteins from cDNA recourses (see **Fig. 1**). For the first step, PCR products are generated by the primer pairs containing in vitro recombination sites (*att*B1 and *att*B2) in the flanking regions using a cDNA clone as a template. For the second step, the BP reaction was performed to create an entry clone from the PCR products and donor vector. The resultant entry clone containing the PCR fragment instead of *ccd*B-Cm^r was used for subsequent LR reaction. These reactions were performed in a single-tube format in principle according to the

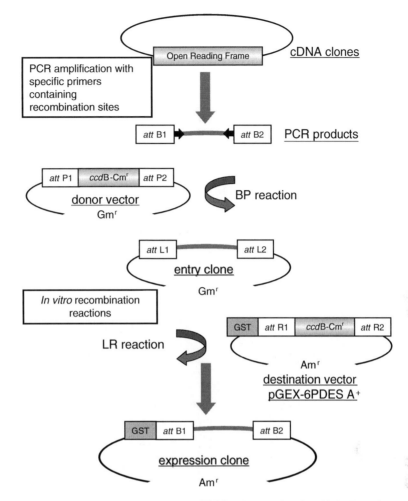

Fig. 1. Outline of the strategy to construct GST-fused expression plasmids by the in vitro recombination-assisted method. Am^r, Gm^r, and Cm^r are abbreviations for ampicillin-, gentamicin-, and chloramphenicol-resistance, respectively. The figure also indicates the *ccd*B gene encoding a toxin targeting the *E. coli* essential DNA gyrase and the phage λ recombination sites (*att*B, *att*P, *att*L, and *att*R).

manufacturer's instructions (Invitrogen). A destination vector, designated pGEX-6PDES A⁺for LR reaction, was constructed by inserting an *att*R1-*ccd*B-Cm^r-*att*R2 fragment (Invitrogen) into an *Sma* I site of a pGEX-6P-1 vector (GE Healthcare Bio-Sciences) (*see* **Fig. 2a**). Protein tags for affinity purification greatly affect the stability, solubility, and yield of the bacterially expressed proteins. We thus first established a system to produce GST-fused recombinant proteins, since GST is a widely used tag for soluble recombinant production in *E. coli* *(7, 8)*. Thus far we have also generated a destination vector for maltose-binding protein (MBP)-fused protein expression in *Escherichia coli* derived from pET30a(+) (Novagen) (*see* **Fig. 2b**). From our preliminary

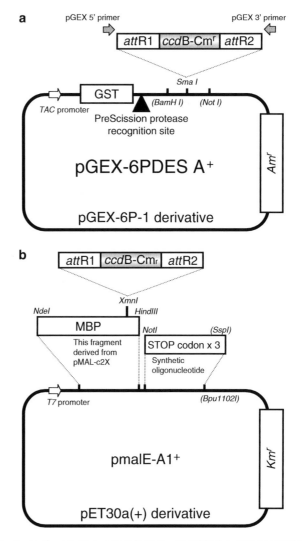

Fig. 2. Structures of expression vectors for N-terminal GST-fused (**a**) and MBP-fused (**b**) proteins. Km^r is an abbreviation for kanamicin resistance. The figure also indicates the location of the primer pair used for DNA sequencing and colony PCR.

experiences, MBP-fused proteins are more soluble than GST-fused proteins. This supports previous findings regarding the solubility of recombinant fusion proteins *(9, 10)*.

PCR and in vitro recombination reactions are quite simple and straightforward for generating multiple expression plasmids in parallel, e.g., in a 96-well plate (*see* **Fig. 3a**). The first preliminary expression experiment was done to evaluate the production level of each GST-fused protein. In this step, we compared the staining patterns of *E. coli* proteins harboring expression plasmids with the patterns of proteins harboring empty vectors on sodium dodecyle sulfate-polyacrylamide gel electrophoresis (SDS-PAGE) under the same culture conditions (*see* **Fig. 3b**). In addition to

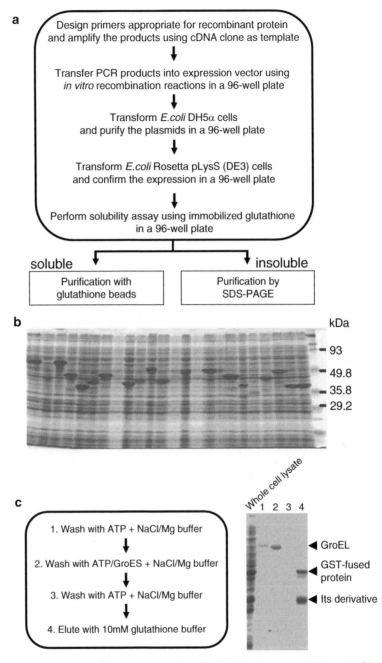

Fig. 3. Flow diagram of the expression and purification (**a**) and a representative result of the first preliminary expression experiment (**b**) of GST-fused recombinant proteins. Flow diagram (**c left**) and the representative result (**c right**) of the removal of GroEL directly binding expressed GST-fused proteins on glutathione sepharose beads. The whole cell lysate of expressed bacteria and each wash and elution fraction are loaded on 12% SDS-PAGE (the numbers at the top of the panel are identical to the numbers in the left diagram).

the expression level, this experiment also elucidates the appropriate expression of the fused protein based on a comparison of the sizes of the predicted proteins.

In the second evaluation step, the solubility of preliminarily expressed GST-fused protein was measured. The results provide important information to determine subsequent purification steps: glutathione-based affinity purification applied to soluble protein or electro-elusion of excised protein bands on SDS-PAGE applied to insoluble protein. To unambiguously determine purification method, we established a "solubility assay" that enabled us to quantitate solubility in a high-throughput manner *(3, 5)*. The solubility assay is less time-consuming in its experimental steps than conventional immunoblotting using an anti-GST antibody *(11)*. Another advantage of the solubility assay is that it more precisely reflects the binding specificity of GST-fused protein to glutathione than does the conventional immunoblotting *(12)*. This is because solubilized GST-fused proteins are initially captured on a glutathione immobilized on a solid phase, in principle *(13, 14)*.

3.1. Construction of Expression Plasmids

1. A diagram for the construction of an expression clone is shown in **Fig. 1**.

2. A cDNA clone encoding the target gene for recombinant protein is selected from among cDNA resources, and primers are designed for the amplification of an appropriate region of the gene (*see* **Note 2**).

3. Prepare a BP reaction component (*see* **Table 1**). The cocktail is gently mixed by pipetting and centrifuged briefly in a 96-well plate. The cocktail is incubated at 25°C overnight.

4. Add 2.5 μL of LR reaction components (*see* **Table 1**). The cocktail is gently mixed by pipetting and centrifuged briefly in an identical plate. The cocktail is further incubated at 25°C for 7 h.

5. Add 0.8 μL Proteinase K. The cocktail is further incubated at 37°C for 15 min.

6. Transform 1 μL of the cocktail into 10 μL of *E. coli* DH5α-competent cells. The *E. coli* is incubated on ice for 30 min in a 96-well plate, transferred at 42°C for 30 s, and then placed on ice for 2 min.

7. Spread on an LB plate containing 200 μg/mL of ampicillin. The LB plate is incubated at 37°C overnight.

8. Perform colony-direct PCR using pGEX5′ and pGEX3′ primers (*see* **Table 1**). The annealing temperature is 55°C and the cycle is maintained at 25.

9. Check the size of the PCR products by agarose gel electrophoresis with 5 μL of PCR mixture.

10. Pretreat excess primers and remaining dephosphorylate dNTPs in the PCR mixture (*see* **Table 1**) for the subsequent sequencing reaction. The mixture is incubated at 37°C for 30 min, after which the enzymes are inactivated by heating at 80°C for 30 min.

Table 1
Buffer components in each reaction

att B DNA: 50 ng/μL PCR products	2.0 μL
att P DNA: 150 ng/μL pDONR207	0.5 μL
5× BP reaction buffer	1.0 μL
Sterilized distilled water	0.5 μL
BP CLONASE Enzyme Mix	1.0 μL
total	5.0 μL
att L DNA: BP reactions	5.0 μL
att R DNA: 150 ng/μL pGEX-6PDES	0.75 μL
0.75 M NaCl	0.25 μL
LR CLONASE Enzyme Mix	1.5 μL
Total	7.5 μL
10× LA buffer	1.5 μL
2.5 mM dNTP	3.0 μL
5 μM pGEX5′ primer	0.5 μL
5μM pGEX3′ primer	0.5 μL
Sterilized distilled water	9.3 μL
LA Taq (5 units/5 μL)	0.2 μL
Total	15.0 μL
PCR reaction product	10 μL
Shrimp alkaline phosphatase (1 U/μL)	0.025 μL
Exonuclease I (20 U/μL)	0.050 μL
Sterilized distilled water	9.925 μL
Total	20 μL

11. The DNA sequence of the PCR product is determined by the ABI3130 DNA sequencer using a pGEX5′primer and a pGEX3′primer.

12. Pick up a single colony of the transformant and incubate the *E. coli* in 0.5 mL of Plusgrow containing 100 μg/mL of ampicillin in a 96-well plate at 37°C overnight.

13. Purify the plasmid DNA using MagExtracter MFX-9000 in the same format.

14. Dry up the DNA using SpeedVac SPD1010 for 2 h.

15. Add 50 μL of distilled water and dissolve with Voltex (Scientific Industries, Bohemia, NY, USA) for 30 min.

3.2. Small-Scale Production of Recombinant Protein

1. Transform 1 μL of the DNA into 10 μL of *E. coli* Rosetta(DE3) pLysS-competent cells. The *E. coli* is incubated on ice for 30 min in a 96-well plate, transferred at 42°C for 30 s, and then placed on ice for 2 min.

2. Add 100 μL of SOC medium and incubate at 37°C for 1 h.

3. Spread the *E. coli* onto LB plates containing 200 μg/mL of ampicillin and 25 μg/mL of chloramphenicol and incubate at 37°C overnight.

4. Pick up a single colony of the transformant and incubate the *E. coli* in 0.5 mL of LB medium containing 200 μg/mL of ampicillin and 5 μg/mL of chloramphenicol in a 96-well plate at 30°C overnight.

5. Dilute one-tenth in 0.5 mL of the same medium containing 0.2 mM IPTG and culture for another 2 h at 37°C.

6. Centrifuge the plate at 5600 *g* for 10 min and discard the supernatant.

7. Suspend the *E. coli* cell pellet in 75 μL of 1× SDS sample buffer.

8. Homogenize the pellet with ultrasonic Bioruptor for 15 min.

9. 7.5 μL of each sample is resolved on 12% SDS-PAGE.

10. Stain SDS-polyacrylamide gels with stain solution.

11. Check the production level and compare the predicted molecular weights of each GST-fused protein (*see* **Fig. 3b** and **Note 3**).

3.3. Solubility Assay

1. Pick up a single colony of the transformant and incubate the *E. coli* in 0.5 mL of LB medium containing 200 μg/mL of ampicillin and 5 μg/mL of chloramphenicol in a 96-well plate at 30°C overnight.

2. Dilute one-tenth of the bacterial supernatant in 0.5 mL of the same medium containing 0.1 mM IPTG and culture for another 1.5 h at 25°C.

3. Centrifuge the plate at 5600 *g* for 10 min and discard the supernatant.

4. Suspend the *E. coli* cell pellet in 100 μL of CelLytic B II.

5. Shake the plate on a MicroIncubator M-36 (Taitec, Saitama, Japan) for 10 min at room temperature.

6. Centrifuge the plate at 5600 *g* for 10 min.

7. Prepare a 1/100th dilution of supernatant in TBST.

8. Transfer 100 μL of diluted solubilized protein fraction onto immobilized glutathione on a 96-well plate. To capture GST-fused recombinant protein onto immobilized glutathione, the plate is incubated for 1 h at room temperature. For the control, 1 μg of purified GST is also analyzed.

9. Wash three times with TBST.

10. Prepare a 1:2,000 dilution of peroxidase-conjugated anti-GST antibody in TBST.

11. Add 100 μL of diluted antibody and incubate for 1 h at room temperature.

12. Wash three times with TBST.

13. Add 100 μL of ABTS and incubate for 6 min at room temperature for visualization by colorimetric reaction.

14. Measure absorbance at 405 nm using a microplate reader (*see* **Note 4**).

3.4. Purification of Soluble Recombinant Proteins

1. Inoculate the transformant in 10 mL of LB medium containing 200 μg/mL of ampicillin and 10 μg/mL of chloramphenicol and incubate at 37°C overnight.

2. Transfer to 500 mL of the same medium and culture at 25°C for 7 h.

3. Add 0.1 mM IPTG and culture at 18°C for 15 h.

4. Centrifuge 5600 *g* for 10 min and discard the supernatant.

5. The *E. coli* cell pellet is disrupted by a Multi-beads shocker (setup conditions: 1400 *g*, on 30 s, off 30 s, 12 cycles) with glass beads in 25 mL of sonication buffer.

6. Centrifuge the lysate at 22400 *g* at 4°C for 30 min.

7. Transfer the supernatant to a new tube.

8. Add 1 mL of glutathione beads (50% slurry) (*see* **Note 5**) and rotate gently at 4°C for 1 h.

9. Wash three times with TBST.

10. Elute the GST-fused protein by adding 5 mL of glutathione buffer (*see* **Note 6**).

11. The purity of recombinant protein could be evaluated by SDS-PAGE (*see* **Note 7**).

3.5. Purification of Insoluble Recombinant Proteins

1. Inoculate the transformant in 2 mL of LB medium containing 200 μg/mL of ampicillin and 10 μg/mL of chloramphenicol; incubate at 37°C overnight.

2. Transfer to 50 mL of the same medium and culture at 37°C for 3.5 h.

3. Add 1 mM IPTG and culture at 37°C for 4 h.

4. Centrifuge at 5600 g for 10 min and discard the supernatant.

5. The cell pellet is disrupted by Bioruptor (setup conditions: on 50 s, off 10 s, 5 cycles) in 4 mL of Bug Buster.

6. Mix in a shaker at room temperature for 30 min.

7. Centrifuge at 22400 g for 30 min.

8. Wash the inclusion with TX wash buffer twice.

9. Wash the inclusion with water once.

10. Residual pellet is suspended in 1× SDS sample buffer.

11. To estimate the amount and purity of the protein, a small quantity of insoluble protein fraction is loaded on SDS-PAGE and stained.

12. An adequate insoluble protein fraction is electrophoresed on SDS-PAGE using a wide range of combs (sample volume: $15 \times 120 \times 2$ mm^3).

13. After negative staining, the band corresponding to the GST-fused protein is excised from the gel by using a surgical knife.

14. The recombinant protein is eluted from the gel by using electroeluter Model 422.

15. The purity of the recombinant protein can be evaluated by SDS-PAGE.

4. Notes

1. To minimize the misincorporation of different nucleotides during PCR reaction, PCR amplification is performed using *LA Taq* polymerase (Takara) since this has relatively high fidelity, and the number of PCR cycles is kept to 20. Excess primers and dNTPs are treated with shrimp alkaline phosphatase and Exonuclease I.

2. The region for protein production is selected in order to satisfy the following criteria: (1) high surface exposure, relatively high negative charge, and low occurrence of modifications; (2) the hydrophilic value of the selected region is –0.3–0.9, as calculated by the Hopp and Woods formula, the most commonly used formula for predicting protein hydrophilicity (15); (3) the region should not be involved in any membrane-spanning region predicted by SOSUI (16); (4) the region is designed to contain 100–300 amino acid residues, and the isoelectric point (pI) is kept between 4 and 11.

3. The apparent molecular mass of the protein in the unusually strong band deviated considerably from the predicted one, and the produced protein was excluded from further experiments.

4. When the solubility assay gave an A_{405nm} value larger than 0.125, the GST-fused protein extracted in a soluble fraction was purified on glutathione-sepharose beads.

5. The glutathione sepharose supplied by GE Healthcare is approximately 75% slurry, and the storage solution contains 20% ethanol. Therefore, the glutathione sepharose should be washed with TBS and replaced by TBS.

6. To remove GST-tag, PreScission protease can be used for elution instead of glutathione buffer.

7. Bacterial heat-shock proteins such as dnaK and GroEL tend to bind inducibly expressed proteins *(17, 18)*. We therefore also established a simple method for removing such bacterial proteins. Briefly, GST fusion proteins attached to glutathione-sepharose beads are washed with buffer consisting of 20 mM $MgSO_4$, 300 mM NaCl, 10 mM adenosine 5′ triphosphate (ATP), and 2.5 μM recombinant GroES at 37°C for 10 min *(19)*. We confirmed that this simple procedure could efficiently remove GroEL before the elution with 10 mM glutathione buffer (*see* **Fig. 3c**).

Acknowledgments

We are grateful to Dr. Takahiro Nagase for his truly helpful discussions, invaluable suggestions, and encouragement. The author also thanks Miss Tomomi Tajino and Mr. Kazuhiro Sato for their technical assistance. This study was supported by grants from the CREATE Program (Collaboration of Regional Entities for the Advancement of Technological Excellence) from JST (Japan Science and Technology Corporation); by the Genome Network Project of the Ministry of Education, Culture, Sports, Science, and Technology of Japan; and by the Kazusa DNA Research Institute.

References

1. Kawasumi M, Nghiem P. (2007) Chemical genetics: elucidating biological systems with small-molecule compounds. *J Invest Dermatol* **127**, 1577–84.

2. Nagase T, Yamakawa H, Tadokoro S, et al. (2008) Exploration of human ORFeome: high-throughput preparation of ORF clones and efficient characterization of their protein products. *DNA Res* **15**, 137–49.

3. Shimada K, Nagano M, Kawai M, Koga H. (2005) Influences of amino acid features of glutathione S-transferase fusion proteins on their solubility. *Proteomics* **5**, 3859–63.

4. Koga H. (2006) Establishment of the platform for reverse chemical genetics targeting novel protein–protein interactions. *Mol Biosyst* **2**, 159–64.

5. Hara Y, Shimada K, Kohga H, Ohara O, Koga H. (2003) High-throughput production of recombinant antigens for mouse KIAA proteins in *Escherichia coli*: computational allocation of possible antigenic regions, and construction of expression plasmids of glutathione-S-transferase-fused antigens by an in vitro recombination-assisted method. *DNA Res* **10**, 129–36.

6. Schenk PM, Baumann S, Mattes R, Steinbiss HH. (1995) Improved high-level expression system for eukaryotic genes in *Escherichia coli* using T7 RNA polymerase and rare ArgtRNAs. *Biotechniques* **19**, 196–8, 200.

7. Smith DB, Johnson KS. (1988) Single-step purification of polypeptides expressed in *Escherichia coli* as fusions with glutathione S-transferase. *Gene* **67**, 31–40.

8. Smith DB. (2000) Generating fusions to glutathione S-transferase for protein studies. *Methods Enzymol* **326**, 254–70.

9. Nallamsetty S, Waugh DS. (2007) Mutations that alter the equilibrium between open and closed conformations of *Escherichia coli* maltose-binding protein impede its ability to enhance the solubility of passenger proteins. *Biochem Biophys Res Commun* **364**, 639–44.

10. Kapust RB, Waugh DS. (1999) *Escherichia coli* maltose-binding protein is uncommonly effective at promoting the solubility of polypeptides to which it is fused. *Protein Sci* **8**, 1668–74.

11. Braun P, Hu Y, Shen B, et al. (2002) Proteome-scale purification of human proteins from bacteria. *Proc Natl Acad Sci U S A* **99**, 2654–9.

12. Murray AM, Kelly CD, Nussey SS, Johnstone AP. (1998) Production of glutathione-coated microtitre plates for capturing recombinant glutathione S-transferase fusion proteins as antigens in immunoassays. *J Immunol Methods* **218**, 133–9.

13. Rabin DU, Palmer-Crocker R, Mierz DV, Yeung KK. (1992) An ELISA sandwich capture assay for recombinant fusion proteins containing glutathione-S-transferase. *J Immunol Methods* **156**, 101–5.

14. Sehr P, Zumbach K, Pawlita M. (2001) A generic capture ELISA for recombinant proteins fused to glutathione S-transferase: validation for HPV serology. *J Immunol Methods* **253**, 153–62.

15. Hopp TP, Woods KR. (1981) Prediction of protein antigenic determinants from amino acid sequences. *Proc Natl Acad Sci U S A* **78**, 3824–8.

16. Hirokawa T, Boon-Chieng S, Mitaku S. (1998) SOSUI: classification and secondary structure prediction system for membrane proteins. *Bioinformatics* **14**, 378–9.

17. Thain A, Gaston K, Jenkins O, Clarke AR. (1996) A method for the separation of GST fusion proteins from co-purifying GroEL. *Trends Genet* **12**, 209–10.

18. Sherman MY, Goldberg AL. (1991) Formation in vitro of complexes between an abnormal fusion protein and the heat shock proteins from *Escherichia coli* and yeast mitochondria. *J Bacteriol* **173**, 7249–56.

19. Yasukawa T, Kanei-Ishii C, Maekawa T, Fujimoto J, Yamamoto T, Ishii S. (1995) Increase of solubility of foreign proteins in *Escherichia coli* by coproduction of the bacterial thioredoxin. *J Biol Chem* **270**, 25328–31.

Chapter 8

An Insect Cell-Free System for Recombinant Protein Expression Using cDNA Resources

Takashi Suzuki, Toru Ezure, Masaaki Ito, Masamitsu Shikata, and Eiji Ando

Summary

The Transdirect *insect cell* is a newly developed in vitro translation system for mRNA templates, which utilizes an extract from cultured *Spodoptera frugiperda* 21 (Sf21) insect cells. An expression vector, pTD1, which includes a 5′-untranslated region (UTR) sequence from a baculovirus polyhedrin gene as a translational enhancer, was also developed to obtain maximum performance from the insect cell-free protein synthesis system. This combination of insect cell extract and expression vector results in protein productivity of about 50 µg per mL of the translation reaction mixture. This is the highest protein productivity yet noted among commercialized cell-free protein synthesis systems based on animal extracts.

Key words: Translation, *Spodoptera frugiperda* 21, Cell-free protein synthesis system, pTD1 vector, Insect cell extract

1. Introduction

In reverse chemical genetics, it is crucial to synthesize proteins of interest using appropriate foreign gene expression systems and cDNA resources. Since cell-free protein synthesis systems have the potential to synthesize any desired proteins, including both native proteins and those that are toxic to cells *(1)*, with high throughput, they can be powerful tools for this objective. We developed a cell-free protein synthesis system from *Spodoptera frugiperda* 21 (Sf21) insect cells, which are widely used as the host for baculovirus expression systems, and commercialized it as the Transdirect *insect cell*.

Hisashi Koga (ed.), *Reverse Chemical Genetics*, Methods in Molecular Biology, vol. 577
DOI 10.1007/978-1-60761-232-2_8, © Humana Press, a part of Springer Science+Business Media, LLC 2009

We have demonstrated that this insect cell-free protein synthesis system is one of the most effective protein synthesis systems among those based on animal extracts *(2)*. Furthermore, it has the potential to perform eukaryote-specific protein modifications such as protein *N*-myristoylation and prenylation *(3, 4)*. Thus, we expect that the insect cell-free protein synthesis system will be a useful method for target protein production in the reverse chemical genetics era, as well as for postgenomic studies. In this chapter, we describe standard protocols to synthesize proteins of interest using the insect cell-free protein synthesis system.

2. Materials

2.1. Construction of an Expression Clone

1. Primers for amplification of the target cDNA (*see* **Subheading 3.1**): Store at –20°C.
2. KOD-plus DNA polymerase (TOYOBO, Kyoto, Japan): Store at –20°C (*see* **Note 1**).
3. Agarose S (Nippon Gene, Tokyo, Japan): Store at room temperature.
4. *50× TAE buffer*. Mix 242 g of Tris base, 57.1 mL of glacial acetic acid, and 100 mL of 0.5 M EDTA (pH 8.0), and adjust to 1,000 mL with water. Store at room temperature.
5. 1 Kb DNA Ladder (BIONEER, Korea): Store at –20°C.
6. Ethidium Bromide (Nippon Gene): Store at 4°C.
7. Phenol:Chloroform:Isoamyl Alcohol 25:24:1 saturated with 10 mM Tris–HCl, pH 8.0, 1 mM EDTA: Store at 4°C.
8. Chloroform: Store at room temperature.
9. 3 M sodium acetate, pH 5.2: Store at room temperature.
10. Ethanol: Store at room temperature.
11. 70% (v/v) ethanol: Store at room temperature.
12. T4 polynucleotide kinase (TOYOBO): Store at –20°C.
13. Restriction endonucleases (*Eco*RV, *Eco*RI, *Sac*I, *Kpn*I, *Bam*HI, and *Xba*I). Store at –20°C.
14. MinElute PCR Purification Kit (QIAGEN, Maryland, USA): Store at room temperature.
15. pTD1 vector, a component of the Transdirect *insect cell* kit (Shimadzu, Kyoto, Japan). Store at –20°C or below. The map of the pTD1 vector is shown in **Fig. 1**.
16. Quick Ligation™ Kit (NEW ENGLAND BioLabs, Ipswich, MA): Store at –20°C.

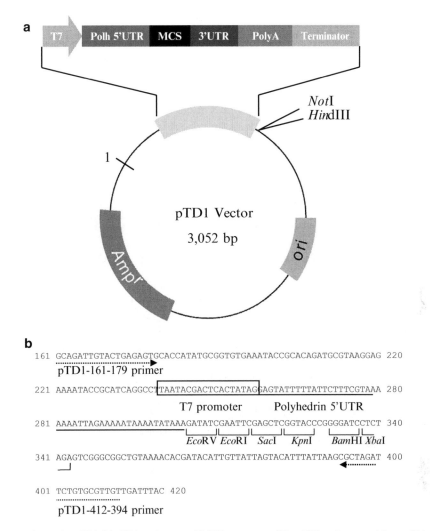

Fig. 1. The expression vector pTD1. (**a**) pTD1 vector map. (**b**) DNA sequence of the pTD1 vector around the multiple cloning sites.

17. Chemically competent cells *Escherichia coli* DH5α (TAKARA Bio, Shiga, Japan): Store at –80°C.

18. Ampicillin sodium salt (SIGMA) is dissolved in distilled water at 100 mg/mL and stored at –20°C.

19. Luria–Bertani (LB, 1.0% polypeptone, 0.5% yeast extract, 1.0% NaCl, pH 7.0) medium containing 100 μg/mL ampicillin (LB-amp) and LB-amp agar medium (LB containing 1.0% agar): Store at 4°C.

20. *GenElute plasmid miniprep kit (SIGMA).* Store at room temperature. Resuspension solution should be stored at 4°C after the addition of RNase A.

21. BigDye Terminator v3.1 Cycle Sequencing Kit (Applied Biosystems, Warrington, UK): Store at –20°C.

22. Primers for DNA sequencing (*see* **Subheading 3.1**): Store at –20°C.

2.2. Preparation of mRNA

1. Restriction endonucleases (*Hin*dIII and *Not*I) are stored at –20°C.

2. T7 RiboMAX™ Express Large Scale RNA Production System (Promega, Madison, WI) (*see* **Note 2**): Store at –20°C.

3. NICK Columns (GE Healthcare, Buckinghamshire, UK): Store at room temperature.

4. 3 M potassium acetate, pH 5.5 (Ambion, Austin, TX): Store at room temperature.

5. TE buffer: 10 mM Tris–HCl, pH 8.0, 1 mM EDTA: Store at room temperature.

6. *MOPS buffer (20×).* 400 mM MOPS, 100 mM NaOAc, 20 mM EDTA (adjust to pH 7.0 by NaOH): Store at 4°C in the shade.

7. 37% formaldehyde: Store at room temperature.

8. Deionized formamide: Store at –20°C.

2.3. In Vitro Transla-tion and Detection of Synthesized Proteins

1. Transdirect *insect cell* (Shimadzu): Store at –80°C.

2. Purified mRNA (*see* **Subheading 3.2**). Store at –80°C.

3. FluoroTect™ Green$_{Lys}$ in vitro Translation Labeling System (Promega): Store at –80°C.

4. *SDS-PAGE running buffer (10×).* 250 mM Tris base, 1.92 M glycine, 1% SDS: Store at room temperature.

5. *SDS-PAGE loading buffer (4×).* 200 mM Tris–HCl, pH 6.8, 8% SDS, 32% glycerol, 0.008% bromophenol blue, 8% 2-mercapto ethanol: Store at room temperature.

6. *Precast gel.* c-PAGEL (ATTO, Tokyo, Japan): Store at 4°C.

7. *Prestained molecular weight markers.* Full range RAINBOW (GE Healthcare): Store at –20°C.

3. Methods

The Transdirect *insect cell* kit is an in vitro translation system for mRNA templates. We developed and optimized a method to prepare the insect cell extract, the concentrations of the reaction components, and an expression vector pTD1 *(2, 5)*. The pTD1 vector contains all factors involved in mRNA and protein synthesis, including the T7 promoter sequence required for mRNA synthesis, the polyhedrin 5'- UTR which enhances the translation reaction, and multiple cloning sites (MCS) (*see* **Fig. 1**). The complete DNA sequence of the pTD1 vector is registered in the following DNA databank: DDBJ/GenBank®/EMBL Accession Number AB194742.

To obtain maximal protein productivity, it is necessary to construct an expression clone in which a protein coding region (open reading frame, mature region, domain, etc.) obtained from a cDNA of interest is inserted into the MCS of the pTD1 vector. Typically, expression of the target protein at about 35–50 μg per mL of the translation reaction mixture can be obtained by using mRNA transcribed from the expression clone and the Transdirect *insect cell* kit. Furthermore, the expression clone can be effectively combined with other eukaryotic cell-free protein synthesis systems, such as rabbit reticulocyte lysate and wheat germ systems (*see* **Note 3**).

3.1. Construction of the Expression Clone for the Insect Cell-Free Protein Synthesis System

1. Procedures for construction of the expression clone follow classical molecular cloning methods. The overall cloning strategy is shown in **Fig. 2**.

2. Design and synthesize two primers, an N-terminal primer and a C-terminal primer, for amplification of protein coding region of the target cDNAs. The N-Terminal primer should have the initiation codon at its 5'-terminus. In the case of the C-terminal primer, the restriction endonuclease recognition sequence should be introduced upstream of the stop codon, and an additional sequence (at least two bases) should be added to the 5'-end (*see* **Note 4**).

3. Perform PCR using these primers, KOD-plus, and cDNA of the target gene as the template and check the size of amplified DNA by gel electrophoresis.

4. Purify the amplified DNA fragment by phenol/chloroform extraction and ethanol precipitation.

5. Treat the purified DNA fragment by T4 polynucleotide kinase at 37°C for 1 h, then purify the DNA fragment by ethanol precipitation.

6. Suspend the precipitate in distilled water, and digest the DNA fragment using the restriction enzyme that recognizes the appropriate sequence in the C-terminal primer at 37°C for 2 h.

7. Purify the DNA fragment using the MinElute PCR Purification Kit.

8. Quantitate the DNA fragment by absorbance at 260 nm using a spectrophotometer, and use it as an insert.

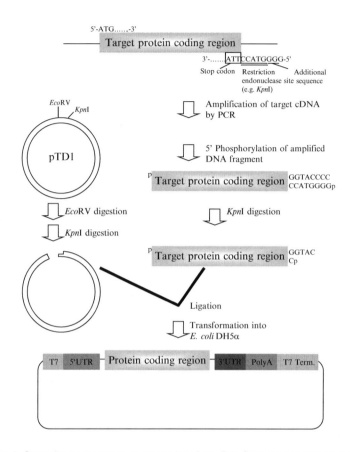

Fig. 2. Strategies to construct an expression clone. This figure shows procedures to construct an expression clone when a *Kpn*I site is introduced into a C-terminal primer.

9. Digest the pTD1 vector with *Eco*RV at 37°C for 2 h (*see* **Note 5**).

10. After ethanol precipitation, digest the pTD1 vector with another restriction endonuclease to produce the same cohesive end as that introduced in the C-terminal primer.

11. Purify the digested pTD1 vector using a MinElute PCR Purification Kit.

12. Quantitate the DNA concentration using a spectrophotometer, and use it as the vector.

13. Mix the vector and the insert at a ratio of about 1:10 (mol:mol), and incubate them with T4 DNA ligase at 25°C for 5 min.

14. Transform the ligation sample into *E. coli* DH5α and incubate on LB-amp agar plates at 37°C overnight (*see* **Note 6**).

15. Cultivate single colonies of the transformants in LB-amp medium at 37°C overnight.

16. Extract the plasmids using a GenElute plasmid miniprep kit, linearize them with an appropriate restriction enzyme, and check their size by agarose gel electrophoresis.

17. Confirm the plasmid DNA sequence using a pTD1–161–179 primer (5′-GCAGATTGTACTGAGAGTG-3′) for N-terminal sequencing and a pTD1–412–394 primer (5′-ACAACGCACAGAATCTAGC-3′) for C-terminal sequencing. The annealing temperature of these primers is 50°C (*see* **Note** 7 and **8**).

3.2. Preparation of mRNA

1. Linearize the expression clone using an appropriate restriction endonuclease downstream from the T7 terminator sequence (*see* **Notes** 9 and **10**).

2. Purify the digested expression clone by phenol/chloroform extraction and ethanol precipitation (*see* **Note 11**).

3. Dissolve the pellet in sterilized distilled water and quantitate the DNA concentration by spectrophotometer, then use as the template for mRNA synthesis (*see* **Note 12**).

4. Perform the in vitro transcription reaction using the T7 RiboMAX™ Express Large Scale RNA Production System (*see* **Note 13**) at 37°C for 30 min (*see* **Note 14**). Use 5 μg of DNA template for 100 μL of transcription reaction. Typically, about 500 μg of purified mRNA is obtained from 100 μL of transcription reaction. This yield corresponds to about 1.5 mL of translation reaction.

5. After the incubation, the synthesized mRNA should be purified immediately using NICK™ Columns, which are gel filtration columns. This purification step is necessary to remove salts and unincorporated NTPs. We recommend performing this treatment in order to achieve stable and highly reproducible translation reactions.

6. Procedures to set up the NICK™ Columns are as follows. First, remove the column cap and pour off the excess liquid. Rinse the column with 3 mL of sterilized distilled water. Remove the bottom cap and place it in a column stand. Equilibrate the gel with 3 mL of sterilized distilled water and flush completely. These procedures should be carried out during the in vitro transcription reaction.

7. Apply 100 μL of the transcriptional reaction mixture on top of the gel, and flush completely. If the reaction scale of the in vitro transcription is less than 100 μL, fill up the reaction mixture to 100 μL with sterilized distilled water before applying to the column.

8. Add 400 µL of sterilized distilled water, and then flush completely. Discard the eluate.

9. Before elution of the mRNA fraction, place a new 1.5 mL tube under the column.

10. Add 400 µL of sterilized distilled water, and collect the eluate.

11. Add 40 µL of 3 M potassium acetate (*see* **Note 15**) and 950 µL of ethanol to the eluate. Mix thoroughly and centrifuge for 20 min at $21,500 \times g$, 4°C.

12. Discard the supernatant and then rinse the pellet with 70% ethanol. Do not dry the pellet completely, so it will dissolve mRNA in water easily. Dissolve the pellet in 100 µL of sterilized distilled water. If the reaction scale of the in vitro transcription is less than 100 µL, dissolve the pellet with sterilized distilled water in an equal volume of the in vitro transcription reaction.

13. After the purification, measure the absorbance at 260 nm of the purified mRNA solution using a spectrophotometer. Dilute 2 µL of the purified mRNA solution into 500 µL of TE buffer, and then measure the absorbance. Use TE as the blank. The mRNA concentration is determined by the following equation: mRNA concentration (mg/mL) = A_{260} value $\times$ 0.04 $\times$ 250.

14. About 3–6 mg/mL mRNA is usually obtained by the above method.

15. Confirm the purity and size of synthesized mRNA by gel electrophoresis as described in the following protocols.

16. Prepare a 1.0% agarose gel in 1× TAE (*see* **Note 16**).

17. Mix 10 µL of 20× MOPS buffer, 30 µL of 37% formaldehyde, and 80 µL of deionized formamide, and use this as an RNA sample buffer.

18. Mix 8 µg of the mRNA sample and 11 µL of the RNA sample buffer, and adjust to 20 µL with sterilized distilled water.

19. Treat the mRNA sample at 65°C for 15 min, and immediately place it on ice.

20. Perform electrophoresis, and visualize the mRNA sample by ethidium bromide staining. If the RNA band is smeared or not visible, possible causes may be degradation of mRNA by RNase contamination.

3.3. In Vitro Translation

1. Kit components of the Transdirect *insect cell* kit are the Insect Cell Extract (yellow cap) (*see* **Note 17–19**), Reaction Buffer (blue cap), 4 mM Methionine (red cap), pTD1 vector (green cap), and the Control DNA (white cap).

Table 1
Reaction components

mRNA		16 μg
4 mM Methionine		1 μL
Reaction buffer		15 μL
Insect cell extract		25 μL
Sterilized distilled water	adjust to	50 μL

2. Procedures to set up a translation reaction mixture should be carried out on ice.

3. Thaw the Reaction Buffer, 4 mM Methionine, and Insect Cell Extract. The reaction Buffer and 4 mM Methionine can be thawed at room temperature.

4. Assemble the reaction components (*see* **Table 1**) (*see* **Note 20**). Gently mix by pipetting up and down. If necessary, centrifuge briefly to return the sample to the bottom of the tube.

5. Incubate the translation reaction mixture at 25°C for 5 h.

6. The protein productivity of the Transdirect *insect cell* kit is about 50 μg per mL of the translation reaction mixture (*see* **Note 21**).

3.4. Detection of a Synthesized Protein

1. Generally, it is difficult to detect synthesized proteins by CBB staining. To confirm the expression of the target protein, we usually perform fluorescent labeling of the in vitro translation products using the FluoroTect™ Green$_{Lys}$ in vitro Translation Labeling System (FluoroTect) (*see* **Note 22**).

2. Add 1 μL of the FluoroTect solution to 50 μL of the translation reaction mixture described in **Table 1**, and incubate at 25°C for 5 h.

3. After the translation reaction, add 2 μL of SDS-PAGE loading buffer (4×) to 6 μL of the reaction mixture. Incubate at 70°C for 3 min.

4. Resolve the sample by SDS-PAGE.

5. Detect the fluorescent-labeled protein using a laser-based fluorescent scanner. An experimental example is shown in **Fig. 3** (*see* **Note 23**).

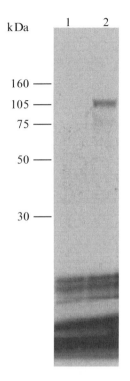

Fig. 3. Detection of a synthesized protein by fluorescent labeling. Cell-free protein synthesis was carried out with or without the use of mRNA transcribed from a linearized expression clone containing the β-galactosidase gene, and the synthesized protein was labeled by FluoroTect. The translational reaction mixtures were resolved by 12.5% SDS-PAGE. Detection of labeled protein was performed using a laser-based fluorescent scanner (FX pro, Bio-Rad, Hercules, CA). Lanes 1 and 2 represent negative control (absence of mRNA) and β-galactosidase, respectively.

4. Notes

1. Other DNA polymerases, which are high fidelity enzymes that do not have terminal transferase activity, also can be used.

2. It has been confirmed that protein synthesis can be performed effectively using mRNA prepared using the following kits: AmpliScribe™ T7-*Flash*™ Transcription Kit (Epicentre), AmpliScribe™ T7 Transcription Kit (Epicentre), CUGA®7 in vitro Transcription Kit (Nippon Genetech), MEGA script® T7 High Yield Transcription Kit (Ambion), RiboMAX™ Large Scale RNA Production System-T7 (Promega), RNAMaxx™ High Yield Transcription Kit (Stratagene), and the Script-MAX™ Thermo T7 Transcription Kit (Toyobo).

3. The pTD1 vector should not be used as the expression vector for an *E. coli* cell-free protein synthesis system because this vector does not contain Shine–Dalgarno sequence.

4. We recommend introducing the *Kpn*I recognition sequence into the C-terminal primer if the target cDNA does not have a *Kpn*I site, because this strategy has been shown to have the highest cloning efficiency.

5. Generally, translation efficiency gradually decreases depending on the length between the initiating codon of the target cDNA and the polyhedrin 5′ untranslated region (UTR), which contains a translational enhancer sequence. To obtain the highest translation efficiency, the initiating codon of the target cDNA should be inserted into the *Eco*RV site of the pTD1 vector.

6. This system does not utilize blue-white selection.

7. Deletion mutation of the initiating codon (especially "A") has sometimes been observed for this cloning strategy.

8. To clarify whether mutations occur during PCR, the overall nucleotide sequence of the insert DNA should be confirmed.

9. For linearization of expression clones, we recommend using *Hin*dIII or *Not*I. Restriction enzymes, *Cfr* 10I, *Eco* 52I, *Eco* T14I, *Nde* I, *Pvu* II, *Sca* I, and *Stu* I may be used.

10. PCR-generated DNA templates can be used in transcription reactions. In such cases, the following primers are recommended: A pTD1–161–179 primer (5′-GCAGATT-GTACTGAGAGTG-3′) and a pTD1–845–827 primer (5′-GGAAACAGCTATGACCATG-3′). Their annealing temperature is 50°C.

11. This step is very important to avoid RNase contamination.

12. At least 125 µg/mL of the linearized DNA template is required for in vitro transcription reactions.

13. Before use, RiboMAX™ Express T7 2× Buffer must be dissolved completely by warming the buffer at 37°C and mixing well.

14. The suggested incubation times should be adhered to. In the case of a long template (more than about 2 kb), an excessive reaction time may cause precipitation. In this case, mRNA will not be collected. To avoid this problem: I: shorten the reaction time to 20 min, II: decrease the quantity of DNA template to 70–80%, III: use a PCR-generated DNA template.

15. Do not use sodium acetate for the precipitation of synthesized mRNA. Sodium ion inhibits the translation reaction.

16. We usually use a nondenaturing agarose gel.

17. We confirmed that the Insect Cell Extract is stable against freeze-thawing up to eight times. After use, the extract should be immediately stored at –80°C.

18. Insect Cell Extract is sensitive to CO_2. After opening the package, avoid prolonged exposure to CO_2 (e.g., dry ice).

19. We confirmed that the Insect Cell Extract has the ability to perform eukaryote-specific protein modifications, such as N-myristoylation *(3)* and prenylation *(4)*. To obtain such modified proteins effectively, specific substrates for each protein modification should be added to the translation reaction mixture.

20. The addition of RNase inhibitor (50 units) to the translation reaction mixture (50 μL) may improve translational efficiency (Recommended products: Promega Code No. N2611).

21. Generally, it is difficult to synthesize membrane proteins having multiple transmembrane domains.

22. Radio-isotope labeling or western blotting may also be used to detect synthesized proteins.

23. For detection of proteins having molecular masses less than 20 kDa, it is necessary to treat the translation reaction mixture with RNase A because unincorporated FluoroTect tRNA migrates at about 20 kDa.

Acknowledgments

We wish to thank Dr. Osamu Ohara and Dr. Takahiro Nagase, Kazusa DNA Research Institute, for valuable discussions. We also thank Dr. Sumiharu Nagaoka, Kyoto Institute of Technology, Dr. Toshihiko Utsumi, University of Yamaguchi, and Dr. Susumu Tsunasawa, Shimadzu Corporation, for helpful discussions.

References

1. Sakurai, N., Moriya, K., Suzuki, T., Sofuku, K., Motiki, H., Nishimura, O., and Utsumi, T. (2007) Detection of co- and post-translational protein N-myristoylation by metabolic labeling in an insect cell-free protein synthesis system. *Anal. Biochem.* **362**, 236–244.

2. Ezure, T., Suzuki, T., Higashide, S., Shintani, E., Endo, K., Kobayashi, S., Shikata, M., Ito, M., Tanimizu, K., and Nishimura, O. (2006) Cell-free protein synthesis system prepared from insect cells by freeze-thawing. *Biotechnol. Prog.* **22**, 1570–1577.

3. Suzuki, T., Ito, M., Ezure, T., Shikata, M., Ando, E., Utsumi, T., Tsunasawa, S., and Nishimura, O. (2006) N-Terminal protein modifications in an insect cell-free protein synthesis system and their identification by mass spectrometry. *Proteomics* **6**, 4486–4495.

4. Suzuki, T., Ito, M., Ezure, T., Shikata, M., Ando, E., Utsumi, T., Tsunasawa, S., and Nishimura, O. (2007) Protein prenylation in an insect cell-free protein synthesis system and identification of products by mass spectrometry. *Proteomics* **7**, 1942–1950.

5. Suzuki, T., Ito, M., Ezure, T., Kobayashi, S., Shikata, M., Tanimizu, K., and Nishimura, O. (2006) Performance of expression vector, pTD1, in insect cell-free translation system. *J. Biosci. Bioeng.* **102**, 69–71.

Chapter 9

Recombinant Protein Production by a Kaiko–Baculovirus System

Hidekazu Nagaya

Summary

Nucleopolyhedrovirus, a baculovirus, generates many intranuclear polyhedra in lepidopterous insects. The replacement of the polyhedra gene with a target gene, under a potent polyhedrin promoter, is widely used to express recombinant proteins. In this chapter, we describe the application of a highly efficient and reproducible baculovirus expression system with high throughput using Kaiko (silkworm).

Key words: Recombinant, Protein, Silkworm, Kaiko, Baculovirus

1. Introduction

Chemical biology is a new area of research in the postgenome era, representing a fusion of chemistry with life science, and is regarded as a promising direction for life science research in the twenty-first century. In this field of research, reverse chemical genetics provides a method for the elucidation of gene function by examining the binding activities of low-molecular compounds with target proteins.

The progress of reverse chemical genetics research is influenced by the efficiency of generation of active recombinant proteins. In recent years, numerous systems for the expression of the recombinant proteins have been developed. Of these, the baculovirus system is considered to be the most efficient. Typically in the baculovirus system, an insect cell line (for example, Sf9) is used as a host for the expression of recombinant proteins. In the present report, we describe the novel application of Kaiko as a host in the baculovirus system for the expression of recombinant

Hisashi Koga (ed.), *Reverse Chemical Genetics*, Methods in Molecular Biology, vol. 577
DOI 10.1007/978-1-60761-232-2_9, © Humana Press, a part of Springer Science+Business Media, LLC 2009

proteins. The Kaiko has several advantages over the traditional insect cells as hosts in the baculovirus system, including high productivity, high reproducibility (stable expression), and rapid and simultaneous production.

2. Materials

2.1. Cell Culture

1. BmN cell line (RIKEN Bio Resource Center, Japan) *(1)*.
2. TC-100 supplemented with 10% fetal bovine serum (FBS) *(2)* (*see* **Note 1**).

2.2. Construction of Recombinant Plasmid

1. PCR-related reagents and restriction enzymes.
2. 2% agarose.
3. UltraClean (MO BIO Laboratories, Inc. CA USA).
4. Transfer vector pM series.
5. Alkaline phosphatase (calf intestine).
6. DNA Ligation Kit Ver2.1 (TAKARA BIO INC., Japan).
7. Competent *E. coli* DHα cells.
8. SOC medium (2% tryptone, 0.5% yeast extract, 10 mM NaCl,, 2.5 mM KCl, 10 mM $MgCl_2$, 10 mM $MgSO_4$, 20 mM glucose).

2.3. Preparation of Viral DNA

1. 10 mM Tris–HCl (pH 7.5), 1 mM EDTA.
2. 40% sucrose solution, stored at room temperature.
3. 10% SDS solution, stored at room temperature.
4. Protease K.

2.4. Cotransfect Ion

1. Lipofectin reagent stored at 4°C.

2.5. Infection of Silkworms

1. Silkworm larvae or pupae (or both).
2. Artificial food (Katakura Industries Co., Ltd., Japan).

2.6. Homogenization

1. *Homogenization buffer.* 20 mM Tris–HCl, 150 mM NaCl, 10 mM benzamidine, 1 mM PMSF, 1 mM DTT, 1 mM EDTA, 1 mM EGTA, 10% (v/v) glycerol, phenylthiourea powder.

2.7. Sds-PAGE

1. e-PAGEL for SDS-PAGE.
2. *Sample buffer (1×).* 50 mM Tris–HCl, pH 6.8, 4% (w/v) SDS, 10% (w/v) glycerol, 0.02% (w/v) BPB, 10% (v/v) 2-mercaptoethanol. Store at room temperature.
3. *Running buffer (10×).* 250 mM Tris–HCl, 1,920 mM glycine, 1% (w/v) SDS. Store at room temperature.
4. Prestained molecular weight markers: Kaleidoscope markers.

2.8. Western Blotting

1. *Transfer buffer (1×).* 10 mM Tris–HCl, 190 mM glycine, 10% (v/v) methanol. Store at room temperature.

2. *TTBS.* Prepare 10× stock with 1.37 M NaCl, 27 mM KCl, 250 mM Tris–HCl, pH 7.4, 1% Tween-20. Dilute 100 mL of stock with 900 mL water just before use.

3. *Blocking buffer.* 5% (w/v) skim milk in TTBS.

4. *First antibody* For example, anti-His probe (Santa Cruz Biotechnology, Inc., USA).

5. *Secondary antibody.* For example, anti-rabbit antibody.

6. Filter paper.

7. PVDF membrane.

8. ECL detection reagent.

9. X-ray film.

3. Methods (Diagram of Protocol Shown in Fig. 1)

1. Quickly thaw frozen stock cells at 25°C in a water bath and then seed into a 25-mL flask with 4 mL of fresh medium.

3.1. Cell Culture

2. Once the cells are attached to the surface, replace the medium with 4 mL of fresh medium at 25°C.

3. When the cells are deemed to be overconfluent, the medium is removed by using a pipette.

4. The cells are removed from the surface of the flask by tapping the flask lightly.

5. The cells are transferred to a new flask containing fresh medium.

6. The cells in the new flask are immediately mixed to ensure uniform distribution of cells and then cultured at 25°C for 4 d (*see* **Note 2**).

3.2. Construction of the Recombinant Plasmid

1. The target gene DNA is prepared by PCR amplification or by excision from the cloning vector by using appropriate restriction enzymes (*see* **Notes 3** and **4**).

2. Target gene DNA is identified by agarose gel electrophoresis.

3. After electrophoresis of all samples, the band containing the target gene is excised from the agarose gel.

4. Target gene DNA is recovered and purified from the gel by using Ultraclean (MO BIO Laboratories, Inc. CA USA).

5. The transfer vector (pM series) is cut with the appropriate restriction enzymes for insertion of the target gene DNA.

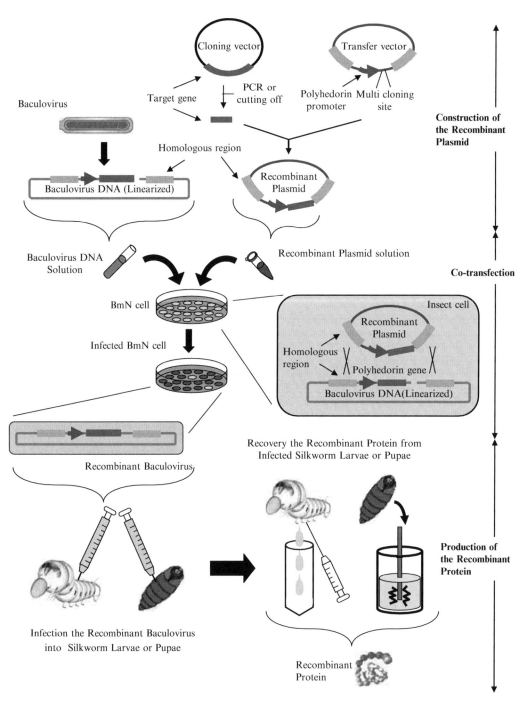

Fig. 1. Protocol of the recombinant protein production system by the Kaiko–baculovirus.

6. After linearization of the transfer vector with alkaline phosphatase, the target gene DNA is ligated into the linearized transfer vector by using DNA Ligation Kit Ver 2.1 (TAKARA BIO INC., Japan) (*see* **Note 5**).

7. The ligation solution is incubated at 16°C for 30 min (*see* **Note 6**).

8. After the incubation, the ligation solution is added to DH5α competent cells.

9. The ligation solution and competent cell mixture is incubated on ice for 30 min.

10. The tube containing the above mixture is placed in a rack in a circulating water bath, preheated at 42°C, for exactly 45 s (*see* **Note 7**).

11. The tube is then rapidly transferred to ice and the mixture cooled for 2 min.

12. SOC medium is added to the tube, and the cultures are incubated at 37°C for 60 min.

13. The transformed competent cells are poured onto an agar plate and distributed by swirling.

14. The plate coated with the transformed competent cells is incubated in an inverted position at 37°C for 12–16 h.

15. Colonies harboring the recombinant plasmid are confirmed by using PCR-based colony identification methods.

16. The confirmed recombinant plasmid is sequenced in the connecting region or in all regions.

3.3. Preparation of Viral DNA

1. For infection, BmN cell monolayers are cultured to confluence in a bottle with a surface area of 225 cm^2.

2. The medium is removed and 1 mL of diluted viral solution containing approximately 2×10^8 PFU of BmNPV is added.

3. After incubation for 60 min with rocking at 10-min intervals, 19 mL of growth medium is added.

4. The cellular fluids are collected at about 6 d (*see* **Note 8**) after inoculation and centrifuged at 3,000 rpm for 20 min at 4°C.

5. The low-speed supernatants then are loaded onto 40% (w/w) sucrose prepared in a 40-mL tube for the SW28 rotor (*see* **Note 9**).

6. After the centrifugation at 20,000 rpm for 30 min, the supernatants are removed by wiping away the water droplets on the surface of the tube.

7. The resultant precipitates are suspended in about 2 mL of 10 mM Tris–HCl (pH 7.5) and 1 mM EDTA, and 200 µL of each solution is transferred into a 1.5-mL microtube.

8. For protease digestion, 10 µL of 10% SDS and 20 µL of 20 mg/mL of protease K are added to a microtube and mixed gently by flicking the tube with a finger (*see* **Note 10**).

9. After incubation at 56°C for 1 h, phenol–chloroform extraction is performed by extracting the mixture 2–3 times with an equal volume of phenol (*see* **Note 11**), an equal volume of phenol:chloroform (1:1), and then twice with an equal volume of chloroform.

10. Each extraction is performed by inverting the tube very slowly. With the exception of the final extraction with chloroform, the lower organic layer is removed by using a pipette.

11. The aqueous layer containing the DNA is transferred to a new microfuge tube and stored at 4°C (*see* **Note 12**).

3.4. Cotransfection

1. Confluent BmN cell monolayers are prepared in a 35-mm dish (5×10^5 cells in 2 mL medium).

2. For cotransfection, the transfer plasmid, baculovirus DNA, and Lipofectin (Invitrogen, CA USA) are mixed with TC-100 medium without FBS.

3. The transfection mixture is incubated at room temperature for 15 min.

4. TC-100 medium without FBS is added to the transfection mixture.

5. The growth medium is removed from the confluent BmN cell monolayers and the cells are washed with TC-100 without FBS.

6. After removal of all TC-100 without FBS, the transfection mixture is added gently.

7. For BmN cells, co-transfection is also performed at 25°C over 5 h (*see* **Note 13**).

8. After cotransfection, the mixture solution is removed, and fresh TC-100 medium is added.

9. After transfection, the BmN cells are cultured for approximately 6 d.

10. After the BmN cells have started to float, the cell culture fluid containing the recombinant baculovirus is harvested for silkworm infection and stored at 4°C or −80°C (*see* **Note 14**).

3.5. Infection of Insects

1. The recombinant baculovirus solution is diluted to 50 times with distilled water.

2. For secretary proteins, the diluted baculovirus solution is injected into the body cavity of silkworm larvae at the 5-instar stage (*see* **Notes 15** and **16**). For nonsecretary proteins, including intracellular proteins, membrane proteins, and nuclear proteins, the diluted baculovirus solution is injected into silkworm pupae (*see* **Note 17**).

3. Infected silkworm larvae or pupae are incubated at 25°C for 6 d (*see* **Note 18**).

3.6. Recovery of Recombinant Protein

1. For recovery of secretary proteins, the legs of the infected silkworms are scratched 6 d after infection, and haemolymph is collected on ice.

2. Haemolymph is collected in a 50-mL tube containing phenylthiourea.

3. Phenylthiourea can inhibit melanization (*see* **Note 19**).

4. The recovered haemolymph samples are centrifuged at $100,000 \times g$ for 60 min.

5. For recovery of nonsecretary proteins, infected silkworm pupae are collected and stored below –80°C.

6. The frozen infected silkworm pupae are homogenized in homogenization buffer.

7. If solubilization is necessary, the homogenized samples are solubilized with the detergent, for example, Triton X-100.

8. Homogenized solutions are centrifuged at $100,000 \times g$ for 60 min, and the supernatant and precipitate are separated.

3.7. SDS-PAGE

1. Sample buffer (1×) is added in equal volumes to the samples (haemolymph or aliquot of the homogenization solution).

2. The samples then are boiled with the sample buffer at 100°C for 2 min.

3. The samples are then immediately cooled on ice and stored at 4°C.

4. The ATTO electrophoresis mini slab-type system is used for SDS-PAGE.

5. Gel unit A is assembled with a ready-made gel, and running buffer diluted 10 times with distilled water is added to the electrophoresis tank.

6. The wells then are rinsed with running buffer.

7. After adding running buffer to the upper chamber, 20 μL of sample is loaded in each well, include 1 well for prestained molecular weight markers.

8. The gel is run at 20 mA for 80 min.

3.8. Western Blotting

1. The PVDF membrane is rinsed in 100% MeOH.

2. The membrane is washed once in distilled water.

3. Filter paper (six sheets) and PVDF membrane are soaked in transfer buffer for 30 min.

4. Once electrophoresis is completed, the gel is removed from the gel unit and soaked in transfer buffer for about 5 min.

5. The Bio-Rad Trans-Blot Semi-Dry system is used for Western blotting.

6. Initially, three sheets of filter paper soaked in the transfer buffer are stacked on the anodic electrode plate.

7. The membrane then is placed exactly over the top sheet of the filter paper.

8. The gel is laid precisely on top of the membrane.

9. The remaining three sheets of filter paper soaked in transfer buffer are placed on top of the gel, ensuring that no bubbles are trapped between each layer.

10. The cathode electrode plate is placed on top of the stack and the safety cover is added.

11. Transfer is performed at 20 V and 0.16 A/gel for 60 min.

12. Once the transfer is completed, the blotting system is carefully disassembled. The filter paper and gel are removed and the membrane is placed in TBS buffer for 10 min. Finally, the membrane is soaked in blocking buffer for 60 min.

13. The blocking buffer is discarded and the membrane is then incubated with primary antibody in blocking buffer for 1 h at room temperature.

14. The primary antibody is removed and the membrane washed 3 times for 5 min each with TTBS (*see* **Note 20**).

15. The membrane is incubated with secondary antibody in blocking buffer for 60 min at room temperature. The secondary antibody is freshly prepared for each experiment as a 1:10,000-fold dilution in blocking buffer.

16. The secondary antibody is discarded, and the membrane is washed 3 times for 10 min each with TTBS.

17. For the final wash, the membrane is washed in TBS and then soaked in TBS.

18. Protein expression is visualized by the ECL Plus Western Blotting Detection Kit (GE Healthcare).

19. The A and B solutions in the kit are mixed together at room temperature and then added directly to the membrane, which is rotated by hand to ensure even coverage.

20. The membrane is picked up from ECL reagents, wiped with a Kim-wipe, and then wrapped in plastic kitchen wrap.

21. The wrapped membrane then is placed in an X-ray film cassette with film in the darkroom for a suitable exposure time, typically about 5 min. An example of the results produced is shown in **Fig. 2**.

3.9. Conclusion

High throughput production of recombinant proteins can be achieved by removing the virus screening step and enhancing the rate of transfection by using linearized baculovirus DNA *(3)*. Knock-down of the cysteine protease gene from the baculovirus

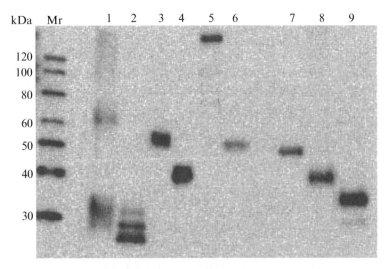

Fig. 2. Expression of the recombinant proteins by the Kaiko–baculovirus. (1) Insulin-like growth factor binding protein 6 (IGFBP6) from the silkworm lavae haemolymph (2) Mouse interferon beta (mIFNβ) from the silkworm lavae haemolymph (3) c-Jun N-terminal kinases (JNK3) from homogenization of the silkworm puae (4) Mitogen-activated protein kinase kinase 3 (MAP2K3) from homogenization of the silkworm puae (5) Sentrin specific peptidase 6 (SENP6) from homogenization of the silkworm puae (6) Caspase 1 from homogenization of the silkworm puae (7) UDP-glucose dehydrogenase (UGDH) from homogenization of the silkworm puae (8) Interleukin 8 receptor, beta (IL8RB) from homogenization of the silkworm puae (9) G protein-coupled bile acid receptor 1 (GPBAR1) from homogenization of the silkworm puae.

genome inhibits degradation of recombinant target proteins (4) and has improved the production and total yield of proteins.

Silkworm larvae or pupae can be selected as hosts according to the localization of the target protein. Silkworm larvae are used as hosts for secretary proteins, whereas silkworm pupae are used as hosts for nonsecretory proteins. **Figure 2** shows the expression of nine proteins by using silkworm larvae and pupae. Bands specific for cytokines IGFBP6 (insulin-like growth factor binding protein 6) and mouse IFN (interferon) β indicate the expression of these proteins in silkworm haemolymph. The multiple bands in the case of mouse IFNβ were perhaps due to variable glycosylation (5). The intracellular kinase proteins JNK3 and MAP2K3 are shown in lanes 3 and 4, respectively. These proteins were expressed in silkworm pupae and were detected after homogenization of the pupae. The high-molecular weight protein SENBP6, a protease of 130 kDa, was expressed normally. The GPCR membrane proteins IL8RB and GPBAR1 migrated at the predicted molecular weights.

The Kaiko–baculovirus protein production system has many advantages, including high productivity, high reproducibility (stable expression), rapid production, and the capacity for simultaneous production of several proteins. Furthermore, this system can be adapted to scale-up production and provides excellent cost performance when compared with insect cell production systems.

To date, complex proteins with biological activity *(6)*, for use in X-ray crystal structure analysis *(7)* and ELISA systems *(8)*, and for the development of animal drugs *(9)* have successfully been produced by using this system. Therefore, the Kaiko–baculovirus protein production system has broad applicability across the field of reverse chemical genetics for the analysis of protein function on the basis of interactions with chemical compounds.

4. Notes

1. The quality of FBS varies by lot number. Therefore, testing of cell morphology and growth is recommended for selection of an optimal batch of FBS.
2. In general, cells progress through one cycle every 4–5 d. When the medium contains many dead cells, replacement with fresh medium is strongly recommended.
3. Target genes and transfer vectors should be purified by large-scale preparation procedures for rapid and efficient digestion by restriction enzymes.
4. Restriction enzyme digestions should be performed by using a 10–20-fold dilution of the DNA.
5. The molar ratio of the target DNA to plasmid vector in the ligation reaction should be 1:1 to 1:10.
6. Perform ligation reactions overnight in cases when ligation is inefficient.
7. Heat-shock treatment is a crucial step. It is very important that cells be raised to exactly the right temperature at the correct rate.
8. For the preparation of viral DNA, the cultured medium should be made with a high concentration of viral particles to provide 200–500 µg viral genome DNA from 50 mL of culture medium.
9. A tube for ultracentrifuge with a much bigger volume than the sample should be used.
10. The baculovirus genome is about 130 kb and unable to withstand shearing. For this reason, it is strongly suggested that vigorous stirring and pipetting be avoided once SDS is added.
11. Use fresh phenol to avoid degradation of DNA due to oxidation products.
12. The concentration of viral DNA should not be less than 0.3 µg/ml.

13. Overnight cotransfection is permitted.

14. Recombinant rates are very high due to the use of linearized viral DNA. According to circumstances, viral screening should be performed.

15. Silkworm larvae can be anesthetized in ice water for 3–5 min in cases when the injection of silkworm larvae is difficult.

16. Take care not to damage the enteric canal with the syringe when performing injections and when harvesting the haemolymph.

17. Silkworm pupae can be stored at low temperature for about 3 mo. When needed for injection, silkworm pupae are removed from the refrigerator and sterilized by using a disinfectant.

18. The cap placed on the container should have tiny holes to prevent the build-up of excessive moisture in the container.

19. A reducing reagent such as DTT or 2-ME can be used instead of phenylthiourea.

20. The primary antibody can be stored at 4°C for subsequent experiments by adding sodium azide to final concentration a 0.02%.

Acknowledgments

I would like to thank Dr. Susumu Maeda of the University of California Davis and Dr. Hisashi Koga of the Kazusa DNA Research Institute and Dr. Kouhei Tsumoto of the University of Tokyo for their help in editing the manuscript. I also thank all the staff of the Research Institute of Biological Science of Katakura Industries Co., Ltd.

References

1. Maeda, S. (1984) A plaque assay and cloning of *Bombyx mori* nuclear polyhedrosis virus. *J. Seric. Sci. Jpn.* **53**, 547–548.

2. Maeda, S. *Invertebrate Cell system applications* 1(J. Mitsuhashi, ed.) (1989) CRC, Boca Raton, Vol. I., p.167.

3. Paul A. K., Martin D. A., and Robert D. P. (1990) Linearization of baculovirus DNA enhances the recovery of recombinant virus expression vectors. *Nucleic Acids Res.* **18**, 5667–5672.

4. Suzuki T., Kanaya T., Okazaki H., Ogawa K., Usami A., Watanabe H., Kadono-Okuda K., Yamakawa M., Sato H., Mori H., Takahashi S. and Oda K. (1997) Efficient protein production using Bpmbyx mori nuclear polyhedrosis virus lacking the cysteine protease gene. *J. Gen. Virol.* **78**, 3073–3080.

5. Misaki R., Nagaya H., Fujiyama K., Yanagihara I., Honda T. and Seki T. (2003) N-linked glycan structures of mouse interferon-β produced by *Bombyx mori* larvae. *Biochem. Biophys. Res. Commun.* **311**, 979–986.

6. Kobayashi M., Morita T., Ikeguchi K., Yoshizaki G., Suzuki T. and Watabe S. (2006) In vivo biological activity of recombinant goldfish gonadotropins produced by baculovirus in silkworm larvae. *Aquaculture.* **256**, 433–442.

7. Matsumoto K., Kondo K., Ota T., Kawashima A., Kitamura, K, Ishida T. (2006) Binding model of novel 1-substituted quinazoline derivatives to poly (ADP-ribose) polymerase-catalytic domain, revealed by X-ray crystal structure analysis of complexes. *Biochi. et Biophy. Acta.* **1764**, 913–919.

8. Suzuki T., Kaki H., Naya S., Murayama S., Tatsui A., Nagai A., Takai S. and Miyazaki M. (2002) Recombinant human chymase produced by silkworm-baculovirus expression system: Its application for a chymase detection kit. *Jpn. J. Pharmacol.* **90**, 210–213.

9. Ueda Y., Sakurai T., Kasama K., Satoh Y., Atsumi K., Hanawa S., Uchino T. and Yanai A. (1993) Pharmacokinetic properties of recombinant feline interferon and its stimulatory effect on 2′–5′-oligoadenylate synthetase activity in the cat. *J. Vet. Med. Sci.* **55**, 1–6

Chapter 10

Pulse-Chase Experiment for the Analysis of Protein Stability in Cultured Mammalian Cells by Covalent Fluorescent Labeling of Fusion Proteins

Kei Yamaguchi, Shinichi Inoue, Osamu Ohara, and Takahiro Nagase

Summary

We used HaloTag® labeling technology for the pulse labeling of proteins in cultured mammalian cells. HaloTag® technology allows a HaloTag-fusion protein to covalently bind to a specific small molecule fluorescent ligand. Thus specifically labeled HaloTag-fusion proteins can be chased in cells and observed in vitro after separation by sodium dodecyl sulfate polyacrylamide gel electrophoresis (SDS-PAGE). The Fluorescent HaloTag® ligand allows quantification of the labeled proteins by fluorescent image analysis. Herein, we demonstrated that the method allows analysis of the intracellular protein stability as regulated by protein-degradation signals or an exogenously expressed E3 ubiquitin ligase.

Key words: Covalent labeling, E3 ubiquitin ligase, Fluorescence, Imaging, Intracellular, Protein degradation signal, Protein stability, Pulse chase

1. Introduction

Pulse-chase experiments by metabolic labeling of cultured cells are used for time course profiling of newly synthesized proteins undergoing intracellular transport, post-translational modification, or degradation *(1–3)*. [35S]methionine has often been used in pulse-chase experiments because it is relatively stable with high specific activity and is not modified by transamination or interconversion in cells *(4)*. However, the use of [35S]methionine has some disadvantages; i.e., it is rather time-consuming, and a specific antibody against the protein of interest is needed to isolate the protein from the labeled cell extract.

Hisashi Koga (ed.), *Reverse Chemical Genetics*, Methods in Molecular Biology, vol. 577
DOI 10.1007/978-1-60761-232-2_10, © Humana Press, a part of Springer Science+Business Media, LLC 2009

Recently, several technologies have emerged for labeling specific fusion proteins in vivo. These technologies are based on the covalent binding of small molecules containing a functional moiety such as fluorophores or affinity molecules *(5–7)*. One of these technologies utilizes the 33 kD HaloTag® protein, which is an engineered haloalkane dehalogenase designed to rapidly form a stable covalent bond with ligands composed of aliphatic chloride and fluorophore *(7)*. It is possible to utilize the specific fluorescent-labeling characteristic of HaloTag-fusion proteins for pulse-chase experimentation. The HaloTag® ligands are useful tools for these experiments because they have a high degree of cell permeability and a rapid labeling activity in living cells. Moreover, the labeling is specific for the HaloTag protein, and the resultant labeled proteins can be observed after the protein separation of cell lysates by sodium dodecyl sulfate polyacrylamide gel electrophoresis (SDS-PAGE). The labeled ligands also allow quantification of the labeled proteins through fluorescent image analysis. Therefore, pulse-chase experiments using this method would be useful in the field of chemical genomics, e.g., in the screening of chemical compounds that affect the stability of the proteins of interest.

2. Materials

1. HaloTag® pHT2 vector (Promega, Madison, WI) was used for the construction of pHT2NF vector. pFC8A (HaloTag) CMV vector (Promega) was used for the construction of SMAD1-HaloTag expression clone.

2. pcDNA-DEST47 and pcDNA-DEST53 (Invitrogen, Carlsbad, CA) were used for the construction of pcDNA-DEST47 GFP.

3. HEK293 (HSRRB, Osaka, Japan; No. JCRB9068) cells were grown in Dulbecco's Modified Eagle's Medium (DMEM) (Gibco/Invitrogen) supplemented with 10% Fetal Bovine Serum (FBS) (BD Biosciences, Franklin Lakes, NJ) and 1× Antibiotic–Antimycotic reagent (100 U/mL penicillin + 100 μg/mL streptomycin + 0.25 μg/mL amphotericin B; Invitrogen).

4. Tissue Culture Plate, 96 well (BD Biosciences).

5. FuGENE6 Transfection Reagent (Roche Diagnostics, Basel, Switzerland).

6. PBS.

7. 37°C cell culture CO_2 incubator.

8. HaloTag® tetramethylrhodamine (TMR) ligand (Promega).

9. HaloTag® succinimidyl ester (O4) ligand (Promega) was used for the preparation of blocking ligand.

10. 100 mM Tris–HCl (pH 8.0).

11. MDG-267 Real Gel Plate (Biocraft, Tokyo, Japan) was used for SDS-PAGE.

12. *2× sample buffer.* 100 mM Tris–HCl (pH 6.8), 20% glycerol, 4% SDS, 2% β-mercaptoethanol, and 0.1% (w/v) bromophenol blue. β-mercaptoethanol was added to the buffer just before use.

13. *SDS-PAGE buffer.* 25 mM Tris, 200 mM glycine, 0.1% (w/v) SDS.

14. Fluoro image analyzer FLA-3000GF (Fujifilm, Tokyo, Japan).

15. MultiGauge image analyzing software (Fujifilm).

16. PVDF membrane (FluoroTrans W; PALL, Portsmouth, UK).

17. *Transfer buffer.* 25 mM Tris, 192 mM glycine, 10% (V/V) methanol, 0.1% (W/V) SDS.

18. BE-300 semidry transfer device (Biocraft).

19. *TBS.* 20 mM Tris–HCl (pH 7.5), 150 mM NaCl.

20. Tween-20.

21. Skim milk (BD Biosciences).

22. Anti-HaloTag rabbit IgG antibody (Promega).

23. HRP-conjugated anti-rabbit IgG antibody (Promega).

24. Amersham™ ECL plus Western blotting detection system (GE Healthcare, Buckinghamshire, UK).

25. Luminescent image analyzer LAS3000 (Fujifilm).

26. MagicMark™ XP Western Protein Standard (Invitrogen).

27. 8-well chambered coverglass (Nalgen Nunc International/ Thermo-Fisher Scientific, Waltham, MA).

28. DMEM without phenol red (Gibco/Invitrogen).

29. Hoechst 33342 (Sigma-Aldrich, St. Louis, MO).

30. BioZero fluorescent microscope (KEYENCE, Osaka, Japan).

3. Methods

3.1. Expression Plasmid

pHT2NF vector was constructed by inserting synthetic double-stranded oligonucleotides (5′-GAGCTCGATCTGATCGAAGG TCGTGGTATCCCTCGTAACTCTCGTGTTGAT-GCGATCGCGAATTCGTTTAAAC-3′) at the *Nae* I site of pHT2 vector to create *Sgf* I and *Pme* I sites after the HaloTag coding sequence. pHT2CF vector was constructed by inserting synthetic double-stranded oligonucleotides (5′-GCGATCGCAA-GCTTGAATTCGAGCTCCA-3′) at the *Eco*R V site of pHT2 vector to create *Sgf* I and *Eco*ICR I sites before the HaloTag coding sequence. The DNA fragments containing PEST or CL1 sequences which are known to be protein-degradation signals were obtained from pGL4.19[luc2CP/Neo] (Promega) by PCR with each primer appended by *Sgf*I or *Pme* I sites at the 5′ end: CL1, 5′-GCGATCGCCATGGCTTGCAAGAACTGGTTCAGTAGCT-TAAGCCACTTTGTGATCCACCTTAACAGCGTTTAAAC-3′; PEST,5′-GCGATCGCCATGCACGGCTTCCCTCCCGAGGT-GGAGGAGCAGGCCGCCGGCACCCTGCCCATGAGCT-GCGCCCAGGAGAGCGGCATGGATAGACACCCTGCT-GCTTGCGCCAGCGCCAGGATCAACGTCGTTTAAAC-3′. The fragments were then inserted into the *Sgf* I and *Pme* I sites of pHT2NF vector for the construction of HaloTag-CL1 and HaloTag-PEST expression clones. To create a SMAD1-HaloTag fusion protein expression clone, Smad1 ORF was recovered from pF1KB5319 *(8)* and inserted into the *Sgf* I and *Eco*ICR I sites of pFC8A (HaloTag) vector. pcDNA-DEST47ΔGFP was constructed by the ligation of a 1,460 bp *Pst* I fragment of pcDNA-DEST53 with a 5,772 bp *Pst* I fragment of pcDNA-DEST47. N-terminal Myc-tagged Smurf1 was constructed using pcDNAnMyc-DEST, which was prepared by inserting double-stranded oligonucleotides including the Myc tag sequence into the *Hind* III site of pcDNA-DEST47ΔGFP, using the Gateway LR recombination reaction (Invitrogen) *(9)*.

3.2. Blocking of Continuous Labeling of HaloTag Protein in Cultured Mammalian Cells

We first optimized the amount of HaloTag blocking ligands for a pulse-chase experiment to prevent continuous labeling of the target proteins (**Fig. 1a**). Fifty nanomolar of TMR ligand was used for the labeling, because an excess amount of TMR ligands results in an increase in the residual free ligands in cells and culture medium (*see* **Note 1**). We also show fluorescent images of TMR-labeled HaloTag proteins in living cultured cells under different conditions by pulse labeling (with blocking ligand) or continuous labeling (without blocking ligand) (**Fig. 1b**).

3.2.1. Effects of Blocking Ligand for Continuous Labeling of HaloTag Protein

1. To prepare HaloTag blocking ligand, HaloTag Succinimidyl Ester (O4) Ligand (20 mM) was incubated with 100 mM Tris–HCl (pH 8.0) for 60 min at 25°C to mask the functional groups.
2. HEK293 cells were plated in a 96-well Tissue Culture Plate (100 μL; 4.5×10^4 cells/well) with DMEM supplemented with 10% FBS and incubated for 24 h at 37°C with 5% CO_2.
3. The cells were transfected with 50 ng of HaloTag expression plasmid with 150 ng of pcDNA-DEST47 GFP as a carrier

DNA using FuGENE6 Transfection Reagent according to the manufacturer's instructions and cultured for 36 h in DMEM with 10% FBS.

4. The HaloTag proteins were labeled for 10 min with the growth medium containing 50 nM HaloTag TMR ligands (Pulse), and the cells were washed free of TMR ligands by a 4-time rinse with 100 μL of the growth medium (*see* **Note 2**).

5. The cells were continuously incubated in the growth medium including a different amount of HaloTag blocking ligands (500 nM, 5 μM, and 50 μM) for the indicated time period (Chase) except for the sample at the zero time point **(Fig. 1a)**.

6. The cells were carefully washed with PBS and dissolved in 40 μL of 2× sample buffer at the indicated time point of the chase **(Fig. 1a)**.

7. TMR-labeled proteins were separated by SDS-PAGE after boiling for 5 min at 95°C, and amounts of the labeled proteins were measured as fluorescence intensities of the TMR by the Fluoro Image Analyzer FLA3000 and MultiGauge software (*see* **Note 3**).

3.2.2. Western Blotting

1. HaloTag-fusion proteins separated by SDS-PAGE were electrophoretically transferred onto a PVDF membrane using the transfer buffer with the semidry transfer device (2 mA/cm², 60 min).

2. The resultant PVDF membrane was washed with TBS including 0.05% Tween-20 (TBST) for 10 min with gentle agitation (incubation was done with gentle agitation thereafter).

3. After preincubation of the membrane with TBST containing 5% skim milk for 60 min, the membrane was incubated with 1:4,000 anti-HaloTag rabbit IgG antibody (Promega) in TBST containing 1% skim milk for 60 min.

4. After being washed with TBST for 5 min four times, the membrane was further incubated with 1:5,000 horseradish-peroxidase-conjugated anti-rabbit IgG antibody (Promega) in TBST containing 1% skim milk for 60 min.

5. After the membrane was washed with TBST for 5 min four times, HaloTag-fusion proteins were finally detected using ECL plus according to the manufacturer's instructions.

6. The luminescent images were recorded by the Luminescent Image Analyzer LAS3000 **(Fig. 1a)**.

7. MagicMark™ XP Western Protein Standard was used for estimation of the apparent molecular masses of the HaloTag-fusion proteins.

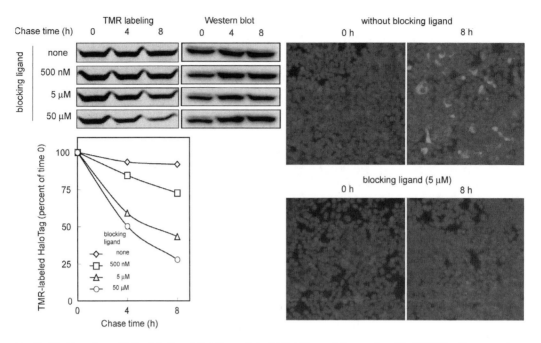

Fig. 1. Blocking of constitutive labeling of HaloTag protein. (a) HaloTag proteins produced in HEK293 cells were pulse-labeled by 50 nM TMR ligand and chased at the indicated times with or without HaloTag blocking ligands (0, 500 nM, 5 μM or 50 μM). Fluorescent images of TMR ligand covalently bound to HaloTag were recorded after SDS-PAGE of cell lysates (*upper*), and the fluorescent intensities are plotted relative to the amount present at the zero time point (*lower*). (b) Fluorescent images of TMR ligand-labeled HaloTag protein in HEK293 cells at the indicated times after the labeling with or without blocking ligand (TMR-labeled proteins and Hoechst-labeled nuclei are shown in *light-gray* and *gray* colors, respectively).

3.2.3. Fluorescent Imaging of HaloTag Protein in Living Mammalian Cultured Cells

1. HEK293 cells (200 μL; 4×10^4/well) were plated in an 8-well chambered coverglass with DMEM supplemented with 10% FBS and incubated for 24 h at 37°C with 5% CO_2.

2. The cells were transfected with 50 ng of HaloTag expression plasmid with 150 ng of pcDNA-DEST47 GFP as a carrier DNA using FuGENE6.

3. The HaloTag proteins were labeled 36 h after the transfection by adding 100 μL of DMEM containing 150 nM TMR ligand (the final concentration of the TMR ligand was 50 nM) for 10 min.

4. The unreacted TMR ligands were carefully removed from the growth medium by exchanging 200 μL of the medium for 500 μL of DMEM without phenol red medium. The cells were further washed by exchanging 400 μL of the culture medium for 400 μL of the colorless DMEM three times. Finally, 100 μL each of colorless DMEM with or without 15 μM blocking ligand was added to the respective wells of the cultured cells after 400 μL of the medium was removed (the final concentration of the blocking ligand was 5 μM) (*see* **Note 2**).

5. The TMR-labeled HaloTag proteins were observed and recorded in the cultured cells using the fluorescent microscope BioZero in the growth medium with or without 5 μM blocking ligand at the time points indicated in **Fig. 1b**.

3.3. Pulse-Chase Experiments of Halo-Tag-Fusion Proteins

The HaloTag® technology is suitable for experiments intended to elucidate differences in the cellular degradation rates of exogenously expressed HaloTag-fusion proteins. However, the results of these types of experiments do not necessarily reflect the intrinsic half-life of the corresponding native protein. To determine if we can effectively monitor differences in the degradation rates of HaloTag fusion proteins based on the expected properties of the fusion partner, we utilized HaloTag proteins fused with known C-terminal protein-degradation sequences such as PEST and CL-1 *(10, 11)* (**Fig. 2a**). In further studies, to examine the degradation rates of HaloTag fusion protein, we evaluated the degradation of C-terminal HaloTag-fused Smad1 (SMAD1-HaloTag) protein. Smad1 is a target protein of the E3 ubiquitin ligase, Smurf1. Targeted ubiquitination and degradation of ectopically expressed Smad1 by coexpressed Flag-tagged hSmurf1 was originally reported in a pulse-chase labeling experiment using [^{35}S]methionine and immunoprecipitation with an anti-Smad1

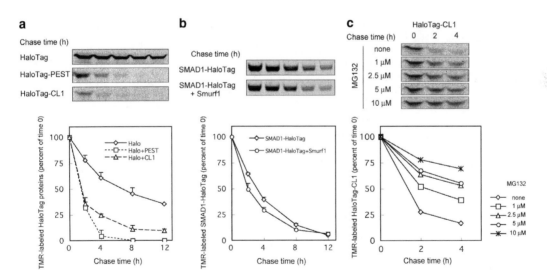

Fig. 2. Pulse-chase experiments of HaloTag-fusion proteins regulated by protein-degradation signals or an E3 ubiquitin ligase. (**a**) HaloTag, HaloTag-PEST, or HaloTag-CL1 produced in HEK293 cells were pulse-labeled by 50 nM TMR ligand and chased at the indicated times with 5 μM blocking ligand. (**b**) SMAD1-HaloTag fusion was expressed in HEK293 with or without Myc-tagged Smurf1 expression clone. SMAD1-HaloTag proteins were pulse-labeled by 50 nM TMR ligand and chased at the indicated times with 5 μM blocking ligand. (**c**) HaloTag-CL1 produced in HEK293 cells was pulse-labeled by 50 nM TMR ligand and chased at the indicated times with 5 μM blocking ligand in the presence or absence of MG132 (0, 1 μM, 2.5 μM, 5 μM, and 10 μM). In these experiments, fluorescent images of TMR were obtained after SDS-PAGE of cell lysates (upper in **a**, **b**, and **c**), and the fluorescent intensities are plotted relative to the amount present at the zero time point as an average of two independent experiments (lower in **a** and **b**) or a single experiment (lower in **c**).

polyclonal antibody *(12)*. To test whether we could monitor this regulation using a HaloTag fusion, we coexpressed Myc-tagged Smurf1 in HEK293 cells with the SMAD1-HaloTag fusion (**Fig. 2b**). We also show the effect of a proteasome inhibitor, MG132, on the protein degradation rate of HaloTag-CL1, since CL1 is a target sequence for degradation by the ubiquitin–proteasome system *(11)* (**Fig. 2c**).

3.3.1. Analysis of Intracellular Protein Stability of HaloTag-Fusion Proteins

1. HEK293 cells were plated on the 96-well Tissue Culture Plate (100 μL, 4.5×10^4 cells/well) with DMEM supplemented with 10% FBS and incubated for 24 h at 37°C with 5% CO_2.

2. The cells were transfected with 50 ng of HaloTag-PEST or HaloTag-CL1 expression plasmid with 150 ng pcDNA-DEST47ΔGFP as a carrier DNA for the pulse-chase experiments involving the protein-degradation signal using FuGENE6 Transfection reagent. The cells were then cultured for 36 h in DMEM with 10% FBS. For the experiments with E3 ubiquitin ligase, HEK293 cells were transfected with Halo-Tag-SMAD1 expression clone (50 ng) in combination with pcDNA-DEST47ΔGFP (control) or pcDNA-DESTmyc-tagged-Smurf1 (150 ng).

3. The HaloTag-fusion proteins were labeled for 10 min with the growth medium containing 50 nM HaloTag TMR ligands, and the cells were washed by a 4-time rinse with 100 μL of the growth medium.

4. The cells were continuously incubated in the growth medium including 5 μM of HaloTag blocking ligands for the indicated time period except for the sample at the zero time point.

5. The cells were washed with PBS and dissolved in 40 μL of 2× sample buffer at the indicated time point of the chase (**Figs. 2a, b**).

6. TMR-labeled proteins were separated by SDS-PAGE after boiling for 5 min at 95°C, and the amounts of the labeled proteins were measured as fluorescence intensities of the TMR by FLA3000 and MultiGauge software.

3.3.2. Blocking of Protein Degradation of HaloTag-CL1 by a Proteasome Inhibitor MG132

1. The HaloTag-CL1 expression plasmid was used for the transfection of HEK293 cells in the 96-well plate according to the method described in **Subheading 3.3.1.**

2. The cells were labeled with 50 nM TMR ligand and washed according to the methods described in **Subheading 3.2**, except for a 2 h-incubation with or without MG132 (0, 1 μM, 2.5 μM, 5 μM, and 10 μM) before the labeling and during the chase-times as indicated in **Fig. 2** (*see* **Note 4**).

3. The cells were continuously incubated in the growth medium including 5 μM of HaloTag blocking ligands for the indicated time period except for the sample at the zero time point.

4. The cells were washed with PBS and dissolved in 40 μL of 2× sample buffer at the indicated time point of the chase (**Fig. 2c**).

3.4. Conclusions

Increased degradation rates were observed with the HaloTag protein fused to the PEST or CL1 sequences (half-lives of less than 2 h) when compared with unfused HaloTag (a half-life of approximately 6 h) (**Fig. 2a**). At the zero time point, the levels of the TMR-labeled HaloTag-PEST and HaloTag-CL1 were considerably lower than that of the unfused HaloTag protein (17% and 9% relative to the amount of unfused HaloTag, respectively). This finding is likely the result of a reduction in the steady-state level of the protein due to the increase in the degradation rate of the PEST and CL-1 fused proteins. The HaloTag technology also allowed us to observe the degradation of labeled Smad1 that was induced by the coexpression of Smurf1 in these experiments. Although these results were not identical to the previously reported data *(12)*, they indicate that the HaloTag technology could allow monitoring of the regulation of SMAD1 degradation.

In conclusion, the experiments suggest that a pulse-chase labeling technique using HaloTag technology based on non-radioisotopic labeling of the target protein can provide a useful alternative to conventional methods. This technique provides an easy, accurate, and safe method of pulse-chase experimentation. In addition, protein-coding sequence (conventionally termed ORF) expression clones have been collected by many groups *(13–15)*. We have also started to prepare a set of human ORF clones in the form of expression plasmids for HaloTag fusion proteins *(8)*. The ORF clones thus prepared would serve as versatile reagents not only for the studies of protein stability but also for a wide variety of studies in chemical genomics using the advanced protein-labeling technology.

4. Notes

1. Although 50 nM of TMR ligand is sufficient to label the HaloTag-fusion proteins in these studies, an appropriate amount of TMR ligand used for the labeling might be optimized because the expression levels and/or TMR ligand-binding efficiencies of HaloTag-fusion proteins are different from gene to gene. To avoid continuous labeling of the target protein in a pulse-chase experiment, blocking ligand in a molar ratio to TMR ligand of more than 100-fold should be added after the cells are washed.

2. HEK293 cells are easy to unstick from the bottom of the plate, especially from a glass bottom, by washing. The washing manipulation should be carefully performed so that the cells are not removed.

3. The results of similar experiments using four other HaloTag-fusion proteins indicated that 5 μM blocking ligand is sufficient to completely prevent continuous labeling of newly synthesized HaloTag fusions by residual TMR ligand remaining in cells (data not shown).

4. Although no morphological changes of HEK293 cells were observed in the above conditions, an appropriate exposure length to MG132 besides an appropriate amount of the reagent should be determined for the cells to be used because long-term exposure to MG132 is toxic for cultured cells.

Acknowledgments

This project was supported by a grant from the Chiba prefectural government. We are grateful to B. Bulleit for his valuable comments. We thank K. Ozawa, T. Watanabe, and K. Yamada for their technical assistance.

References

1. Zhao, Z., Li, X., Hao, J., Winston, J. H., and Weinman, S. A. (2007) The ClC-3 chloride transport protein traffics through the plasma membrane via interaction of an N-terminal dileucine cluster with clathrin *J Biol Chem* **282**, 29022–29031.

2. Magee, A. I., Wootton, J., and de Bony, J. (1995) Detecting radiolabeled lipid-modified proteins in polyacrylamide gels *Methods Enzymol* **250**, 330–336.

3. Mosteller, R. D., Goldstein, R. V., and Nishimoto, K. R. (1980) Metabolism of individual proteins in exponentially growing *Escherichia coli J Biol Chem* **255**, 2524–2532.

4. Bonifacino, J. S. (1999) Metabolic labeling with amino acids P. 3.7.1–3.7.10. In J. E. Coligan, B. M. Dunn, D. W. Speicher, P. T. Wingfield, and G. P. Taylor (Eds.), *Current Protocols in Protein Science* **1**, Wiley, Hoboken, NJ.

5. Gronemeyer, T., Godin, G., and Johnsson, K. (2005) Adding value to fusion proteins through covalent labeling *Curr Opin Biotechnol* **16**, 453–458.

6. Keppler, A., Gendreizig, S., Gronemeyer, T., Pick, H., Vogel, H., and Johnsson, K. (2003) A general method for the covalent labeling of fusion proteins with small molecules *In Vivo Nat Biotechnol* **21**, 86–89.

7. Los, V. G., and Wood, K. (2007) The HaloTag™ p. 195–208. In D. L. Taylor, J. R. Haskins, and K. Giuliano (Eds.), *Methods in Molecular Biology* **356**. Human Press, Totowa, NJ.

8. Nagase, T., Yamakawa, H., Tadokoro, S., Nakajima, D., Inoue, S., Yamaguchi, K., Itokawa, Y., Kikuno, F. R., Koga, H., and Ohara, O. (2008) Exploration of human ORFeome: High throughput preparation of ORF clones and efficient characterization of their protein products *DNA Res* **15**, 137–149.

9. Yamaguchi, K., Nagase, T., Ando, A., and Ohara, O. (2008) Smurf1 directly targets hPEM-2, a GEF for Cdc42, via a novel combination of protein interaction modules in ubiquitin–proteasome pathway *Biol Chem* In press.

10. Rogers, S., Wells, R., and Rechsteiner, M. (1986) Amino acid sequences common to rapidly degraded proteins: The PEST hypothesis *Science* **234**, 364–368.

11. Gilon, T., Chomsky, O., and Kulka, R. G. (1998) Degradation signals for ubiquitin system

proteolysis in *Saccharomyces cerevisiae EMBO J* **17**, 2759–2766.

12. Zhu, H., Kavsak, P., Abdollah, S., Wrena, J. L., and Thomsen, G. H. (1999) A Smad ubiquitin ligase targets the BMP pathway and affects embryonic pattern formation *Nature* **400**, 687–693.

13. Rual, J. F., Hill, D. E., and Vidal, M. (2004) ORFeome projects: gateway between genomics and omics *Curr Opin Chem Biol* **8**, 20–25.

14. Nakajima, D., Saito, K., Yamakawa, H., et al. (2005) Preparation of a set of expression-ready clones of mammalian long cDNAs encoding large proteins by the ORF trap cloning method *DNA Res* **12**, 257–267.

15. Temple, G., Lamesch, P., Milstein, S., et al. (2006) From genome to proteome: developing expression clone resources for the human genome *Hum Mol Genet* **15**, R31–R43.

Part III

**The Refinement of Established
Methods by Recent Innovations**

Chapter 11

Application of 2D-DIGE in Cancer Proteomics Toward Personalized Medicine

Tadashi Kondo and Setsuo Hirohashi

Summary

Two-dimensional difference gel electrophoresis (2D-DIGE) is an advanced variation of two-dimensional polyacrylamide gel electrophoresis (2D-PAGE); protein samples are labeled with different fluorescent dyes, mixed and separated by 2D-PAGE. 2D-DIGE solves major inherent drawbacks of 2D-PAGE, demonstrating great utility in biomarker studies. Biomarker development requires quantitative, reproducible, highly sensitive and high-throughput experimental platforms, and 2D-DIGE meets these criteria. Here we demonstrate the advantages of 2D-DIGE and discuss the possibilities 2D-DIGE offers for further, more comprehensive proteome studies.

Key words: Cancer, Personalized medicine, Biomarker, Proteome, Database

1. Introduction

Biomarker identification is a key technology in the effort to improve the clinical outcome of patients with cancer. Cancer is a diverse disease. The response to treatment and prognosis after therapy vary between patients, and existing diagnostic technologies do not always demonstrate such important disease features accurately. The patients diagnosed as being at the same clinical stage often demonstrate different response to treatment and have varying survival periods. Pathologic grading does not always correlate with clinical outcome either. For these reasons, treatment with the best-optimized therapy for each individual patient, namely personalized medicine, has long required the development of the

Hisashi Koga (ed.), *Reverse Chemical Genetics*, Methods in Molecular Biology, vol. 577
DOI 10.1007/978-1-60761-232-2_11, © Humana Press, a part of Springer Science+Business Media, LLC 2009

next level of diagnostic tools. Cancer is a disease of the genome. Genomic aberrations result in the transformation of normal cells into fully malignant tumor cells, and the type of these aberrations determines cancer phenotypes. Many lines of evidence suggest that specific molecules and pathways govern the malignant behaviors of tumor cells, such as unexpected early metastasis after curative surgery and disease progress after chemotherapy. By monitoring such molecules or pathways, we can use them as biomarkers to predict life-threatening events after therapy and to individual treatment (**Fig. 1**).

Recent technological advances have enabled the performance of comprehensive studies at the genome, transcriptome, and proteome level. The application of novel technologies to DNA, RNA, and protein samples of tumor tissues provided us new insights into the molecular background of cancer. Global studies revealed that cancer phenotypes demonstrate distinctive genome, transcriptome, and proteome profiles, allowing the possibility of novel cancer classification *(1)*. At the same time, these global studies shed light on curious relations between the genome, transcriptome, and proteome. Aberrations in the genomic content of cancer cells are not always reflected in the transcriptome, and, similarly, aberrations in the transctiptome are not necessarily reflected in the proteome *(2, 3)*. Many lines of evidence suggest that the copy number of DNA sequences is not always

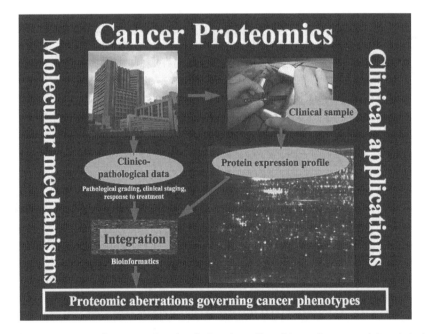

Fig. 1. Work flow and purpose of cancer proteomics. Proteomic profiles of tumor tissues are integrated with clinico-pathological data to identify the proteomic aberrations governing cancer phenotypes. The goals of cancer proteomics are understanding of the molecular mechanisms of cancer diversity and developing applications of potential clinical benefit.

parallel with the expression level of the corresponding mRNA, and that the expression level between mRNAs and corresponding proteins may show discordance *(4, 5)*. In addition, proteins do not function in the form that they are translated from mRNA; they are post-translationally modified by small molecules such as phosphates, acetylates, lipids, and glycans. The functionality of proteins largely depends on their localization in the cells and tissues, and is determined by their association with other proteins or nucleic acids. These properties are aberrantly regulated in cancer cells. The aberrant proteome may also generate cancer-specific autoantibodies in the cancer patients *(6–14)*. Considering that the functional translation of the genome is the proteome, these observations suggest that genomic aberrations do not directly determine the process of carcinogenesis and cancer phenotypes. As reading DNA sequences and measuring RNA levels alone do not presently predict the status of the proteome, it is proteomic studies that will provide the unique information about the molecular mechanisms underlying cancer. By examining the proteomic features, we may be able to identify the molecules directly regulating the phenotypes of individual cancers. Therefore, we consider that the proteome is a rich source for biomarkers for personalized medicine.

With this notion, we conduct cancer proteomics studies to develop biomarkers for personalized medicine. Using large-scale clinical sample sets and linking the acquired proteome data to clinicopathological data, we try to identify the proteomic aberrations which may govern cancer phenotypes **(Fig. 1)**. We have found protein groups or specific proteins the expression of which correlates highly with response to treatment *(15)*, the development of unexpected metastases after surgical operation *(16)*, the number of lymph node metastases *(17)*, and shorter survival *(18)*, all of which should be good biomarker candidates for personalized medicine.

To identify biomarker candidates by global studies, we need a technology with the following technical characteristics. First, it must measure protein expression levels in a quantitative way. Most oncogene products and their downstream molecules exist in the cells of the different cancer types, and their expression level often determines the characteristics of malignant cells. Therefore, we need the quantitative data to determine the cut-off value to distinguish samples from certain tumor types from others. Second, the data should be generated in a reproducible way. We need to examine proteome data across many clinical samples to obtain conclusive results in a statistically valid way. The reproducibility of the proteome data is indispensable for the statistical analysis. Third, it should uncover as much proteome data as possible; the more proteins are detected, the more likely it is to succeed in identifying biomarkers. Fourth, data should be generated in a high-throughput way. Measuring the expression level of proteins is only the very first phase of biomarker development, and thus may need to be concluded within a reasonable time frame. Fifth, biomarkers should be identified so that they can then be measured using other, simpler, and less costly tools, since comprehensive technologies are not always suitable for application in a clinical setting.

In this manuscript, we reviewed a novel gel-based proteomics technology, two-dimensional difference electrophoresis (2D-DIGE). 2D-DIGE is an advanced variation of two-dimensional gel electrophoresis (2D-PAGE). In 2D-DIGE, the protein samples are labeled with different fluorescent dyes, mixed together, and separated according to isoelectric points and molecular weights. 2D-DIGE solves many drawbacks of gel-based proteomics and facilitates cancer proteomics. We found that 2D-DIGE meets the above-mentioned criteria for a biomarker development tool. In the National Cancer Center Research Institute, approximately 2,000 large format 2D-DIGE gels are annually ran to identify biomarker candidates. The detailed protocols were published in our previous report *(19)*. We will describe the advantages that, based on our experience, we believe 2D-DIGE offers with respect to biomarker identification studies, and discuss the critical issues relating to biomarker development.

2. 2D-PAGE in Cancer Proteomics

2D-PAGE is the most popular proteomics tool *(20–22)*. In 2D-PAGE, proteins are separated according to the individual physiological characteristics of proteins, namely their isoelectric point and molecular weight. Following the colorimetric staining of gels, the expression level of proteins is quantified by measuring the staining intensity of the corresponding protein spots. Alternatively, the cellular proteins are labeled with either ^{35}S-methionine *(23)*, ^{32}P-phosphate *(24)*, ^{14}C-containing amino acids *(25)* or ^{125}I-Na *(26)* in tissue culture conditions, and the isotope-labeled proteins are subjected to 2D-PAGE and then detected by exposing the gel to an X-ray film. Protein expression can be quantified by measuring the intensity of the protein spots on X-ray film. The identification of the proteins is nowadays achieved by mass spectrometry and database search. A series of proteomic experiments using 2D-PAGE has been established with innovative improvements such as the application of immobilized pH gradient gels, detergents for membrane proteins and sample application methods *(27–32)*, and many relevant protocols have been published *(20, 33)*. There have also been many reports in the last three decades regarding its application to cancer research *(34–36)*. However, besides its popular use and fruitful academic results, there are a number of limitations inherent in 2D-PAGE.

First, in 2D-PAGE, single gels separate single samples, so that gel-to-gel variations can affect the apparent expression level of proteins. Because the intensity of protein spots reflects both the amount of corresponding proteins and experimental variations, it may not be exactly the same for identical proteins in different gels. We can somehow compensate for the experimental variations by running multiple gels. However, the compensation is not perfect, and running multiple gels multiplies labor intensity. Second, silver staining was known to be the most sensitive detection method next to radioisotope labeling method, and widely used in 2D-PAGE experiments. However, the protein detection by silver staining is the most rate-limiting and labor intense step in 2D-PAGE. Silver staining takes at least several hours, uses large quantities of water, and requires well-trained operators and a considerable amount of laboratory space for staining trays. Moreover, to store the gel images for further analysis, the gel needs to be scanned by an optical scanner or photographed, requiring additional time. Silver staining enhances the other inherent problems of 2D-PAGE as follows. Third, 2D-PAGE does not uncover the entire proteome; similar to other proteomic tools, and despite many efforts to increase the number of observable proteins *(20)* only a limited number of proteins can be visualized. The number of protein spots is almost parallel to the area of gel; the larger the gel, the higher the number of protein spots on the gel. Thus, the large format gel is one of the most powerful solutions to increase proteome coverage *(37)*. However, polyacrylamide gels are very fragile and are often damaged during the multistep procedures of the colorimetric protein detection methods such as silver staining. Multiple fractionations *(38)* and the use of narrow range isoelectric focusing gels *(39)* also increase the number of observable proteins, but these approaches multiply the number of gels used and thus labor intensity, particularly when colorimetric gel staining is used. Fourth, in 2D-PAGE with conventional silver staining, 100 µg of protein are usually needed for single gels; the study of the proteome of tumor tissues requires higher sensitivity. Tumor tissues consist of heterogenous populations of cells that include nontumor cells, and each cell population probably has different proteome content. Once they are homogenized together for the purpose of protein extraction, the expected proteome pattern would reflect both the ratio of the number of cells of the different populations and the different protein contents in the individual cells. It is hard to know which factors more dominantly affect the intensity of protein spots, and accurate protein profiling requires the separate collection of specific cell populations before protein extraction. One possible remedy is laser microdissection (LMD), by which the cells are recovered under microscopic observation *(40)*. LMD has been used in conjunction with 2D-PAGE to specifically study tumor cells in tumor tissues *(41)*. However, because of the limited sensitivity of silver staining, several hours or days were required in order to recover adequate numbers of cells by LMD *(42)*, suggesting that LMD was not a practical tool for biomarker studies in which a relatively large number of tumor tissues was examined to generate conclusive results. When the tissues are histologically homogeneous and the use of LMD is not required, samples may be homogenized for protein extraction. However, in many cases, the amount of tumor tissues obtained from the hospital is very limited, and higher sensitivity is required. The isotope-labeling method has much higher sensitivity than silver staining, but requires a special laboratory set up to reduce the risk of exposure to hazardous materials and may not be suitable for routine experiments. In addition, metabolic labeling needs living cells, meaning that frozen tissues cannot be used. Fifth, the identification of proteins corresponding to protein spots has been sometimes very difficult using Edman degradation. However, this limitation has largely been solved with the recent use of mass spectrometry and database searching. Taken all together, classical 2D-PAGE had obvious limitations, mainly in the associated spot detection methods. We have thus long needed a novel technology to address the problems inherent in 2D-PAGE.

3. Advanced 2D-PAGE, 2D-DIGE, and its Application for Biomarker Development

Recently, two-dimensional difference gel electrophoresis (2D-DIGE) *(43)* was introduced as an innovative 2D-PAGE technology that can solve its afore-mentioned problems. **Figure 2** demonstrates the basic application of 2D-DIGE in the comparison of two protein samples. In this application, each individual protein sample is labeled with Cy3 and Cy5 dye respectively. The fluorescent dyes are designed so that the electrophoretic mobility of proteins labeled with different fluorescent dyes is almost identical. After stopping the labeling reaction, the samples are mixed together and separated in one 2D-PAGE gel. After gel electrophoresis, the 2D-PAGE images of the two samples are obtained by scanning the gel with a laser for Cy3 and Cy5 respectively. As these protein samples are separated on the same gel, there are no gel-to-gel variations. This protocol can be used for multiple protein samples depending on the number of different fluorescent dyes used. Three fluorescent dyes with different emission and excitation wavelengths are currently commercially available for

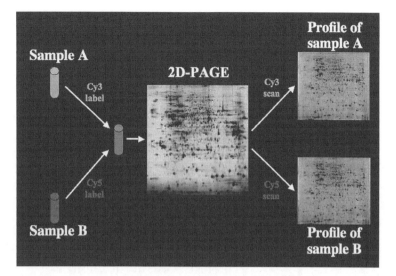

Fig. 2. Basic protocol of 2D-DIGE for two protein samples. The different protein samples are labeled with different fluorescent dyes (Cy3 and Cy5), mixed together and separated on the same 2D gel. After gel electrophoresis, the gels are scanned with laser at the appropriate wavelength for Cy3 and Cy5. A single gel can generate two 2D images, so that gel-to-gel variations are canceled out. We can compare as many protein samples as the number of available fluorescent dyes.

Table 1
Fluorescent dyes used in 2D-DIGE

Name of dye	Dyes commercially available[1]	Amino acids labeled	Sensitivity[2,3]
CyDye DIGE Fluor minimal dye[2]	Cy2, Cy3, Cy5	A small % of lysine residues	Equivalent to silver staining
CyDye DIGE Fluor saturation dye[3]	Cy3, Cy5	100% of cystein residues	One hundred times higher than silver staining

[1]GE Healthcare
[2]Ref. 43
[3]Ref. 45

2D-DIGE, (Cy2, Cy3, and Cy5; **Table 1**), meaning that three samples can be compared using this 2D-DIGE application. This way, 2D-DIGE can address the most major problem inherent in 2D-PAGE, gel-to-gel variations. In addition, the spot intensity is measured as a fluorescent signal, the nature of fluorescence allowing the data obtained to have wide dynamic range.

3.1. 2D-DIGE Allows Multiple Sample Comparisons

Cancer is, however, a genetically diverse disease and therefore more than three samples need to be examined in cancer proteomics to compensate for the genetic variations. In general, results from one-by-one comparisons do not provide any meaningful information in clinical studies. The application shown in **Fig. 3** can be used to examine more protein samples than the number of fluorescent dyes used. In this application, a mixture of a small portion of all protein samples is used as the internal control sample. The internal control sample is alliquoted into small tubes and stored in a deep freezer until use. This internal control sample is labeled with Cy3, while the individual samples are labeled with Cy5. These two differently labeled protein samples are mixed together and separated by 2D-PAGE. All gels thus generate the 2D image of the internal control sample as the Cy3 image. Therefore, by normalizing Cy5 intensity with that of Cy3 intensity for all protein spots, we can cancel out gel-to-gel variations. **Figure 3** shows that 100 protein samples can be examined using the same number of gels. Gel-to-gel variations can be further decreased by running each sample in multiple gels and then using the mean or median of the obtained normalized intensity values. Using this

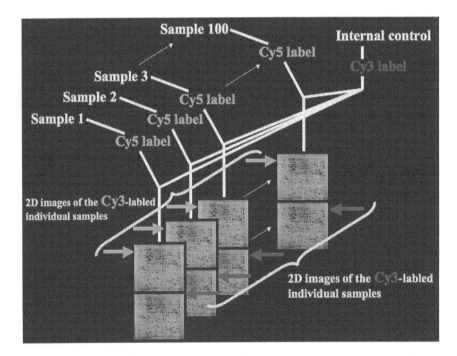

Fig. 3. Advanced protocol of 2D-DIGE for a number of protein samples larger than the available fluorescent dyes. The internal control sample and individual samples are labeled with Cy3 and Cy5, respectively. The differently labeled protein samples are mixed together and separated on individual gels. After gel electrophoresis, the gels are scanned with laser at the appropriate wavelength for Cy3 and Cy5. As all gel scans generate the Cy3 image that represents the proteomic profile of the internal control sample, gel-to-gel variations are compensated by normalizing Cy5 images with Cy3 images for each gel. We can compare more protein samples than the available fluorescent dyes.

protocol, we can perform 2D-DIGE using two fluorescent dyes and as many protein samples as necessary *(19)*.

3.2. 2D-DIGE Facilitates High-Throughput Gel-Based Proteomics Applications

Studies in which several hundred clinical samples need to be examined by 2D-PAGE require a large number of gels to be run. The most popular method to detect proteins separated by conventional 2D-PAGE is silver staining, that is time consuming and labor intensive. In contrast, in 2D-DIGE, because all proteins are labeled with fluorescent dyes, simply laser scanning the gel generates a gel image within 1 h and much less laboriously. By using multiple laser scanners in a parallel way, many gels are run in a high-throughput way. At the National Cancer Center, we achieve such high-throughput proteomics results by using multiple electrophoresis devices and six laser scanners (Typhoon Trio, GE Healthcare), enabling us to annually run approximately 2,000 large format 2D gels for biomarker studies *(19)*.

We found that this high-throughput facilitated the use of not only a large number of surgical specimens, but also of fractionated samples *(44)*. We fractionated plasma samples in order to detect low-abundance plasma proteins, by subjecting them to multiple chromatograms such as the immuno-affinity column and the ion-exchange column, and then examined the fractionated samples by 2D-DIGE. Multidimensional fractionation is widely used in plasma proteomics to reduce the complexity of protein samples and increase the number of detectable proteins. Single samples were separated into eight fractions, and then separated on 2D-DIGE gels containing 3,890 protein spots. In this experiment, we found that laser scanning enabled high-throughput experiments while also decreasing labor intensity.

3.3. 2D-DIGE Enables More Comprehensive Proteomics Applications

The fragility of gels is not of substantial consequence in 2D-DIGE, because the gels are scanned sandwiched between the two low-fluorescent glass plates that were used for electrophoresis. Therefore, we can run a gel as large as the scanning area of the laser scanner. We found that the number of protein spots detected was parallel with that of the gel area, probably because the increased resolution increases the visualization of the protein spots that were behind neighboring protein spots in small format 2D gels. We constructed a large format 2D electrophoresis device for the purpose of increasing the number of protein spots. The gel area of this device is twice that of the second largest electrophoretic device, EttanDalt II (GE Healthcare) and allows us to observe approximately 5,000 protein spots on single gel images using the DeCyder software (GE Healthcare) *(19)*.

3.4. 2D-DIGE Allows Highly Sensitive Proteomics Applications

Currently, two types of fluorescent dyes are available from GE Heathcare (**Table 1**) *(43, 45)*. We first reported that the use of an ultra highly sensitive fluorescent dye (CyDye DIGE Fluor saturation dye, GE Healthcare) enabled protein expression profiling even when using samples with scarce protein amounts such as those from laser microdissected tissues *(46)*. As proteins cannot be amplified like DNAs, highly sensitive detection systems such as protein-labeling with highly sensitive fluorescent dyes are the only remedy for samples with low-protein content. The high sensitivity of the CyDye DIGE Fluor saturation dye means that few cells are needed for proteomics applications, and microdissection does not take a long time. We applied this method to study adenoma in min mice *(46)*, lung cancer *(47)*, esophageal cancer (*(17)* and Uemra et al, manuscript in preparation) and hepatocellular carcinoma (Orimo et al, manuscript in preparation), while other research groups later followed with studies using tissues of pancreatic cancer *(48)*, gastric cancer *(49)*, and transgenic mice *(50)*. The manufacturer (GE Healthcare) has released a basic protocol for protein-labeling, and we have published the detailed protocol for laser microdissection, protein extraction from microdissected tissues, and labeling of the extracted proteins *(19)*. Currently, two types of CyDye DIGE Fluor saturation dyes are commercially available, Cy3 and Cy5 **(Table 1)**. By using the protocol for multiple samples as mentioned above **(Fig. 3)**, we can compare multiple microdissected samples using these two dyes *(17)*. One noticeable character of the CyDye DIGE Fluor saturation dye is that it changes the electrophoretic mobility of proteins after labeling. Therefore, we cannot compare the 2D image generated by the CyDye DIGE Fluor saturation dye with that by the CyDye DIGE Fluore minimal dye or silver staining.

We found that the use of samples with minute protein content can improve the quality of 2D gel images. In routine experiments with silver staining, 100 μg of protein are applied to 2D-PAGE. Protein samples include the substances that may interfere with 2D-PAGE; those include lipids, glycans, nucleic acids and salts. As they hinder the reproducibility of the 2D image, their amount should not exceed a critical interference threshold. Although they can be removed by precipitating proteins, low-abundance proteins are lost during the precipitation procedure. In 2D-DIGE with CyDye DIGE Fluor saturation dye, only 1 μg of protein is enough when using EttanDalt II size gels (24 cm × 20 cm). Because 1 μg of protein sample includes 1/100 of the interfering substances contained in the protein amount used for 2D-PAGE, we obtained high-quality 2D images in a constant way.

The problems inherent to 2D-PAGE that are solved with the use of 2D-DIGE are summarized in **Table 2**.

Table 2
Drawbacks of classical 2D-PAGE addressed by 2D-DIGE

Drawbacks of classical 2D-PAGE	Solution by 2D-DIGE
Low reproducibility due to gel-to-gel variations	Mixing the differently labeled protein samples cancels the experimental variations
Time-consuming and labor-intensive spot detection method	The gel image is produced by laser scanning within 1 h in a less labor-intensive way
Limited proteome coverage	Large-format gel, multi-fractionation, combined narrow range pI gels
Requires large protein content	Saturation dye is 100 times more sensitive than silver staining requiring significantly lower protein content
Difficult protein identification	Fluorescently labeled proteins are compatible with mass spectrometry

4. Data-Mining for Cancer Proteomics Using 2D-DIGE Data and Clinicopathological Information

2D-DIGE generates a huge amount of proteome data that have to be collected and analyzed. For instance, for a lung cancer proteomics study, we are currently examining 250 tumor tissues to develop biomarkers to predict lymph node metastasis and survival of lung cancer patients; each sample is applied on gels in triplicate, and each gel generates approximately 5,000 protein spots that produce quantitative data. These protein expression data are to be examined in relation to clinicopathological parameters such as TNM grading, histological classification, and the patients' response to treatment and survival period. With this method, visual inspection of the gels would not be of any benefit.

Image-analysis software for 2D-DIGE, such as DeCyder (GE Healthcare) and Progenesis SameSpot (Nonlinear Dynamics) are commercially available. The software is used to normalize Cy5 images with Cy3 images, then export the image data as numerical data in the format of an xml file or an xls file. Data-mining software that were basically developed to study DNA microarray data, such as Expressionist (GeneData, Switzerland), are then used to identify proteomic signatures that correlate with certain clinicopathological parameters and to rank these protein spots for further validation studies. In addition, proteome-based cancer classification can be achieved using clustering algorithms (51).

The use of these tools enables the collection of novel information that could not be achieved via visual inspection of the gels.

Image analysis is one of the rate-limiting steps of 2D-DIGE experiments as the different gel images have to be matched by manual inspection. We found that the use of the Progenesis SameSpot software dramatically shortens the image analysis process. Progenesis SameSpots transforms the gel images so that focal gel distortions are corrected and the groups of protein spots in every small area are aligned between the different gels. For more details the reader is referred to the Nonlinear Dynamics homepage (http://www.nonlinear.com). The image analysis software for 2D-DIGE has improved significantly in the last several years, providing an added advantage to the use of 2D-DIGE, as it enables the quantitative study of a large number of 2D gels with ease. Inclusion of optimized-multivariate analysis tools will be the next challenge in the refinement of image analysis software.

5. Protein Identification from 2D-DIGE Gels

Proteins corresponding to the protein spots of interest are identified by mass spectrometry *(19)*. By comparing the 2D image generated for analytical purpose using a sample with low-protein content with that generated for preparative purposes using a sample containing 100 µg of protein, we can identify the target protein spots on the 2D image from a preparative gel. The target protein spots are then collected into 96-well PCR plates using an automated spot recovery machine. Before subjecting the recovered proteins to mass spectrometry, the proteins in the gel are digested by specific protease into peptides. It is generally hard to extract proteins from polyacrylamide gels. However, once the proteins are digested to peptides, it is easy to extract them from the gel. The protocol of digesting the proteins in a gel matrix and extracting the digested peptides was established with the name of "in-gel digestion" *(52)*. In this protocol, the recovered gels are extensively washed with a buffer to remove the remaining detergent, and are then repeatedly shrunk and reswollen with treatment with organic solvent and buffer. By overnight treatment with trypsin, the proteins in the gel plug are digested to peptides. The peptides are then extracted with an organic solvent. We have extensively optimized the in-gel digestion protocol so that protein identification can be successfully achieved for most protein spots *(19)*.

In our experience, the identification of proteins with MALDI TOF MS (oMALDI Q-STAR, ABI) can be achieved when they are labeled with the CyDye DIGE Fluor minimal dye but is very hard when they are labeled with the CyDye DIGE Fluor saturation dye. The two dyes have different characteristics; the former labels a small portion of lysine residue while the latter labels all reduced cystein residue. Therefore, the proteins labeled with the CyDye DIGE Fluor saturation dye include more fluorescent dye. We speculate that the fluorescent dye may have a suppressive effect on the ionization of peptides. The tryptic digests spotted on the MALDI plates include both labeled and nonlabeled peptides, and the ionization of nonlabeled peptides is also hindered by the presence of neighboring dyes. In the case of the CyDye DIGE Fluor minimal dye, protein identification can be achieved by MALDI TOF MS because only a limited number of lysine residues is labeled and the peptide samples may contain a lower amount of fluorescent dye. In contrast, the peptide samples labeled with CyDye DIGE Fluor saturation dye may contain a larger amount of fluorescent dye, resulting in reduced ionization efficiency. Alternative to MALDI TOF MS, we found that efficient protein identification can be achieved with the use of LC-MSMS even for proteins labeled with CyDye DIGE Fluor saturation dye. We speculate that the labeled peptides are separated from the unlabeled ones by LC separation, and then ionized by MS, so that the fluorescent dye does not hinder protein identification using the unlabeled peptides. Using the in-gel digestion protocol and LC-MSMS, we have already identified more than 3,000 protein spots labeled by the CyDye DIGE Fluor saturation dye *(19)*.

6. Practical Biomarker Discovery Using 2D-DIGE Data

2D-DIGE is a powerful technology for biomarker discovery. We found that even beginners in basic research can master it in a short period following an adequate training program. However, it will be hard to optimize 2D-DIGE in terms of cost performance so that it is used as a clinical examination tool. After a small number of biomarker candidates is identified, one does not have to run large format gels; instead, we need a tool to survey these specific proteins across a large number of clinical samples in a reproducible, cost-effective, and less labor-intensive way. Therefore, desirably, the developed biomarkers can be used in hospitals using the existing equipment without or with minimal modifications. Such applications are also required at the validation phase in biomarker development. To establish the candidates as novel biomarkers, we may need to demonstrate their diagnostic or prognostic value in several hundred clinical samples, in collaboration with clinicians, in which case we are expected to examine the candidates in a high throughput and more cost-effective way.

To validate the candidate biomarkers, specific antibodies against the identified proteins are used. As immunohistochemical examinations and enzyme-linked immuno assays (ELISA) are performed routinely in hospitals, once the relevant antibodies are obtained, the existing devices can be utilized for the examination. Indeed, we have successfully validated 2D-DIGE results in immunohistochemical *(16)* and ELISA *(15)* studies. However, the antibodies do not always work in the expected way. This is due to the fact that in 2D-DIGE experiments a specific protein may repeatedly appear in different protein spots owing to post-translational modifications. As a consequence, each protein spot may represent a particular protein isoform and not the total amount or all isoforms of each protein, and thus some isoforms may alone be identified as biomarker candidates, even when the total expression level of that particular protein is constant between sample groups. In this case, as the antibodies used are not specific to the protein isoform identified as the candidate but recognize all isoforms of the particular protein, the immunohistochemical and ELISA results are not consistent with those of 2D-DIGE. We are developing monoclonal antibodies to use our research results as diagnostic tools. The development of antibodies is now one of the most rate-limiting steps in biomarker studies and is a challenge that requires novel technologies or methods to be addressed.

7. 2D-DIGE Data Proteome Database

One of the unique characteristics of 2D-PAGE is that the data can be integrated in a database which in turn will facilitate biomarker development in the validation phase. In transcriptome studies, the expression data are deposited in public cyber space such as the Gene Expression Omnipus (GEO, www.ncbi.nlm.nih.gov/geo) and Oncomine databases (http://www.oncomine.org) *(53)* and are freely downloaded to validate the results of individual small-scale studies. This way, so-called metaanalysis enables large-scale expression studies *(54)*. These research tools are compatible with studies that have common experimental platforms, such as DNA microarrays. In contrast, we do not have common experimental platforms in proteomic studies. Although there are many proteome databases using 2D-PAGE data (http://www.expasy.org/world-2dpage), they cannot be used as tools for biomarker development without problems. Most 2D databases include the intensity value for only a small number of protein spots. The number of annotated protein spots is generally very small and is often less than 100. Each sample group usually consists of only one sample, and biological and clinical information is not provided in most cases. The experimental methods such as that for protein extraction, isoelectric focusing in the first dimension separation, size of gel in the second dimension separation, and staining protocol vary between the databases. Because of its high reproducibility, 2D-DIGE may provide a common experimental platform for biomarker development studies. We consider that the construction of a proteome database using 2D-DIGE data is the next challenge in our project.

For this reason, we are currently constructing a public proteome database named GeMDBJ Proteomics (Genome Medicine Database of Japan Proteomics, http://gemdbj.nibio.go.jp). GeMDBJ is an integrative database that includes genome and transcriptome data. Our database will include the quantitative proteome data generated by 2D-DIGE from tumor tissues of different cancer types such as lung, esophageal, liver, and colon cancer, soft-tissue sarcoma, bone tumors, and malignant mesothelioma. Annotation data acquired by LC-MSMS will be added to as many protein spots as possible. We have published the beta-version, which includes 2D-DIGE data from nine pancreatic cancer cell lines and two normal pancreatic duct cell lines. The database includes annotations for approximately 1,100 protein spots. Proteome data from tumor tissues from studies conducted in our laboratory will be constantly up-loaded to the database.

8. Further Possibilities of 2D-DIGE

Using the present large format 2D gel device without prior fractionation, we can observe up to 5,000 protein spots with the DeCyder software, which may correspond to up to 2,500 unique proteins as identified by mass spectrometry *(19)*. We have already identified many interesting proteins the expression of which correlates in a statistically significant way with important clinico-pathological parameters of tumors. However, the protocol still needs to be improved to expand the proteome coverage while keeping the advantageous characteristics of 2D-DIGE.

Such future modifications may include enlarging the gel size, fractioning the protein samples prior to electrophoresis, and using narrow range isoelectric focusing gels. These steps have been applied in the classical 2D-PAGE to increase the number of observable protein spots, and can therefore be employed to 2D-DIGE experiments. Because of the afore-mentioned advantages of 2D-DIGE, we believe it will be easier to carry out these modifications in 2D-DIGE compared with the classical 2D-PAGE.

9. Collaboration Between Basic Researchers, Clinicians, Pathologists, and Industry is Critical in Biomarker Studies

Needless to say that technology alone does not develop biomarkers. We believe that collaboration between basic researchers, clinicians, and industry is critical in biomarker development. Basic researchers may know the details of the technological aspects of proteomics and how to investigate the proteome. They can develop novel technologies and establish novel concepts in biology using proteome data. However, they may not evaluate the results from a clinical perspective or select biomarkers that can best benefit cancer patients. Clinicians, in contrast, have a better understanding of what may improve the clinical outcome for the patients and can collect the required clinical samples and information. They can suggest the types of biomarkers that can optimize existing therapeutic protocols based on their experience. More importantly, they are the potential users of novel biomarkers, and biomarkers should be developed in the way that the final products can be accepted in a clinical setting. In addition to the medical benefits from the use of biomarkers, one may need to consider whether industry will be interested in commercializing the proposed novel diagnostic tools. Basic researchers and clinicians may not be familiar with the business aspects of biomarker development. Therefore, the involvement of industry partners in the project from an early phase is also critical to the successful development of biomarkers.

For these reasons, our research group includes basic researchers including a bioinformatics specialist, clinicians, pathologists, and industry partners, in a way that best-optimizes the use of 2D-DIGE related methods for biomarker development studies (**Fig. 4**).

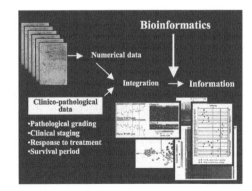

Fig. 4. Application of bioinformatics tools to 2D-DIGE data analysis. Proteome data consisting of the normalized spot intensity values are exported from the image analysis software and their correlation with clinicopathological data examined. Using informatics tools including clustering algorithms and machine-learning methods, a novel cancer classification based on proteome data is established, and key proteomic features and proteins corresponding to biomarker candidates are identified.

10. Conclusions

This chapter demonstrates the benefits of the use of 2D-DIGE in cancer proteomics for biomarker development. **Table 1** lists the commercially available fluorescent dyes for 2D-DIGE. **Table 2** summarizes the major drawbacks of the classical 2D-DIGE and how 2D-DIGE addresses them. **Table 3** shows how 2D-DIGE meets the criteria for a biomarker development tool. All detailed protocols were published in our previous paper *(19)*. We should keep in mind that although 2D-DIGE is one of the most advanced versions of 2D-PAGE, additional modifications can further improve its performance. Finally, we would like to emphasize that a practical research strategy and a translational research mind are the most important factors to make the best use of 2D-DIGE for biomarker development.

Table 3
Advantageous characteristics of 2D-DIGE for biomarker studies

Technical requirements for proteomic tools to identify biomarker candidates	How 2D-DIGE meets the requirements
Quantitativity	1. The use of a common internal control sample enables normalization of gel-to-gel variations so that spot intensity directly reflects the protein expression level 2. The fluorescent signal that measures spot intensity has wide dynamic range
Reproducibility	The use of a common internal control cancels out the gel-to-gel variation, which hinders reproducibility
Coverage	The use of large format gels, pre-fractionation and multiple use of narrow range isoelectric focusing gels enable more comprehensive proteomic studies
Throughput	Gel images are produced by laser scanning within a short time and less laboriously
Transactivity	The proteins corresponding to protein spots are identified by mass spectrometry

Acknowledgments

This work was supported by a grant from the Ministry of Health, Labor, and Welfare and by the Program for Promotion of Fundamental Studies in Health Sciences of the National Institute of Biomedical Innovation of Japan. We appreciate Dr. Hisao Asamura (National Cancer Center Hospital) for an excellent photograph of surgical operation.

References

1. Rhodes DR, Chinnaiyan AM. (2005) Integrative analysis of the cancer trasncriptome. *Nat Genet* **37**, S31–7.

2. Hanash SM. (2003) Operomics: molecular analysis of tissues from DNA to RNA to protein. *Clin Chem Lab Med* **38**, 805–13.

3. Orntoft TF, Thykjaer T, Waldman FM, Wolf H, Celis JE. (2002) Genome-wide study of gene copy numbers, transcripts, and protein levels in pairs of non-invasive and invasive human transitional cell carcinomas. *Mol Cell Proteomics* **1**, 37–45.

4. Varambally S, Yu J, Laxman B, et al. (2005) Integrative genomic and proteomic analysis of prostate cancer reveals signatures of metastatic progression. *Cancer Cell* **8**, 393–406.

5. Chen G, Gharib TG, Huang CC, et al. (2002) Discordant protein and mRNA expression in lung adenocarcinomas. *Mol Cell Proteomics* **1**, 304–13.

6. Wang X, Yu J, Sreekumar A, et al. (2005) Autoantibody signatures in prostate cancer. *N Engl J Med* **353**, 1224–35.

7. Nam MJ, Madoz-Gurpide J, Wang H, et al. (2003) Molecular profiling of the immune response in colon cancer using protein microarrays: occurrence of autoantibodies to ubiquitin C-terminal hydrolase L3. *Proteomics* **3**, 2108–15.

8. Hanash S. (2003) Harnessing immunity for cancer marker discovery. *Nat Biotechnol* **21**, 37–8.

9. Shin BK, Wang H, Hanash S. (2002) Proteomics approaches to uncover the repertoire of circulating biomarkers for breast cancer. *J Mammary Gland Biol Neoplasia* **7**, 407–13.

10. Le Naour F, Brichory F, Misek DE, Brechot C, Hanash SM, Beretta L. (2002) A distinct repertoire of autoantibodies in hepatocellular carcinoma identified by proteomic analysis. *Mol Cell Proteomics* **1**, 197–203.

11. Le Naour F, Misek DE, Krause MC, et al. (2001) Proteomics-based identification of RS/DJ-1 as a novel circulating tumor antigen in breast cancer. *Clin Cancer Res* **7**, 3328–35.

12. Brichory FM, Misek DE, Yim AM, et al. (2001) An immune response manifested by the common occurrence of annexins I and II autoantibodies and high circulating levels of IL-6 in lung cancer. *Proc Natl Acad Sci U S A* **98**, 9824–9.

13. Brichory F, Beer D, Le Naour F, Giordano T, Hanash S. (2001) Proteomics-based identification of protein gene product 9.5 as a tumor antigen that induces a humoral immune response in lung cancer. *Cancer Res* **61**, 7908–12.

14. Prasannan L, Misek DE, Hinderer R, Michon J, Geiger JD, Hanash SM. (2000) Identification of beta-tubulin isoforms as tumor antigens in neuroblastoma. *Clin Cancer Res* **6**, 3949–56.

15. Okano T, Kondo T, Fujii K, et al. (2007) Proteomic signature corresponding to the response to gefitinib (Iressa, ZD1839), an epidermal growth factor receptor (EGFR) tyrosine kinase inhibitor, and mutation in EGFR in lung adenocarcinoma. *Clin Cancer Res* **13**, 799–805.

16. Suehara Y, Suehara Y, Kondo T, et al. (2008) Pfetin as a prognostic biomarker of gastrointestinal stromal tumors revealed by proteomics. *Clin Cancer Res* **14**, 1707–17.

17. Hatakeyama H, Kondo T, Fujii K, et al. (2006) Protein clusters associated with carcinogenesis, histological differentiation and nodal metastasis in esophageal cancer. *Proteomics* **6**, 6300–16.

18. Yokoo H, Kondo T, Okano T, et al. (2007) Protein expression associated with early intrahepatic recurrence of hepatocellular carcinoma after curative surgery. *Cancer Sci* **98**, 665–73.

19. Kondo T, Hirohashi S. (2006) Application of highly sensitive fluorescent dyes (CyDye DIGE Fluor saturation dyes) to laser microdissection and two-dimensional difference gel electrophoresis (2D-DIGE) for cancer proteomics. *Nat Protoc* **1**, 2940–56.

20. Gorg A, Weiss W, Dunn MJ. (2004) Current two-dimensional electrophoresis technology for proteomics. *Proteomics* **4**, 3665–85.

21. O'Farrell PH. (1975) High resolution two-dimensional electrophoresis of proteins. *J Biol Chem* **250**, 4007–21.

22. Klose J. (1975) Protein mapping by combined isoelectric focusing and electrophoresis of mouse tissues. A novel approach to testing for induced point mutations in mammals. *Humangenetik* **26**, 231–43.

23. Bravo R, Celis JE. (1982) Human proteins sensitive to neoplastic transformation in cultured epithelial and fibroblast cells. *Clin Chem* **28**, 949–54.

24. Fey SJ, Larsen PM, Celis JE. (1983) Evidence for coordinated phosphorylation of keratins and vimentin during mitosis in transformed human amnion cells. Phosphate turnover of modified proteins. *FEBS Lett* **157**, 165–9.

25. Bravo R, Celis JE. (1982) Up-dated catalogue of HeLa cell proteins: percentages and characteristics of the major cell polypeptides labeled with a mixture of 16 14C-labeled amino acids. *Clin Chem* **28**, 766–81.

26. Litin BS, Grimes WJ. (1979) Two-dimensional electrophoresis of membrane proteins from normal and transformed cells. *Cancer Res* **39**, 2595–603.

27. Gorg A, Postel W, Gunther S. (1988) The current state of two-dimensional electrophoresis with immobilized pH gradients. *Electrophoresis* **9**, 531–46.

28. Righetti PG. (1990) Immobiline pH Gradients: Theory and Methodology. Amsterdam: Elsevier.

29. Molloy MP, Herbert BR, Walsh BJ, et al. (1998) Extraction of membrane proteins by differential solubilization for separation using two-dimensional gel electrophoresis. *Electrophoresis* **19**, 837–44.

30. Rabilloud T, Adessi C, Giraudel A, Lunardi J. (1997) Improvement of the solubilization of proteins in two-dimensional electrophoresis with immobilized pH gradients. *Electrophoresis* **18**, 307–16.

31. Herbert B. (1999) Advances in protein solubilisation for two-dimensional electrophoresis. *Electrophoresis* **20**, 660–3.

32. Rabilloud T, Valette C, Lawrence JJ. (1994) Sample application by in-gel rehydration improves the resolution of two-dimensional electrophoresis with immobilized pH gradients in the first dimension. *Electrophoresis* **15**, 1552–8.

33. Carrette O, Burkhard PR, Sanchez JC, Hochstrasser DF. (2006) Stat-of-the-art two-dimensional gel electrophoresis: a key tool of proteomics research. *Nature Protocols* **1**, 812–23.

34. Chen G, Gharib TG, Huang CC, et al. (2002) Proteomic analysis of lung adenocarcinoma: identification of a highly expressed set of proteins in tumors. *Clin Cancer Res* **8**, 2298–305.

35. Gharib TG, Chen G, Wang H, et al. (2002) Proteomic analysis of cytokeratin isoforms uncovers association with survival in lung adenocarcinoma. *Neoplasia* **4**, 440–8.

36. Hanash S. (2001) 2-D or not 2-D – is there a future for 2-D gels in proteomics? Insights from the York proteomics meeting. *Proteomics* **1**, 635–7.

37. Young DA, Voris BP, Maytin EV, Colbert RA. (1983) Very-high-resolution two-dimensional electrophoretic separation of proteins on giant gels. *Methods Enzymol* **91**, 190–214.

38. Gorg A, Boguth G, Kopf A, Reil G, Parlar H, Weiss W. (2002) Sample prefractionation with Sephadex isoelectric focusing prior to narrow pH range two-dimensional gels. *Proteomics* **2**, 1652–7.

39. Wildgruber R, Harder A, Obermaier C, et al. (2002) Towards higher resolution: two-dimensional electrophoresis of Saccharomyces cerevisiae proteins using overlapping narrow immobilized pH gradients. *Electrophoresis* **21**, 2610–6.

40. Emmert-Buck MR, Bonner RF, Smith PD, et al. (1996) Laser capture microdissection. *Science* **274**, 998–1001.

41. Banks RE, Dunn MJ, Forbes MA, et al. (1999) The potential use of laser capture microdissection to selectively obtain distinct populations of cells for proteomic analysis – preliminary findings. *Electrophoresis* **20**, 689–700.

42. Craven RA, Totty N, Harnden P, Selby PJ, Banks RE. (2002) Laser capture microdissection and two-dimensional polyacrylamide gel electrophoresis: evaluation of tissue preparation and sample limitations. *Am J Pathol* **160**, 815–22.

43. Unlu M, Morgan ME, Minden JS. (1997) Difference gel electrophoresis: a single gel method for detecting changes in protein extracts. *Electrophoresis* **18**, 2071–7.

44. Okano T, Kondo T, Kakisaka T, et al. (2006) Plasma proteomics of lung cancer by a linkage

of multi-dimensional liquid chromatography and two-dimensional difference gel electrophoresis (2D-DIGE). *Proteomics* **6**, 3938–48.

45. Shaw J, Rowlinson R, Nickson J, et al. (2003) Evaluation of saturation labelling two-dimensional difference gel electrophoresis fluorescent dyes. *Proteomics* **3**, 1181–95.

46. Kondo T, Seike M, Mori Y, Fujii K, Yamada T, Hirohashi S. (2003) Application of sensitive fluorescent dyes in linkage of laser microdissection and two-dimensional gel electrophoresis as a cancer proteomic study tool. *Proteomics* **3**, 1758–66.

47. Seike M, Kondo T, Fujii K, et al. (2005) Proteomic signatures for histological types of lung cancer. *Proteomics* **5**, 2939–48.

48. Sitek B, Luttges J, Marcus K, et al. (2005) Application of fluorescence difference gel electrophoresis saturation labelling for the analysis of microdissected precursor lesions of pancreatic ductal adenocarcinoma. *Proteomics* **5**, 2665–79.

49. Greengauz-Roberts O, Stoppler H, Nomura S, et al. (2005) Saturation labeling with cysteine-reactive cyanine fluorescent dyes provides increased sensitivity for protein expression profiling of laser-microdissected clinical specimens. *Proteomics* **5**, 1746–57.

50. Wilson KE, Marouga R, Prime JE, et al. (2005) Comparative proteomic analysis using samples obtained with laser microdissection and saturation dye labelling. *Proteomics* **5**, 3851–8.

51. Suehara Y, Kondo T, Fujii K, et al. (2006) Proteomic signatures corresponding to histological classification and grading of soft-tissue sarcomas. *Proteomics* **6**, 4402–9.

52. Rosenfeld J, Capdevielle J, Guillemot JC, Ferrara P. (1992) In-gel digestion of proteins for internal sequence analysis after one- or two-dimensional gel electrophoresis. *Anal Biochem* **203**, 173–9.

53. Rhodes DR, Kalyana-Sundaram S, Mahavisno V, et al. (2007) Oncomine 3.0: genes, pathways, and networks in a collection of 18,000 cancer gene expression profiles. *Neoplasia* 9, 166–80.

54. Rhodes DR, Kalyana-Sundaram S, Tomlins SA, et al. (2007) Molecular concepts analysis links tumors, pathways, mechanisms, and drugs. *Neoplasia* **9**, 443–54.

Chapter 12

Fully Automated Two-Dimensional Electrophoresis System for High-Throughput Protein Analysis

Atsunori Hiratsuka and Kenji Yokoyama

Summary

A fully automated two-dimensional electrophoresis (2DE) system for rapid and reproducible protein analysis is described. 2DE that is a combination of isoelectric focusing (IEF) and sodium dodecyl sulfate polyacrylamide gel electrophoresis (SDS-PAGE) is widely used for protein expression analysis. Here, all the operations are achieved in a shorter time and all the transferring procedures are performed automatically. The system completed the entire process within 1.5 h. A device configuration, operational procedure, and data analysis are described using this system.

Key words: High-throughput assay, Two-dimensional electrophoresis, Automation, System, Simultaneous detection, Protein

1. Introduction

An approach of reverse chemical genetics has become dominant over the past few decades owing to the development of powerful and familiar techniques. Small molecule compounds that intervene in biological systems have been sought as tools to perturb enzymes and signaling pathways and of course as therapeutic agents for disease. It is essential to test the vast number of potential unique carbon-scaffold small molecule compounds. Recently, developing high-throughput screening methods has progressed and facilitated. A high-density microarray which is called a small-molecule microarray (SMM) is used in a high-throughput protein-binding assay *(1, 2)*. A high-throughput cell-based approach which is called cytoblot assay is used any post-translational modifications *(3)*. Recent technical innovations in automated

Hisashi Koga (ed.), *Reverse Chemical Genetics*, Methods in Molecular Biology, vol. 577
DOI 10.1007/978-1-60761-232-2_12, © Humana Press, a part of Springer Science+Business Media, LLC 2009

microscopy also allow image-based small molecule and screening which is called automated cell imaging.

Two-dimensional electrophoresis (2DE) that is a combination of isoelectric focusing (IEF) and sodium dodecyl sulfate polyacrylamide gel electrophoresis (SDS-PAGE) *(4)* is widely used for protein expression analysis.

Protein-binding assays with a small molecule compound for post-translational modifications, e.g., phosphorylation and glycosylation can be applied with a combination of the 2DE and a blotting procedure. Employing the protein-binding assay with the small molecule compound on the blotted proteins can reveal that the number of binding proteins and extent of binding affinities indicate candidates and order of precedence. However, 2DE still have major issues that need to addressed, such as complex time-consuming experimental procedure and poor reproducibility of the result, because several different procedures must be performed to complete 2DE *(5)*.

Previously, we developed a prototype model of automated 2DE system which enabled rapid, highly reproducible, and required minimal maintenance *(6)*. All the 2DE procedures including IEF, on-part protein staining, SDS-PAGE, and in situ protein detection were automatically completed. The system completed the entire process within 1.5 h. Recently, an improved model of this system was capable of reliability *y* and portability, e.g., operational stabilities in both componentry and software, and miniaturization of whole apparatus. Followings are described system components, operational procedure, and data analysis of this 2DE system in a hands-on form.

2. Materials

2.1. Sample Preparation

1. Male ICR mice are used from Charles River, Japan.

2. Mouse liver tissue (0.4 g) is lysed in 2 mL of lysis buffer (50 mM Tris–HCl (pH 7.6), 20% glycerol, 0.3 M NaCl, protease inhibitor cocktail) by homogenization using a homogenizer.

3. The lysate is centrifuged at $1,000 \times g$ for 10 min at 4°C, and the supernatant is centrifuged at $15,000 \times g$ for 30 min at 4°C.

4. The supernatant is collected and filtered using a 0.45 μm pore-sized filter.

5. Chromosomal DNA in the lysate is eliminated using the 2D Clean-Up Kit (GE Healthcare UK Ltd.) (*see* **Note 1**).

6. Protein concentration is measured by using the 2D Quant Kit (GE Healthcare UK Ltd.) with bovine serum albumin as the standard and adjusted to 10 μg/μL at a pH of 9.

**2.2. Fluorescence
Labeling of Protein**

1. A fluorescence labeling reagent (Cydye DIGE fluors, Cy5 Minimal, from GE Healthcare UK Ltd.) is dissolved into N,N-dimethylformamide (DMF) and adjusted to 400 pmol/μL of concentration.

2. 50 μg (5 μL) parts of the lysate is mixed with 400 pmol (1 μL) of the fluorescence reagent using a Vortex Mixer and maintained in a light-resistant container for 30 min at 4°C to employ the labeling reaction.

3. 6 μL parts of the mixture of lysate and reagent is mixed with 10 pmol (1 μL, 10 mM) of L-Lysine using the Vortex Mixer and maintained in a light-resistant container for 10 min at 4°C to terminate the labeling reaction (*see* **Note 1**).

2.3. Solution

1. *Sample buffer.* 8 M urea, 2 M thiourea, 4% w/v 3-[(3-cholamidopropyl)dimethylammonio]propanesulfonic acid (CHAPS), 20 mM dithiothreitol (DTT), 0.5%v/v carrier ampholyte.

2. *Monomer solution for resolving gel.* Tris–HCl buffer (pH 8.8) containing 12.5% (w/v) acrylamide, 0.3% (w/v) N,N'-methylenebisacrylamide, 0.05% (w/v) ammonium persulfate and 0.1% (v/v) N,N,N',N'-tetramethylethylenediamine (TEMED) (*see* **Note 2**).

3. *Monomer solution for stacking gel.* Tris–HCl buffer (pH 6.8) containing 3% (w/v) acrylamide, 0.3% (w/v) N,N'-methylenebisacrylamide, 0.05% (w/v) ammonium persulfate and 0.1% (v/v) TEMED (*see* **Note 2**).

4. *Rehydration buffer.* 8 M urea, 2 M thiourea, 4%w/v CHAPS, 20 mM DTT, 0.5%v/v carrier ampholyte.

5. *Equilibrating buffer.* Sample buffer (2× NuPAGE LDS), 50 mM DTT.

6. *Washing buffer.* 100 mM Sodium carbonate buffer (pH 9.3).

7. *Staining solution.* 0.2 mg/mL Cy5 Mono-reactive Dye, 2%w/v SDS, 100 mM sodium carbonate buffer (pH 9.3).

8. *Dye washing buffer.* 150 mM Tris–HCl (pH 7.5).

9. *Electrode cleaning solution 1.* 0.25%w/v SDS.

10. *Electrode cleaning solution 2.* distilled water.

11. *Electrophoresis buffer.* (cathodic reservoir: 25 mM Tris–HCl, 0.19 M glycine, 0.1%w/v SDS, (pH8.3)) (anodic reservoir: 150 mM Tris–HCl buffer (pH 8.8)).

**2.4. 2D Fluorescence
Detection**

The following detection system is constructed to measure protein spots for the simultaneous detection during SDS-PAGE.

1. A xenon lamp (MAX-300, Asahi Spectra Co., Ltd., Japan) provided the fluorescence excitation light that is focused onto the part by using a 620-nm band pass filter (Asahi Spectra Co., Ltd.).

2. The fluorescence signal is spectrally filtered through a 680-nm band pass filter (Asahi Spectra Co., Ltd.) prior to being detected by a CCD camera (2,048 × 2,048 pixels, DW436, Andor Technology, Northern Ireland) using a 55-mm focal length lens (F number:2.8, Nikon Corporation, Japan).

3. The results are visualized using the Andor-MCD program (Andor Technology).

3. Methods

The fully automated 2DE system is designed to ensure that an operator performs only the following procedures: opening the sealed box, placing the three parts, applying sample and buffer solutions into the grooves on the solution part, closing the box, and clicking the start button of a control program. Even the temperature and humidity are maintained by the Peltiert devices and closed box.

The system comprises a main component and laptop computer. The total system is 33 cm long, 27 cm wide and 29 cm high (**Fig. 1**). The components of the system are shown in **Fig. 2**.

The main component is constructed using the following apparatuses: an IEF part, solution part, SDS-PAGE part, electrodes, electrode storage site, biaxial conveyer, Peltiert devices, high-voltage generating devices, digital input/output (I/O) device, analog I/O device, and thermocouple controller. A positioning arm is constructed on the top of the biaxial conveyer. A charge-coupled device (CCD) detection system is placed above the SDS-PAGE part for simultaneous monitoring.

The biaxial conveyor that moves in only the perpendicular and horizontal directions is applied in this system. Including a solution transfer apparatus might be one option to automate solution handlings. However, applying such a system is expensive because the apparatus comprises several instruments, e.g., tubes, pumps, and solenoid valves for dispensing and discharging solutions. If this apparatus is applied, the system may need to flush unused solutions to prevent clogging and contamination of tubes. Since such an apparatus is extremely complicated, it needs routine maintenance and hence straightforward operation is not possible. Therefore, the conveyer unit is applied by substituting solution transfer with part transfer (*see* **Note 3**).

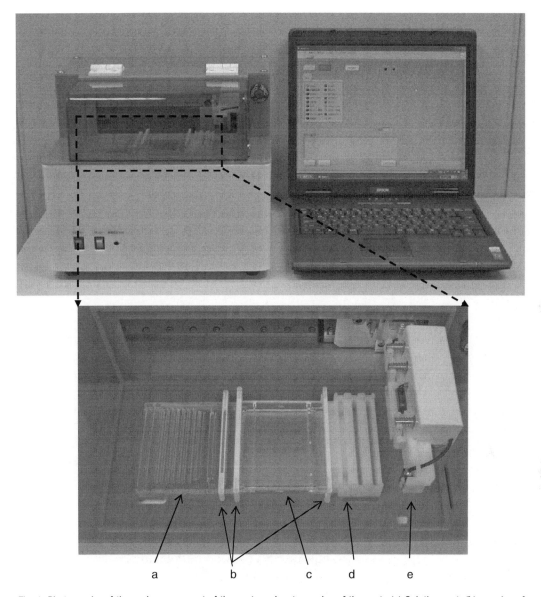

Fig. 1. Photographs of the main component of the system. *Inset:* a series of the parts (**a**) Solution part, (**b**) a series of electrodes, (**c**) SDS-PAGE part, (**d**) electrode storage, (**e**) biaxial conveyer.

The series of disposable parts are merely placed on the stage to achieve simplicity of preparation and disposal prior to and after use of the system (**Fig. 1** inset) (*see* **Note 4**). For reuse, a series of platinum electrode units are fabricated separately. The conveyer automatically set the electrode units in designated positions on the parts at the electrode storage site. The electrode units are washed and returned to the site after the electrophoresis procedures are performed.

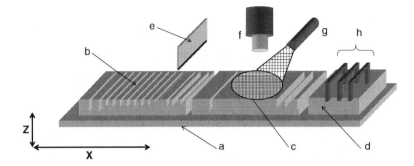

Fig. 2. Schematics of 2DE system (**a**) Stage unit incorporated with peltiert devices, (**b**) Solution part, (**c**) SDS-PAGE part, (**d**) electrode storage, (**e**) IEF part, (**f**) CCD camera, (**g**) fluorescence induced-lights, (**h**) a series of electrodes.

The solution part is a square of 70 mm and 10 mm thick. Grooves for IEF, IEF part storage, spare (optional: p*I* marker part), sample, rehydration, SDS equilibration, two for IPG washing, staining, two for dye washing, and two for electrode cleaning are formed. Grooves for solution reservoirs, the IPG storage site, and IEF chamber are constructed on the PMMA substrate.

The IEF part comprised of a PMMA support board for attaching the conveyer and an IPG gel strip bonded to the edge of the support via a PET backing film. The IPG gel used in this system had a linear pH gradient, pH 3–10. The part is 52 mm long in the pH direction, 1.2 mm wide, and 14 mm high. The IPG gel is 52 mm long in the pH direction, 1.1 mm wide and 0.03 mm thick in dehydrated condition. The size of the gel is smaller than the commercial gel, in particular, the width of the gel is approximately one-third size of the commercial gel. The gel is miniaturized to avoid both higher electric current and heat generated when a higher voltage is applied.

The SDS-PAGE part comprised of two components. The two components are bonded together to form buffer reservoirs and a polyacrylamide gel cavity. The part is constructed with a region for separation gel formation in the center and two grooves for introducing electrophoresis buffers on both the sides. The gel is 60 mm long in the pH direction, 48 mm long in the PAGE direction, and 1 mm thick. The capacities of the electrophoresis buffer are 5.87 and 5.70 mL in the anodic and cathodic terminus sides, respectively.

Monomer solutions for resolving gel and stacking gel are poured in the cavity and polymerized. To minimize the entire size of the part, both the gel dimension and buffer amount are reduced. Rapid separation is performed without an increase in the volume of the buffer solution to maintain the separation mobility by applying a condition of constant current. The automated system requires neither any linking solution such as agarose nor solution sending apparatus. Protein transferring is achieved by attaching only the IPG gel part against a gel with a tapered edge. The edge of the separation gel is exposed to the groove and is tapered.

3.1. Placing the Parts and Introducing Solutions

1. The solution part, SDS-PAGE part, and storage site are placed on the left, center, and right of the Peltiert devices, respectively. The parts are located in a closed box under controlled humidity and thermal conditions.

2. A series of electrodes for IEF and SDS-PAGE are stored in the storage site.

3. Sample solutions are introduced into grooves of the solution part.
Following solutions are introduced into the grooves.
   (a) 10 μL of sample solution is introduced into the groove for sample.
   (b) 80 μL of rehydration buffer is introduced into the groove for IPG rehydration.
   (c) 300 μL of equilibrating buffer is introduced into the groove for IPG equilibration.
   (d) Two of 450 μL of IPG washing buffer are introduced into the grooves for IPG washing, respectively.
   (e) 450 μL of staining solution is introduced into the groove for protein staining.
   (f) Two of 450 μL of dye washing buffer are introduced into the grooves for dye washing, respectively.
   (g) 1,800 μL of electrode cleaning solution 1 is introduced into the groove for the electrodes cleaning
   (h) 1,800 μL of electrode cleaning solution 2 is introduced into the groove for the electrodes cleaning.

4. Two of 4.0 mL of electrophoresis buffers are introduced into the reservoirs of SDS-PAGE part.

3.2. 2DE Operation

Operational procedures are performed automatically as follows:

1. A series of electrodes for IEF and SDS-PAGE are transferred by the conveyer to a predefined position on the solution and SDS-PAGE parts, respectively.

2. The IEF part is transferred into the groove containing 10 μL of sample solution for 5 min.

3. The part is transferred into the groove containing 80 μL of rehydration buffer and incubated for 5 min.

4. The part is transferred into the groove for IEF (see **Note 5**). After the control program detects the contacts between the part and the electrodes, the program applies the voltage as follows. The voltage linearly increased from 0 to 6,000 V for 10 min, and then it is maintained at 6,000 V for 20 min.

5. The part is transferred into the groove containing 300 μL of equilibrating buffer for 5 min.

6. The part is positioned at the tapered surface of PAG on the SDS-PAGE part containing 4.0 mL of each electrophoresis buffer (see **Note 6**).

7. SDS-PAGE is performed at a constant current of 20 mA for 30 min (see **Note 7**).

8. The part is transferred to the initial position.

9. The electrodes are transferred into the two grooves containing cleaning solutions 1 and 2.

10. The electrodes are transferred to the storage site.

Following procedures are performed between the IEF **(step 4)** and equilibration procedure **(step 5)** for the simultaneous protein labeling and detection. A fluorescence labeling is performed between the IEF and equilibration procedures (In-between staining).

1. The part is continuously transferred into two grooves containing 450 μL of IPG washing buffer for 2.5 min, respectively.

2. The part is transferred into a groove containing 450 μL of staining solution for 5 min.

3. The part is continuously transferred into two grooves containing 450 μL of dye washing buffer for 2.5 min, respectively.

3.3. Data Analysis

Mouse liver has been widely used for proteome analysis by the 2DE method. (7, 8) In this study, the extracted proteins from the mouse liver tissue are used as an example. Protein spots are evaluated using the gel analysis software ProFINDER 2D (PerkinElmer Life And Analytical Sciences, Inc., Wellesley, MA) and PDQuest (Bio-Rad Laboratories, Hercules, CA)).

Figure 3 shows the 2D separation images of the extracted proteins by using the automated system. The proteins are separated, and protein spots are visualized over the entire gel region.

The numbers of the spots are automatically counted by using the software. Subsequently, false spots such as dust and dirt are manually removed.

3.3.1. Assignment of 2DE Spot Position

1. Zero point for the length of the gels for separation along the IEF and SDS-PAGE directions is assigned at the acidic end (+) of the terminus of an electrode and at the beginning of the

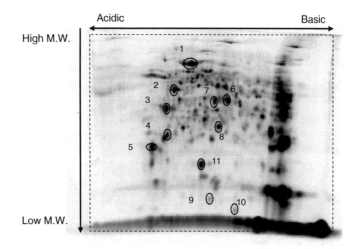

Fig. 3. Representative 2D image The protein sample from mouse liver (2.3 μg) is applied in each system. 11 protein spots (1–11) are selected in each gel image for image analysis.

separation gel region, respectively. The length is described in pixel counts.

2. Position of the protein spot is set at the position of its fluorescence peak signal.

The signals used in these analyses are employed without background corrections.

3.3.2. Resolution of Spot

Resolutions of both IEF and SDS-PAGE directions are calculated as follows:

1. *pI direction*. Pixel value of the width in pI direction at half height of the peak spot is assigned $S1$. Pixel value of the IPG gel length is assigned $L1$.

Then, resolution of pI direction = $L1/S1$

2. *SDS-PAGE direction*. Pixel value of the width in SDS-PAGE direction at half height of the peak spot is assigned $S2$. Pixel value of migration length of the spot for SDS-PAGE direction is assigned $L2$. Then, resolution of SDS-PAGE direction = $L2/S2$.

The resolution of the spots obtained by this method is evaluated. Distinct protein spots are selected from over the entire region of the image for subsequent investigations. The 11 spots are indicated by red circles in each image **(Fig. 3)**. The resolution of each spot is evaluated with regard to its separation along the IEF and molecular weight (M.W.) directions. The results are summarized in **Table 1**.

3.3.3. Reproducibility of Spot Position and Intensity

Relative standard deviations (coefficient of variance (CV)) of the position and the intensity are calculated to demonstrate reproducibility.

Table 1
Resolution of spot

	1	2	3	4	5	6	7	8	9	10	11
p*I* direction (mean value)	55.7	69.1	64.0	52.2	38.8	71.2	70.6	56.9	34.1	15.3	71.0
M.W. direction (mean value)	9.3	15.5	13.6	17.0	19.1	16.0	16.30	19.5	16.3	19.7	22.3

Number: Protein spots, selected spots are indicated in **Fig. 3** condition. Protein sample: mouse liver lysate 2.3 μg, Number of tested times: 5, the values shown in the table are mean values. The data are summarized in p*I* and molecular weight (M. W.) directions

Table 2
Reproducibly of spot position

Spot number	1	2	3	4	5	6	7	8	9	10	11
p*I* direction (CV)	1.6	2.0	2.2	2.6	3.8	1.7	2.8	2.6	2.3	1.3	2.2
M.W. direction (CV)	7.2	4.2	5.2	3.6	3.6	5.0	3.5	3.1	3.4	3.2	5.7

Number: Protein spots; selected spots are indicated in **Fig. 3** condition. Protein sample: mouse liver lysate 2.3 μg, Number of tested times: 5, The values shown in the table are coefficient of variance (CV) (%). The data are summarized in p*I* and molecular weight (M. W.) directions

Table 3
Reproducibility of spot intensity

Spot number		1	2	3	4	5	6	7	8	9	10	11
Automated system	mean value ($\times 10^5$)	25.9	11.9	19.5	10.8	22.9	9.54	7.7	6.8	5.9	5.2	17.8
	CV (%)	26.6	10.1	25.6	14.3	24.0	15.8	13.7	20.6	18.7	15.7	9.4

Number: Protein spots, selected spots are indicated in **Fig. 3** condition. Protein sample: mouse liver lysate 2.3 μg, Number of tested times: 5, the values shown in the table are mean value ($\times 10^5$) and coefficient of variance (CV) (%)

The reproducibility of the positions of the protein spots is evaluated. The position of each protein spot is calculated in the IEF and M.W. directions. The results are summarized in **Table 2**. Reproducibility of the spot amount in association with the spot intensity is evaluated. The results are summarized in **Table 3**.

4. Notes

1. The samples should be stored at –80°C and prepared into small quantity. Only the necessary quantity can be used and unused samples are maintained at –80°C in use.

2. TEMED is stored at room temperature. Use a small bottle and put the undiluted solution in use as it may decline in quality after opening.

3. Although a conveyer unit equipped with a multiaxial controller is expensive, a conveyer with minimized axial controllers and limited working area can be inexpensive.

4. Various protocol changes are possible by using different combinations of the parts constructed in different designs, e.g., changes in the number of the grooves, capacity of the reservoirs, and separation methods.

5. Mineral oil is routinely poured into the IPG gel in commercial minigel systems to prevent water evaporation during IEF. This time-consuming oil removal process is indispensable after IEF. In this system, IEF is performed without pouring the oil by inverting the gel and maintaining the temperature and humidity by including Peltiert devices and a sealing box.

6. The surface of the IPG should be buried into the tapered gel by adjusting 0.5 mm downward from the surface of the tapered gel when the IPG is attached on the surface. Then, the proteins are transferred into the tapered gel without leaking to electrophoresis buffer.

7. Under this condition of reduced solution amounts, the amount of the SDS ions in the electrolyte solution decreases with time and protein mobility during electrophoresis becomes gradually reduced if the applied potential is maintained at a constant voltage. Applying the condition of constant current, the voltage is increased to maintain the separation mobility in the latter half of the process.

Acknowledgments

The authors would like to thank our project members from National Institute of Advanced Industrial Science and Technology (AIST), Toppan Printing Co. Ltd, Sharp Corporation, Astellas Pharma Inc., Tokyo University of Technology and Kumamoto University. This work was financially supported by the New Energy and Industrial Technology Development Organization (NEDO), Japan.

References

1. MacBeath, G., Koehler, A.N., Schreiber, S.L. (1999) Printing small molecules as microarrays and detecting protein.ligand interactions en masse. *J Am Chem Soc.* **121**, 7967–7968

2. Bradner, J.E., McPherson, O.M., Mazitschek, R., Barnes-Seeman, D., Shen, J.P., Dhaliwal, J., Stevenson, K.E., Duffner, J.L., Park, S.B., Neuberg, D.S., Nghiem, P., Schreiber, S.L., Koehler, A.N. (2006) A robust Small-molecule microarray platform for screening cell lysates. *Chem Biol.* **13**, 493–504.

3. Stockwell, B.R., Haggarty, S.J., Schreiber, S.L. (1999) High-throughput screening of small molecules in miniaturized mammalian cell-based assays involving post-translational modifications. *Chem Biol.* **6**, 71–83

4. O'Farrell, P.H. (1975) High resolution two-dimensional electrophoresis of proteins. *J Biol Chem.* **250**, 4007–4021

5. Quadroni, M., James, P. (1999) Proteomics and automation. *Electrophoresis.* **20**, 664–677

6. Hiratsuka, A., Kinoshita, H., Maruo, Y., Takahashi, K., Akutsu, S., Hayashida, C., Sakairi, K., Usui, K., Shiseki, K., Inamochi, H., Nakada, Y., Yodoya, K., Namatame, I., Unuma, Y., Nakamura, M., Ueyama, K., Ishii, Y., Yano, K., Yokoyama, K. (2007) Fully automated two-dimensional electrophoresis system for high-throughput protein analysis. *Anal Chem.* **79**, 5730–5739

7. Tsugita, A., Kawakami, T., Uchida, T., Sakai, T., Kamo, M., Matsui, T., Watanabe, Y., Morimasa, T., Hosokawa, K., Toda, T. (2000) Proteome analysis of mouse brain: two-dimensional electrophoresis profiles of tissue proteins during the course of aging. Electrophoresis. **21**, 1853–1871

8. Park, B., Jeong, SK., Lee, WS., Seong, JK., Paik, YK. (2004) A simple pattern classification method for alcohol-responsive proteins that are differentially expressed in mouse brain. Proteomics. **4**, 3369–3375

Chapter 13

Large-Scale Whole Mount In Situ Hybridization of Mouse Embryos

Hirohito Shimizu, Kenta Uchibe, and Hiroshi Asahara

Summary

Whole-mount in situ hybridization (WISH) is a method to visualize gene expression within a whole organism. Although it is an essential approach in developmental biology to describe the gene expression patterns during embryogenesis, the simultaneous processing of numerous embryos in a large-scale experiment such as a screening assay has been difficult for an individual due to the limited capacity of the experimental setting. This chapter describes the optimal protocol for a WISH assay in a relatively large experimental scale, which allows for more efficient processing of embryos. The major improvement in the efficiency has been achieved by the several refinements such as the introduction of a quick method for probe synthesis, the use of mesh-buckets to facilitate handling samples, and the simplification of the conventional procedures. In combination with publicly accessible gene expression databases, WISH assays will be more favorable for a large-scale assay using mouse embryos.

Key words: In situ hybridization, Mouse, Whole-mount, Gene expression pattern, Large-scale assay, Gene expression database

1. Introduction

Chemical genetics is a highly effective approach in drug discovery, intended to screen for small molecule compounds that are responsible for the specific phenotype of interest and to determine their targets. As opposed to forward chemical genetics, which is a phenotype-driven approach aiming at identifying the small molecules that perturb the molecular pathway responsible by screening a large library, reverse chemical genetics starts off with a particular gene or protein of interest and inactivate it with

Hisashi Koga (ed.), *Reverse Chemical Genetics*, Methods in Molecular Biology, vol. 577
DOI 10.1007/978-1-60761-232-2_13, © Humana Press, a part of Springer Science+Business Media, LLC 2009

a known inhibitor in order to elucidate the biological function of the protein in question *(1, 2)*. In these approaches, it is essential to evaluate the phenotypic alterations as a consequence of chemical compound administration. However, in addition to anatomical alterations, such evaluation can entail a variety of aspects that cannot be observed externally, including physiological and biochemical changes. Although these aspects can be investigated using cell lines, the use of whole organisms is more advantageous in that they allow us to examine numerous biological processes that cannot be reproduced in cultured cells *(3)*. Thus, it is desirable to examine the molecular markers that serve as the indicators of these biological processes in a whole organism.

To this end, whole-mount in situ hybridization (WISH), which enables us to visualize spatiotemporal gene expression, is one of the optimal methods as an initial evaluation of the outcome following chemical compound administration. WISH has been extensively employed in a high throughput manner in large-scale drug screening systems using zebrafish *(4, 5)*. However, it would be valuable to apply this sort of large-scale WISH assay, if not as large as zebrafish chemical genetics, to mouse embryos for several reasons (1) mouse is an excellent model in the field of biomedical sciences due to its highly analogous development and phenotype to human, (2) many functional studies have been performed using mutant mouse models in which the comprehensive gene expression analysis is one of the critical methods to investigate the molecular network that the gene of interest is involved, (3) several gene expression databases are now available as a source of gene expression profiles that can be referenced or compared with the data obtained.

The protocol outlined in this chapter has been optimized for processing a large number of mouse embryos simultaneously. Since a lot of protocols include optional or even unnecessary steps largely for historical reasons, this protocol intends to maximize the efficiency of assays and minimize the temporal and financial burden, which are often the serious issues in a large-scale experiment. For reference, the alternative procedures, which were omitted or simplified in this protocol, are described in **Subheading 4** as potential troubleshooting tips.

2. Materials

2.1. Equipment

1. Hybridization oven.
2. Rocking platform.
3. 12-well plates (Gleiner, cat. no. 665180).
4. Buckets with fine mesh net (Netwell™ 12 well Carrier Kit for 15mm Inserts, Corning, cat. no. 3477).

2.2. Preparation of the Template cDNA

1. Plasmid DNA that contains the gene of interest.
2. RNA polymerase promoter site-tagged PCR primers.
3. DNA polymerase (*see* **Note 1** and **Fig. 1**).
4. PCR buffer and $MgSO_4$/dNTPs (supplied with DNA polymerase).

2.3. Synthesis of the cRNA Probes by In Vitro Transcriprion

1. Diethylpyrocarbonate (DEPC) (*see* **Note 2**).
2. RNA polymerase (T3, T7, or Sp6).
3. *10× DIG RNA Labeling Mix* 10 mM ATP, 10 mM CTP, 10 mM GTP, 6.5 mM UTP, 3.5 mM DIG-11-UTP (Roche).
4. 10× Transcription buffer and 100 mM Dithiothreitol (DTT)/ bovine serum albumin (BSA; supplied with RNA polymerase).

2.4. Embryo Preparation

1. *10× phosphate-buffered saline (PBS)*. Dissolve 80 g of NaCl, 2 g of KCl, 29 g of $Na_2HPO_4 \cdot 12H_2O$, and 2 g of KH_2PO_4 in approximately 800 ml of DEPC-treated ddH_2O. Adjust pH to 7.4 with HCl. Add DEPC-treated ddH_2O to 1 L, and sterilize by autoclaving. Dilute to make 1× PBS as necessary.

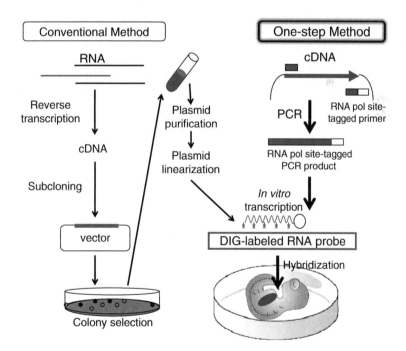

Fig. 1. Synthesis of RNA probes: comparison of the one-step method with the conventional method. A DNA fragment is amplified by PCR using a plasmid as a template. The Sp6 RNA polymerase promoter site is tagged to the 5′ end of the reverse primer. Following the purification of amplified DNA fragments, probes are synthesized with Sp6 RNA polymerase in the presence of digoxigenin (DIG)-conjugated UTP. This method greatly expedites the probe synthesis, which conventionally includes relatively lengthy procedures such as bacteria culture, plasmid purification, and linearization of plasmid.

2. *4% PFA fixative.* Add 4% paraformaldehyde powder to PBS followed by 2–3 drops of 5 M NaOH. Dissolve PFA completely with vigorous shaking at 60°C. Allow to cool on ice before use. Make fresh as required (*see* **Note 2**).

2.5. Prehybridization Treatment and Hybridization

1. *PBT.* 0.1% Tween 20 and PBS. This solution is also referred to as PBST in some protocols. Store at room temperature for up to 1 month and at 4°C for long-term storage. Do not autoclave.

2. *6% H_2O_2 solution.* 1× PBS and 6% H_2O_2. Make fresh as required.

3. *10 μg/ml proteinase K solution.* Dissolve proteinase K powder in ddH$_2$O. Aliquot the solution into microcentrifuge tubes and store at –20°C.

4. *2 mg/ml glycine solution.* Dissolve glycine powder in PBS. Make fresh as required.

5. *PFA-GA fixative.* Prepare 4% PFA in PBS as described above and add 0.2% glutaldehyde (GA). Make fresh as required.

6. *20× SSC.* Dissolve 175.3 g of NaCl and 88.2 g of sodium citrate dihydrate in approximately 800 ml of DEPC-treated ddH$_2$O. Adjust pH to 4.5 with citric acid. Add DEPC-treated ddH$_2$O and sterilize by autoclaving.

7. *tRNA solution.* Add approximately 12 mg of Torula baker's yeast tRNA in 400 μl of TE buffer, and perform typical phenol–chloroform–isoamyl alcohol extraction and ethanol precipitation procedures. Resuspend the pellet in 1 ml of DEPC-treated ddH$_2$O and determine the concentration by spectrophotometer. Store at –20°C.

8. *50 mg/ml Heparin solution.* 50 mg/ml of heparin sodium salt and 4× SSC. Store at –20°C.

9. *Hybridization Mix.* Add 50% formamide (ultrapure is recommended), 5× SSC, 1% SDS, 50 μg/ml heparin, 50 μg/ml tRNA ito DEPC-treated dd H$_2$O. Storable at –20°C up to 3 months.

2.6. Posthybridization Washes and Antibody

1. *WASH1 solution.* 50% formamide, 5× SSC, 1% SDS, and add ddH$_2$O to volume. Make fresh as required.

2. *5% CHAPS solution.* Dissolve CHAPS powder in ddH$_2$O Store at room temperature in dark.

3. *WASH2 solution.* 50% formamide, 2× SSC, 0.05% CHAPS, and add ddH$_2$O to volume. Make fresh as required.

4. *10× Tris-buffered saline (TBS).* Add 500 ml of 1 M Tris–HCl (pH 7.5), 300 ml of 5 M NaCl, and fill up to 1 L with ddH$_2$O. Sterilize by autoclaving and store at room temperature.

5. *10× TBST.* 0.1% Tween 20 and TBS. Store at room temperature for up to 1 month and at –20°C for long-term storage. Do not autoclave.

6. *Sheep serum.* Heat-inactivate by incubating in a water bath at 55°C for 30 min. Store in appropriate amount of aliquots at –20°C. Do not freeze-thaw repeatedly.

7. *Anti-DIG antibody solution.* Anti-DIG antibody (Roche) 1:2,000 ratio, 1% sheep serum in 1× TBST. Centrifuge the stock antibody solution at 14,000 g for 5 min and use the supernatant.

2.7. Postantibody Washes and Color Development

1. *NTMT buffer.* 100 mM NaCl, 100 mM Tris–HCl (pH 9.5), 50 mM $MgCl_2$, 0.1% Tween 20, and add ddH_2O to volume. Filter sterilize the buffer with 0.22 μm filter papers. Make fresh as required.

2. *NBT/BCIP.* Follow the manufacturer's instructions to prepare the solution. Make fresh as required (*see* **Note 3**).

3. 10% neutral-buffered formalin (*see* **Note 2**).

3. Methods

In all procedures prior to hybridization, utmost precautions must be taken to prevent the contamination of ribonucleases, which results in the degradation of cellular RNA. Gloves must be worn throughout the steps. PBS and water must be autoclaved and, if possible, should be treated with DEPC (*see* **Note 4**). All containers must be clean and ribonuclease-free. Particularly, it is important that, if reused, 12-well plates and insert buckets are treated with H_2O_2 and DEPC (*see* **Note 5**).

3.1. Preparation of In Situ Hybridization

3.1.1. Preparation of Template cDNA by PCR

This protocol describes a method to amplify the DNA template for in vitro transcription by using PCR instead of bacteria culture (*see* **Fig. 1**). Because a PCR product can be directly used for in vitro transcription following ethanol precipitation, this method is optimal for a large-scale probe synthesis.

1. Obtain the genes of interest in the plasmids.

2. Amplify an appropriate DNA fragment with an appropriate polymerase according to the manufacturer's instruction (*see* **Note 1** and **6**). Make sure to tag the RNA polymerase promoter site to the 5′ end of the reverse primer (*see* **Fig. 1**).

3. Add 1/10 vol of RNase-free 3 M NaOAc and 2 vol of 100% ethanol, and store at –20°C for 15 min (*see* **Note 7**).

4. Spin in a refrigerated centrifuge at 14,000 g for 15 min and remove supernatant.

5. Rinse the pellet with 70% ethanol.

6. Resuspend the pellet in 6 μl of DEPC-treated ddH$_2$O. Use a 1-μl aliquot to determine the concentration, and use another 1-μl aliquot for electrophoresis on an agarose/TAE gel containing 0.5 μg/ml ethidium bromide (*see* **Note 2**).

3.1.2. Preparation of DIG-Labeled RNA Probes

1. Add the following to a microcentrifuge tube:
   (a) PCR product (template DNA) (500 ng)
   (b) 10× Transcription Buffer 1 μl
   (c) 100 mM DTT 1 μl
   (d) 0.1% BSA 1 μl
   (e) 10× DIG-labeling Mix 1 μl
   (f) 50 U/μl RNA polymerase 1 μl
   (g) DEPC-treated ddH$_2$O up to10 μl

2. Incubate at 37°C for 2 h.

3. Add 90 μl of DEPC-treated ddH$_2$O, mix, and remove a 5-μl aliquot from the reaction mixture to confirm the successful probe synthesis by running on an agarose/TAE gel containing 0.5 μg/ml ethidium bromide (*see* **Note 8**).

4. Add 10 μl of RNase-free 3 M NaOAc and 250 μl of RNase-free 100% ethanol, and store at –20°C for 30 min.

5. Spin in a refrigerated centrifuge at 14,000 g for 15 min and remove supernatant.

6. Rinse the pellet twice with 500 μl of RNase-free 80% ethanol.

7. Resuspend the pellet in 6 μl of DEPC-treated ddH$_2$O. Use a 1-μl aliquot to determine the concentration with a spectrophotometer and check the quality of the RNA probe on an agarose gel (*see* **Note 9**).

8. Add 95 μl of Hybridization Mix (*see* **Subheading 2.3**). RNA probe solution can be stored at –20°C or –80°C up to at least 1 year.

3.1.3. Preparation of Embryos

1. Harvest embryos into cold PBS (*see* **Note 10**).

2. Fix the embryos in a solution of 4% paraformaldehyde in PBS overnight at 4°C.

3. Wash 3 times with PBS for 5 min each on ice.

4. Dehydrate embryos with graded series of methanol washes (25%, 50%, 75%, and twice with 100%) in PBS on ice for 5 min each.

5. Store the embryos in 100% methanol at –20°C until needed (use glass vials or plastic tubes).

**3.2. In Situ
Hybridization Assay**

All further procedures are performed at room temperature and samples are handled in mesh-buckets with a 12-well plate unless otherwise specified (*see* **Fig. 2**). Wear gloves when moving mesh-buckets manually. All the wash steps are conducted with a defined incubation time indicated by moving up and down the buckets softly but occasionally to ensure thorough mixing. To facilitate the transfer of individual embryos, use a pipette fitted with a 200 μl or a 1,000 μl tip that was cut to make a wide opening, but avoid excessive agitation.

*3.2.1. Prehybridization
Treatment and
Hybridization*

1. Put 100% methanol in a 12-well plate, insert the mesh-buckets, and transfer the embryos. At this point, the embryos of the same stage should be put in the same well.

2. Rehydrate the embryos with a 75%, 50%, 25% methanol in PBT series and wash 3 times with PBT for 5 min each on ice.

3. Bleach the embryos with 6% H_2O_2 in PBT for 15–30 min, and wash 3 times with PBT for 5 min each (*see* **Note 11**).

4. Digest the embryos with 10 μg/ml of proteinase K in PBT for stage-dependent/varying durations (*see* **Note 12**).

5. Stop digestion by washing in a solution of 0.2 mg/ml glycine in PBT for 10 min, and wash twice with PBT for 5 min each.

6. Refix the embryos with 4% paraformaldehyde and 0.2% glutaraldehyde in PBT for 20 min, and wash twice with PBT for 5 min each.

7. Replace PBT with Hybridization Mix and incubate at room temperature until the embryos settle on the bottom.

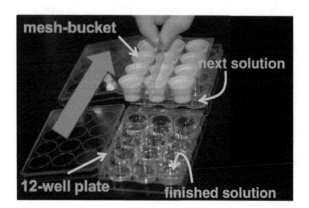

Fig. 2. 12-well plates and buckets with fine mesh net. Embryos are contained within the buckets and solution is contained in the wells. Upon completion of a washing/treatment step, buckets are moved to the new plate, which contains the next solution in each well. A large number of embryos can be processed easily at the same time by using this method.

8. Change Hybridization Mix and incubate the embryos for 1 h at 70°C in the hybridization oven with rocking.

9. Prepare Hybridization Mix containing 500 ng/ml of DIG-labeled RNA probe in a plastic screw-cap tube, and transfer the embryos.

10. Hybridize at 70°C for at least 14 h with gentle rocking (*see* **Notes 13** and **14**).

3.2.2. Posthybridization Washes and Preabsorption of Antibody

1. Prepare WASH1 solution in the 12-well plate, and transfer the embryos with mesh-buckets. Wash 3 times with prewarmed WASH1 solution at 70°C in the hybridization oven for 30 min each (*see* **Note 15**). Probes can be recovered in the screw-cap tubes and stored at –20°C for reuse up to at least 3 times.

2. Wash twice with prewarmed WASH2 solution at 65°C in the hybridization oven for 30 min each.

3. Wash 3 times with TBST.

4. Block the embryos with 10% heat inactivated sheep serum in TBST for 1 h (*see* **Note 16**). Prepare the blocking solution in the screw-cap tubes and transfer the embryos.

5. Replace the blocking solution with the antibody solution (1% heat inactivated sheep serum in TBST containing 1:2,000 dilution of anti-DIG antibody). It is easy to conduct this process by transferring the embryos with pipette after pouring them out into the petri-dish.

6. Incubate the embryos for at least 8 h at 4°C with gentle rocking.

3.2.3. Postantibody Washes and Color Development

1. Prepare TBST in the 15 ml tubes, and transfer the embryos. Wash the embryos 3 times for 10 min each.

2. Wash the embryos twice with TBST for 30 min each.

3. Wash the embryos at least 6 times with TBST for 1 h each. It is sometimes convenient to stop at the end of the series of TBST washes. In this case, incubate the embryos in TBST at 4°C with gentle rocking.

4. Equilibrate the embryos 3 times with NTMT for 5 min each. Make sure that embryos are washed enough with mild rocking; otherwise the developing color will get brownish red rather than blue.

5. Put the embryos into NBT/BCIP solution and incubate in the dark until desired extent of signal is detected (*see* **Note 17**).

6. Wash the embryos 3 times with prewarmed (70°C) PBT.

7. Fix the embryos with 10% neutral-buffered formalin. Embryos can be stored at 4°C up to at least 6 months.

3.3. Photography and Evaluation of Data

Image data of whole mount embryos after WISH assays can be obtained using a computer-controlled display (CCD) camera installed to a dissection microscope. It is advisable to minimize the aperture of the dissection microscope and illuminate the embryo at right angle in order to obtain well-focused images with excellent contrast. When capturing the image from a given angle desired, follow the following steps:

1. Pour 1% agarose into a Petri dish and let the gel set (*see* **Note 18**).

2. Cut grooves (s) in a layer of agarose gel with a scalpel blade or forceps to accommodate the embryo.

3. Immerse the embryo in PBS.

When evaluating the data obtained, it might be worthwhile to compare the photo images with the data stored in the public gene expression databases. We have established, using this WISH protocol, a web-based gene expression database, called EMBRYS (http://www.embrys.jp/beta/html/MainMenu.html), which provides a comprehensive expression atlas of transcription regulating genes (submitted). Additionally, some of the representative gene expression databases are listed below (*6–9*):

EMAGE by Western General Hospital by Edinburg, UK (http://genex.hgu.mrc.ac.uk/Emage/database/emageIntro.html)

EurExpress by EurExpres Consortium (http://www.eurexpress.org/ee/)

Functional Genomic Atlas of the Mouse Brain by Harvard Univesity, Boston, USA (http://mahoney.chip.org/mahoney/database.html)

GenePaint by Max Planck Institute of Experimental Endocrinology, Hannover, Germany (http://www.genepaint.org/)

Mamep by Max Planck Institute for Molecular Genetics, Berlin, Germany (http://mamep.molgen.mpg.de/)

4. Notes

1. Avoid using PCR polymerases that generate 3′ overhangs. This kind of overhang can result in the decreased efficiency of the in vitro transcription reaction.

2. A number of reagents used in this protocol are known or potential toxicants. Be sure to use a fume hood and protective equipment as necessary. In particular extreme care should be exercised when handling DEPC, ethidium bromide, paraformaldehyde, and formalin since they are widely assumed to be carcinogenic.

3. There are several options for the reagents used in color development including solution, powder, and tablets. Among these,

NBT/BCIP ready-to-use tablet (Roche) and BM purple solution (Roche) are highly recommended. Follow the instructions provided by manufacturers.

4. A critical general precaution prior to hybridization is to avoid RNase contamination in the solution. Although autoclave treatment of the glassware is presumably sufficient, dirthyl pyrocarbonate (DEPC) treatment of ddH_2O is known to be effective to inactivate RNase. Particularly, if cell culture plates and inserts are reused, they need to be treated with DEPC-treated ddH_2O after use since they cannot be autoclaved. Water can be DEPC-treated by adding 0.1% of DEPC to distilled water and shaking vigorously at room temperature overnight. Make sure to autoclave at 120°C for 20 min to degrade DEPC.

5. Although cell culture plates and inserts can be reused, the following washing process is highly recommended to maintain an RNase-free condition (1) wash thoroughly with detergent and rinse with ddH_2O, (2) soak in 3% H_2O_2 overnight, (3) rinse with ddH_2O and sonicate, (4) rinse with DEPC-treated ddH_2O, (5) dry at 60°C.

6. When designing a cRNA probe, avoid highly conserved motifs in order to minimize crosshybridization to transcripts of other genes, which leads to higher nonspecific staining. Whether the fragment is highly conserved or not can be checked using public databases such as NCBI BLAST. Likewise, try to select a fragment of the gene that lacks repetitive sequences, A–T rich stretches and a poly(A) tail. In general, a shorter probe gives higher in vitro transcription efficiency and better tissue penetration but results in lower signals and lower hybridization specificity. However, when synthesizing many probes simultaneously, just choose the probe size of 500–1,000 base pairs. If one hopes to optimize the condition, it might be effective to change the size and position of the probe since the performance of each probe differs depending upon the nature of the tissue and extent of cross-linking by the fixative.

7. The amplified cDNA template can be purified via phenol–chloroform–isoamyl alcohol extraction or with commercially available column kit. However, it was found that this purification step is not necessary for the following procedures.

8. While the RNA band is ideally much more intense than the template band on an agarose gel, RNA fragments can frequently appear as a smear as well. However, such probes can often work well. It might be worth trying the probe in a WISH assay to evaluate the quality of the probe. Note that RNA probe can also appear in multiple bands since RNA is single stranded. Check that these bands are present in the proximity of the expected position. If you hope to check the size more precisely, run the probe on a denaturing gel to obtain a single band.

9. Unincorporated nucleotides and short cRNA fragments with DIG label might cause nonspecific hybridization, which results in higher background staining. If the background staining is consistently observed with the same probe, the purification of the labeled probe can be effective to increase the sensitivity. Some purification kits are commercially available such as High Pure PCR Cleanup Micro Kit (Roche)

10. Be sure to remove the extraembryonic membrane. Failure to do this may result in the lower colorimetric detection due to the reduced penetration of the probe. If technically difficult, the extraembryonic membrane should be at least partially torn. Additionally, be sure to puncture the vesicular structures such as brain, heart, and otic vesicles to prevent the false-positive staining caused by trapping of the probe.

11. This step is important if the tissue of interest has intense pigmentation, which will significantly hamper the colorimetric detection. The H_2O_2 treatment might be also effective when older embryos (>E11.0) are assayed because they get tinged as they grow. Even if neither of the above is the case, this step is recommended to inactivate endogenous phosphatase and peroxidase, which can be a cause of nonspecific staining. Although most of the endogenous phosphatase is inactivated by the paraformaldehyde fixation and the following high temperature treatments, this step will supplement these processes.

12. Tissues are permeabilized through a methanol series by removing lipid membranes, but the proteinase K treatment is effective for additional permeabilization by partially digesting cellular proteins, which assists the penetration of the probe to the inner structures. More thorough treatment will enhance the staining but will make embryos more breakable. Thus, the exact conditions are determined largely on an empirical basis. It is highly recommended that the standard condition be tested first and then optimize it according to the colorimetric detection of the probe. In general, embryos are treated with 10 µg/ml of proteinase K at room temperature for various durations depending upon the developmental stages of the embryo. The typical durations of the treatment are: E9.5 – 8 min, E10.5 – 16 min, E11.5 – 24 min. However, when the outer, fragile structures such as epithelium are examined, proteinase K treatment can be omitted, or performed with the reduced concentration of proteinase K to prevent the destruction of the tissues of interest. On the other hand, when deeper structures including musculature, cartilage, and internal organs are examined, the proteinase K concentration, the reaction temperature, and the duration should be increased to facilitate the probe penetration.

13. If the higher background is obtained, it might be better to decrease the concentration of the probe and/or increase the hybridization temperature. In addition, longer incubation (up to 3 days) might help when examining the genes with low expression levels.

14. Some controls should be included in the hybridization step to ensure that the staining is specific and the endogenous mRNA in tissues or RNA probe is not degraded. The sense strand probe is beneficial to distinguish between specific vs. nonspecific staining. The probe that is known to work serves as a positive control to validate the protocol or technique. Also, the probe against the housekeeping gene such as Actin and β-tubulin is useful to test the tissue RNA degradation.

15. It is crucial that the posthybridization washes are stringent and thorough enough to avoid unwanted nonspecific staining. Make sure to perform the washing steps with appropriate agitation without damaging embryos. To reduce nonspecific staining, it might be effective to increase the time, the temperature, and the salt concentration in the buffers for the washing steps. Moreover, as some protocols indicate, RNase treatment is worth testing when the strong background is the problem, although it might even decrease the specific staining.

16. Many protocols use blocking powder with sheep serum for this step. However, the blocking only with sheep serum was found to be appropriate for this particular protocol, although the background staining tends to be higher if the color development is performed for a longer period of time. Presumably, it is beneficial to block with blocking powder and sheep serum if embryos are subject to overnight staining at 4°C or if the background tends to be strong. Likewise, this protocol omits the preabsorption of the antibody with embryo powder, and this step is also an option, which possibly reduces the background staining as indicated elsewhere.

17. Check the staining status occasionally under a dissection microscope since the staining can show up quickly, but minimize exposure of samples to light. Generally, the color develops within 20 min at room temperature if the gene expression level is relatively high.

18. The thickness of the gel can be determined based on the stage of the embryo and the region to be captured. Larger embryos might need thicker gels, but try to make a gel as thin as possible because thicker gels might affect the color balance and the contrast due to refraction and reflection of light.

Acknowledgments

The authors are grateful to Shigetoshi Yokoyama for professional and valuable advice. This work was supported by Genome Network Project 2004–2008 by MEXT, and the Grant of Research on Child Health and Development by Ministry of Health, Labor, and Welfare.

References

1. Kawasumi, M., and Nghiem, P. (2007) Chemical genetics: elucidating biological systems with small-molecule compounds *J Invest Dermatol* **127**, 1577–84.

2. Koga, H. (2006) Establishment of the platform for reverse chemical genetics targeting novel protein–protein interactions *Mol Biosyst* **2**, 159–64.

3. Berger, J., and Currie, P. (2007) The role of zebrafish in chemical genetics *Curr Med Chem* **14**, 2413–20.

4. Lam, S. H., Mathavan, S., Tong, Y., Li, H., Karuturi, R. K., Wu, Y., Vega, V. B., and Liu, E. T. (2008) Zebrafish whole-adult-organism chemogenomics for large-scale predictive and discovery chemical biology *PLoS Genet* **11**, e1000121.

5. Murphey, R. J., and Zon, L. I. (2006) Small molecule screening in the zebrafish *Methods* **39**, 255–61.

6. Sunkin, M. S., and Hohmann, G. J. (2007) Insights from spatially mapped gene expression in the mouse brain *Hum Mol Genet* **16**, R209–19.

7. Christiansen, J. H., Yang, Y., Venkataraman, S., Richardson, L., Stevenson, P., Burton, N., Richard A. Baldock,R. A. and Davidson D. R., (2006)EMAGE: a spatial database of gene expression patterns during mouse embryo development *Nucleic Acids Res* **34**, D637–41.

8. Gray, P. A., Fu H., Luo P., Zhao Q., Yu J., Ferrari A., Tenzen T., Yuk D., Tsung E. F., Cai Z., Alberta J. A., Cheng L., Liu Y., Stenman J. M., Valerius M. T., Billings N., Kim H. A., Greenberg M. E., McMahon A. P., Rowitch D. H., Stiles C .D., and Ma Q. (2004) Mouse brain organization revealed through direct genome-scale TF expression analysis *Science* **306**, 2255–7.

9. Visel, A., Thaller, C., and Eichele, G. (2004) GenePaint.org: an atlas of gene expression patterns in the mouse embryo *Nucleic Acids Res* **32**, D552–6.

Chapter 14

Identification of the Specific Binding Proteins of Bioactive Small Compound Using Affinity Resins

Akito Tanaka

Summary

For preparation of "chemical shotgun (CSG)" affinity resins, bioactive compounds are nonselectively immobilized via one of their functional groups by a simple protocol without the design and synthesis of specific derivatives. The CSG affinity resins have merit of capture of specific-binding proteins through multisurfaces of the compound, compared to the conventional affinity resins in which compound is immobilized only through a designated surface. We have shown that this nonselective immobilization is effective for both natural compounds bearing multifunctional groups such as FK506 and compounds bearing no inherent functional group such as Valdecoxib. We also show versatile and alternative method to widely-used competition method for identification of specific binding protein among binding proteins on affinity resins, because application of the traditional one is often restricted by poor solubility of compounds.

Key words: Affinity resins, Chemical shotgun, FK506, Valdecoxib, Benzensulfonamide, Methotrexate

1. Introduction

Affinity resins bearing bioactive compound have been widely used for identification of the specific-binding proteins *(1, 2)*. However it is still troublesome to identify those proteins using traditional technology. Requirement of high level of synthetic chemistry expertise sometime restricts its application, especially for nonsynthetic chemists. On the other hand, the competition method is not often effective due to the poor solubility of orally active compounds. Some methods to solve these problems will be shown here, exemplified by identifications of the known specific binding proteins without such restrictions.

Hisashi Koga (ed.), *Reverse Chemical Genetics*, Methods in Molecular Biology, vol. 577
DOI 10.1007/978-1-60761-232-2_14, © Humana Press, a part of Springer Science+Business Media, LLC 2009

2. Materials

2.1. Synthesis of Affinity Resins

1. Toyopearl™ (TOSOH, http://www.tosoh.com/, AF-Amino-650M, #08002).

2. The synthesis of a FK506 (**1**) derivative bearing linker moiety (**2, Fig. 1**) in details is described in literature *(3)*.

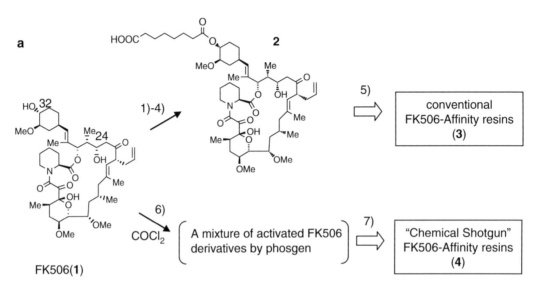

Conditions: 1) TBS-OTf, lutidine/CH$_2$Cl$_2$, 2) *p*-TosOH/MeOH, CH$_2$Cl$_2$, 3) TBDPSOOC(CH$_2$)$_6$COOH, EDC hydrochloride, dimethylaminopyridine/ CH$_2$Cl$_2$, 4) 48%HFaq./acetnitrile, 5) solid material, EDC hydrochloride, HOBt/NMP, 6)20% phosgen/toluene, 7) solid material.

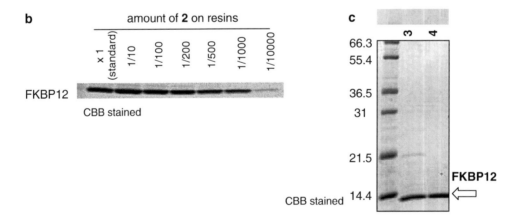

Fig. 1. Compatibility of conventional and "shotgun" FK506-affinity resins. (**a**) Synthesis of conventional and "shotgun" FK506-affinity resins. For synthesis of conventional ones, synthesis of a FK506 derivative *(3)* with linker moiety. On the other hand, "chemical shotgun" affinity resins were prepared by a simple. (**b**) Requisite amount of FK506 for capture of FKBP12, a specific binding protein. 1, 1/10, 1/100, 1/200, 1/500, 1/1,000, and 1/10,000 μmol of **2** were immobilized on 10 μL of Toyopearl resins (TOSHO, 1 μmol amines on them), respectively. FKBP12 was equivalently identified by affinity resins bearing 0.1% FK506 (1/1,000, lane 6) from rat brain lysate, which exhibited that only small amount of active FK506 was enough to capture specific binding protein. (**c**) Compatibility of both FK506-affinity resins. Binding proteins on the both resins were analyzed after mixing with 1 mL of rat brain lysate. Obvious difference was not detected between them.

3. All chemical reagents are commercially available, and used without further purifications.

4. S9 mixture (Kikkoman Co., Ltd., http://www.kikkoman. co.jp/, #S-9 mix).

5. Speed Vac apparatus: centrifugal evaporator (EYELA, http:// www.eyelaworld.com/, #CVE-1000) with a vacuum pump (Leybold Vakuum GmbH, http://www.oerlikon.com/ leyboldvacuum/, #DIVAL 1.2 L).

2.2. Preparation of Lysates

1. *Buffer for preparation of rat brain lysate and THP-1.* 25 mM Tris–HCl pH8.0, 0.1% Tween20, 300 μM N,N-diethylthio-carbamate (DDC).

2. Homogenizer (TAITEC, http://www.e-taitec.com/index. html, #VP-050) with a Potter homogenizer (SOGO LABO-RATORY GLASS WORKS Co., Ltd, Kyoto, JAPAN, http:// www.topsrg.co.jp/, #1099–06).

3. RPMI 1640 with L-Gln (Nacalai Tesque, http://www. nacalai.co.jp/en/index.html, #30264–85) with 10% FBS (Fetal Bovine Serum, biowest, http://www.biowest.net/us/ accueil.php, #S1820).

4. Penicillin–Streptomycin mixed solution (Nacalai Tesque, #26253–84).

5. PBS (Nacalai Tesque, #14249–95).

6. Tissue Grinder (SOGO LABORATORY GLASS WORKS Co., Lt, #2622–02 with #2624–04).

2.3. Capture of Specific Binding Protein and its Analysis

1. SDS sample buffer solution (Nacalai Tesque, Sample Buffer Solution with 2-mercaptoethanol for SDS-PAGE, #30566–22).

2. Running buffer for SDS-PAGE (Bio-rad, http://www. bio-rad.com/, Tris/Glycine/SDS buffer, 10×, #161–0772). Store at room temperature.

3. Precast polyacrylamide gels for SDS-PAGE (Bio-rad, Ready Gel J 5–20%, #161J373V). Store at 4°C.

4. CBB staining (WAKO, http://www.wako-chem.co.jp/english/, Quick-CBB, #299–50101).

5. Antibody against COX-2 and CA2 (Santa Cruz Biotechnology, Inc., http://www.scbt.com/, #sc-19999 and SC-25596, respectively).

6. ECL plus Western Blotting Detection system (Amersham Bio-sciences, http://www.amersham.com/businesses/Biosciences. html, #RPN 2132).

3. Methods

3.1. Overview of Synthesis of Affinity Resins Bearing Bioactive Compound

Synthesis of effective affinity resins is usually troublesome task, especially for nonorganic chemists, due to the difficulty and time-consuming nature of synthesizing such affinity reagents. Convenient method for synthesizing affinity matrices, designated "chemical shotgun (CSG)" affinity resins, is described here. For preparation of CSG affinity resins, bioactive compounds are nonselectively immobilized via one of their functional groups by a simple protocol without the design and synthesis of specific derivatives (**Fig. 1a**). This method was devised based upon a speculation that immobilization of a fraction of each compound through an appropriate linker should be sufficient for identification of the target, since µmol quantities of ligand are usually immobilized on solid support and mass spectrometry-based protein sequencing using SDS-PAGE can be conducted on pico- or femto-molar quantities of protein. For example, only 0.1% purity of FK506 derivative with linker moiety (**2, Fig. 1**) was needed to capture FKBP12, the specific binding protein, from rat brain lysate (**Fig. 1b**). CSG affinity resins have merit of capture of specific binding proteins through multisurfaces of the compound, compared to the conventional affinity resins in which compound is immobilized only through a designated surface. This nonselective immobilization is effective for compounds bearing multifunctional groups such as natural products.

Synthetic medicines usually have few functional groups available for the nonselective immobilization. Therefore, immobilization of such compounds on affinity resins is usually difficult, in contrast with the above example. In this case, a combination of nonselective introduction of functional groups by bioconversion before the phosgene-based immobilization is effective (**Fig. 2a**). Valdecoxib (**5**) *(4)* is a selective cyclooxygenase-2 (COX2) inhibitor that has no inherent functional group for immobilization. In order to generate functional groups, we applied bioconversion reactions using a S9 mixture *(5)*, a mixture of hepatic microsomal enzymes with cofactors, before the nonselective immobilization process. These hepatic microsomal metabolic enzymes are known to play an important role in metabolization of compounds, typically converting hydrophobic moieties into hydrophilic ones by oxidation, reduction, and other chemical reactions, which afford suitable functional groups for the phosgene-based immobilization.

3.2. Preparation of Conventional and Novel Effective Affinity Resins of Natural Product

FK506 *(1)* is a natural product with complex macrolide structure, and an immunosuppressive drug that targets a 12 kDa FK506-binding protein (FKBP12) with a Kd of 0.4 nM *(6)*. FKBP12 was initially identified by affinity resins bearing FK506 *(1, 2)*. For synthesis of conventional FK506-affinity resins, the synthesis of a

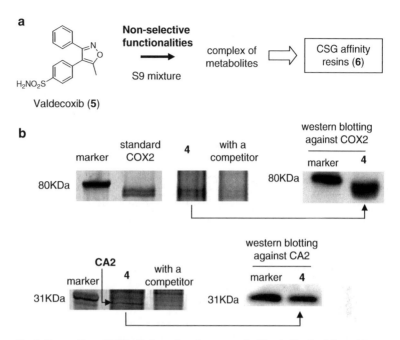

Fig. 2. Preparation of CSG affinity resins of compound without effective inherent functional groups after bioconversion using S9 mixture. (**a**) Preparation of CSG affinity resins of valdecoxib (**5**) that has no effective inherent functional groups for immobilization. (**b**) Capture of COX2 from sheep placenta lysate (**Fig. 2b** upper). Due to previously reported structure–activity relationships *(8)*, we believe that conversion of the methyl group to hydroxymethyl was achieved by the S9 treatment. Moreover carbonic anhydrase type 2 (CA2) was also captured by these resins from THP1, a human leukemic cell line, lysates (**Fig. 2b** lower). CA2 has been recently reported to be specifically inhibited by valdecoxib at 43 nM *(10)*.

FK506 derivative with linker moiety, that has equivalent bioactivity to FK506, is required. FK506 derivative with linker at the 32 position (**2, Fig**. **1a**) has abilities to capture not only FKBP12, but also the target proteins, calcineurin A/B, and calmodulin, from rat brain lysate *(7)*.

3.2.1. Synthesis of Conventional FK506-Affinity Resins

1. Toyopearl™ is used in this chapter since it is chemically stable in most of synthetic conditions and now commercial available while AffiGel™, one of the most widely used solid material for affinity chromatography, is often denatured in such conditions (*see* **Note 2**).

2. A mixture of **2** (38.4 mg, 0.04 mmol), Toyopearl™ (*see* **Note 3**), 1-(3-dimethylaminopropyl)-3-ethylcarbodiimide (EDC) hydrochloride (9.2 mg, 48 μmol), 1-hydroxybenzotriazole (HOBt, 6.5 mg, 48 μmol), and *N*-methylpyrrolidone (NMP, 1 mL) was shaken in a 1.5 mL tube at room temperature for 6 h or overnight.

3. After removal of solvents by filtration or precipitation by flash centrifugation in a microcentrifuge, the resin was carefully washed with NMP (*see* **Note 4**).

4. The Ninhydrin test is useful for monitoring the reaction (*see* **Note 5**).

5. For capping of unreacted amines (*see* **Note 6**), the resin was mixed with 20% *N*,*N*-dimethylforamide (DMF) solution of acetic anhydride (0.5 mL) at room temperature for 30 min, washed with NMP and 20% aqueous solution of EtOH.

6. The resins were kept in 20% aqueous solution of EtOH until the binding experiment.

3.2.2. Synthesis of FK506-Affinity Resins by Nonselective Immobilization Without Specific Skills ("Chemical Shotgun" Method)

1. To a mixture of FK506 (**1**, 27 mg, 34 μmol) and acetonitrile (1 mL), 20% solution of phosgene in toluene (274 μL) was added (*see* **Note 7**), and was mixed in a 1.5 mL tube at room temperature for 1 h.

2. In order to remove excess of phosgene, the mixture was concentrated under reduced pressure for 5 min using Speed-Vac apparatus (*see* **Note 8**). Bubbling with nitrogen gas is also effective for removal of excess phosgene.

3. The resulting mixture was mixed with Toyopearl™ (340 μL, 34 μmol) at room temperature overnight (*see* **Note 9**).

4. After washing with acetonitrile (1 mL, 6 times), the resins were washed with a saturated aqueous solution of sodium bicarbonate (200 μL), and then washed with water (more than 6 times) (*see* **Note 10**). The Ninhydrin test is useful for estimation of the reaction ration.

5. The resulting resins were mixed with 20% acetic anhydride in DMF (200 μL) at room temperature for 10 min, for capping of nonreacted amines. After washing with NMP (6 times), EtOH (1 time), and 20% EtOH (1 time), in series (*see* **Note 11**), the resins were kept at 4°C in an aqueous solution of 20% EtOH until the binding experiment.

3.2.3. Preparation of Tissue Extracts of Rat Brain

All procedure below was performed on ice or at 0–4°C.

1. Fresh rat brain was successfully homogenized using homogenizer with a Potter homogenizer in lysate buffer (1:10, w/v, *see* **Note 1**).

2. The homogenate was centrifuged at $14,170 \times g$ for 10 min. After supernatant was separated, it was centrifuged at $100,000 \times g$ for 30 min again.

3. Obtained supernatant (total proteins; ca. 8 mg/mL) was used for lysate and kept at –80°C before use.

3.2.4. Capture of FKBP12 by Conventional and Shotgun FK506-Affinity Resins

Binding Assay on Affinity Resins

1. 10 µL of the affinity resins was mixed with 1 mL of the lysate buffer at least for 1 h at 4°C to equilibrate them before binding experiment.

2. After removal of buffer, the resulting affinity resins were calmly mixed with 1 mL of rat brain lysate at 4°C for 60 min (*see* **Note 12**).

3. The resins were precipitated by flash centrifugation in a microcentrifuge. The resins were washed 5 times with 1.0 mL of lysate buffer (*see* **Note 13**).

4. The washed beads were then resuspended in 20 µL of SDS sample buffer solution, shaken at 25°C for 10 min (*see* **Note 14**), and centrifuged for 1 min. The supernatant was subjected to SDS-PAGE followed by CBB staining (**Fig. 1c**).

3.3. Preparation of Affinity Resins of Valdecoxib by "Chemical Shotgun" Method

3.3.1. Reparation of CSG Valdecoxib-Affinity Resins

1. A mixture of valdecoxib (12 mg) and methanol (600 µL) was added to 160 mL of the S9 mixture. This reaction mixture was shaken at 37°C for 1 day (*see* **Note 15**).

2. The metabolites were successfully extracted with ethyl acetate, after wash with *n*-hexane (*see* **Note 16**).

3. The extract was concentrated under nitrogen flow or a Speed-Vac apparatus.

4. To this mixture, acetonitrile (1.2 mL) and 20% solution of phosgene in toluene (485 µL) were thereto added, and was shaken at room temperature for 1 h.

5. In order to remove excess of phosgene, the mixture was concentrated under reduced pressure for 5 min using a Speed-Vac apparatus.

6. The resulting mixture was mixed with Toyopearl™ (200 µL, 20 µmol), *N*-diisopropyl-*N*-ethylamine (68 µL, 400 µmol) at room temperature overnight.

7. After washing with acetonitrile (5 mL × 5 times), DMF (5 mL × 5 times), the resins were washed with a saturated aqueous solution of sodium bicarbonate (5 mL), and then washed with water. The Ninhydrin test is useful for estimation of the reaction ration.

8. The resulting resins were mixed with 20% acetic anhydride in DMF (200 µL) at room temperature for 10 min, for capping of nonreacted amines. After washed with NMP (6 times), EtOH (1 time), and 20% EtOH (1 time), in series, the resins were kept at 4°C in an aqueous solution of 20% EtOH until the binding experiment.

3.3.2. Preparation of Lysate from Sheep Placenta

The procedure below was performed on ice or at 0–4°C.

1. Partially thawed sheep placenta (ca. 400 g) were homogenized in 400 mL of lysate buffer (0.1 M phosphate, pH 7.8, containing 10 mM EDTA, 0.25 M mannitol, and 300 µM DDC) using Tissue Grinder.

2. The crude homogenate was subjected to centrifugation at 10,000 × *g* for 20 min. The supernatant was subjected to further centrifugation at 100,000 × *g* for 90 min to obtain the microsomes.

3. The microsomes were solubilized with lysate buffer (10 v/w, 10% CHAPS in 80 mM Tris–HCl pH 8.0, 500 μM EDTA, 300 μM DDC) for 45 min, and was used as lysate for binding experiment.

3.3.3. Preparation of THP1 Lysate

1. THP1 cells were grown at 37°C in RPMI 1640 medium with 10% FBS, penicillin (100 μg/mL), and streptomycin (100 U/mL) until approaching confluency.

2. The cells (ca. 1 × 10^9) were washed with PBS once and collected by centrifugation at 1,000 × *g* for 3 min and resuspended into ice-cooled lysate buffer.

3. After sonication and removal of cellular debris by centrifugation at 3,000 × *g* at 4°C for 10 min, supernatant was used as lysate for binding experiment.

3.3.4. Capture of COX2 or Carbonic Anhydrase II (CA2) by "Chemical Shotgun" Valdecoxib-Affinity Resins

Serial affinity chromatography (SAC) method, described in **Subheading 3.4** in detail, was used for identification of the specific binding protein since solubility of Valdecoxib was too low to perfome the traditional competition method.

1. 10 μL of Valdecoxib-affinity resins was calmly mixed with lysate from sheep (1 mL) at 4°C for about 45 min.

2. The resins were precipitated by flash centrifugation in a microcentrifuge.

3. The resulting supernatant was carefully removed, and mixed with another 10 μL of fresh valdecoxib-affinity resin at 4°C, again for about 45 min.

4. The resins were precipitated by flash centrifugation in a microcentrifuge. The supernatant was removed by precipitation, and was kept as flow through lysate.

5. The resulting resins were washed with the lysate buffer (1 mL × 3 times).

6. Binding proteins were eluted by 30 μL of SDS sample buffer solution, shaken at 25°C for 10 min, and centrifuged for 1 min. The resulting bands were stained with CBB, the silver method, or Western blotting, and then comparatively analyzed to identify COX2 (**Fig. 2b**).

   For capture of CA2, THP1 lysate described above (1 mL) was used instead of that from sheep placenta.

3.3.5. Western Blot Analysis

1. A specific antibody against COX-2 and CA2 were obtained from Santa Cruz Biotechnology, Inc (#sc-19999 and #sc-25596), respectively.

2. Protein bands were detected with the ECL plus Western Blotting Detection system according the manufacture's protocols.

3.4. Overview of Identification of Specific Binding Proteins Among Binding Ones

The isolation of both specific and nonspecific binding proteins on affinity matrices bearing bioactive compounds hinders the identification of drug cellular targets. While solid-phase elution or the competition methods are conventionally used to distinguish between specific and nonspecific receptor–ligand interactions, these approaches are often severely restricted by low ligand solubility and/or slow kinetic dissociation *(8)*. This low solubility of these compounds are not uncommon, since the hydrophobic properties of these compounds are often vital for their bioactivity and/or membrane permeability.

This session describes an alternative and versatile method, in which no competitor is required, termed "SAC" method *(8)*, to identify ligand receptors using affinity resins (**Fig. 3**). Compatibility of SAC method with the competition method for identifying specific binding proteins was exemplified by identifications of the known specific binding proteins, FKBP12, CA2, and DHFR to FK506, benzensulfonamide, and methotrexate, respectively (**Fig. 4**). Affinity resins bearing benzensulfonamide or methotrexate were synthesized by similar method as those for the traditional FK506-affinity resins, described in **Subheading 3.2**.

3.4.1. Traditional Method for the Identification: Competition Method

1. Two tubes including the same FK506-affinity resins (10 μL each) and two tubes including 1 mL of the same lysate from rat brain were prepared in advance.
2. FK506 (1.5 μmol in 10 μL of DMSO) was mixed in one of the lysate (*see* **Note 17**), 40 min before carrying out the binding experiment (*see* **Note 18**). This lysate will be used for the competition (+) (A2 in **Fig. 3**).
3. Solvent effects were offset by adding 10 μL of DMSO into another lysate instead of the FK506 solution. This is for the competition (−) (A1 in **Fig. 3**).
4. Other protocol is the same as that described in **Subheading 3.1**.

3.4.2. Novel Method for the Identification Without Any Restrictions: SAC Method

1. Lysate from rat brain (1.0 mL) was stirred gently with FK506-affinity resin (10 μL) at 4°C for about 40 min.
2. The affinity resins were precipitated by centrifugation in a microcentrifuge at $14{,}170 \times g$ for 1 min. The resulting affinity resins, B1 in **Fig. 3**, were kept at 4°C until analysis.
3. The resulting supernatant was carefully removed and mixed with another 10 μL of fresh FK506 affinity resin at 4°C, again for about 40 min.
4. The supernatant was removed by precipitation, and was kept as flow through lysate.

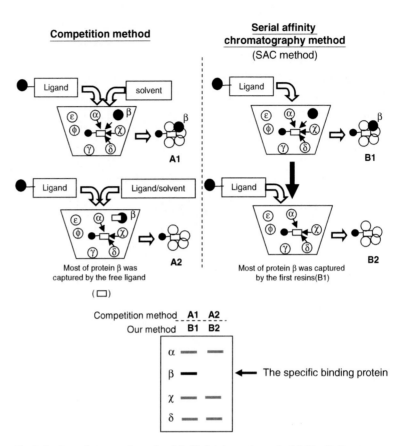

Fig. 3. A schematic comparison of serial affinity chromatography (*right*) with the competition method (*left*). In the competition method, the addition of a bioactive compound or its bioactive derivative disturbs a specific interaction. A comparison of sample without (A1) and with (A2) competitor showed that the amount of a specific binding protein β, is greatly decreased in the latter. The competitor is usually added with solvent to accelerate its dissolution (A2). Thus, the same solvent was added into A1 without competitor to offset solvent effects. In serial affinity chromatography, affinity resins are mixed with lysate, the resins removed and the same amount of fresh affinity resin added to the remaining lysate. Most of the specific binding protein β should be captured by the first resin owing to its high affinity for the ligand. This, in turn, causes a large decrease in the amount of protein β in the remaining lysate. Therefore, the amount of protein β on the second affinity resin (B2) should be much less than the amounts of other proteins present in the lysate. In serial affinity chromatography, it is not necessary to add other reagents, such as solvent, into the mixture, which should minimize artifacts.

5. The resulting resins, B2 in **Fig. 3**, were kept at 4°C until analysis.

6. The both resins were washed 5 times with 1.0 mL lysate buffer, respectively.

7. The resulting resins were resuspended in 20 μL SDS sample buffer, shaken at 25°C for 10 min and then centrifuged for 1 min. The supernatant was subjected to SDS-PAGE. The resulting bands were stained with CBB or the silver method, and then comparatively analyzed to identify specific binding proteins (**Fig. 4**).

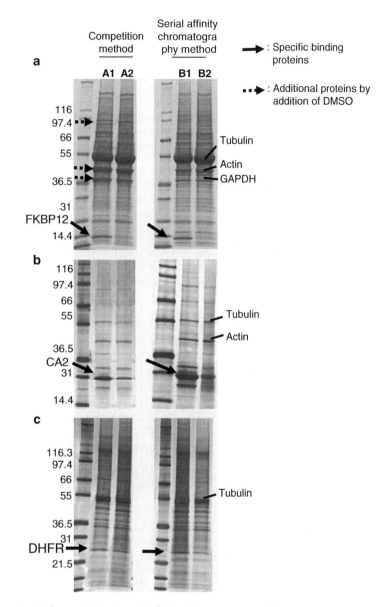

Fig. 4. Compatibility of serial affinity chromatography (*right*) with the competition method (*left*) for identifying specific binding proteins. (**a**) Identification of FKBP12 as a specific binding protein to FK506 affinity resin. FK506 affinity resin bearing 1 μmol of FK506 captured FKBP12 and other proteins from rat brain lysate. To identify FKBP12 as a specific binding protein by the competition method, a solution of FK506 (1.5 μmol) in DMSO was premixed with the lysate and exposed to the resin. In order to identify those proteins using SAC method, the same amount of FK506 affinity resin was mixed twice with the lysate, as illustrated in **Fig**. **3**. A comparison of proteins bound to the first (B1) and second (B2) resins showed that only FKBP12 decreased significantly in amount, indicating that it was a specific binding protein. Comparison of A1 and B1 showed that the amount of some binding proteins in the lysate increased (*blue arrow*), which indicated that the properties of those proteins were modified by the addition of 1% DMSO, since the only difference between the two samples was the presence of 1% DMSO in the mixture. (**b**) Identification of CA2 as a specific binding protein of benzenesulfonamide affinity resin. (**c**) Identification of DHFR as a specific binding protein to MTX affinity resin.

4. Notes

1. Addition of surfactant such as Tween20 is usually effective for reduction of absorption of nonspecific protein bindings.

2. Selection of solid material is vital for target identifications (**Fig. 5**). Tubulin, actin, or Glyceraldehyde-3-phosphate dehydrogenase are frequently appearing proteins as nonspecific binding proteins. Binding of these proteins to affinity resins was generally proportional to hydrophobicity of the resins *(7)*. Therefore, usage of hydrophilic solid material such as AffiGel™ *(9)*, an agarose derivative, is usually preferable. But, these materials are often denatured in several synthetic conditions, and its applications are severely restricted. In contrast, Toyopearl™ *(10)*, a poly(methacrylate) derivative, is stable under most synthetic conditions, which allow the synthesis of

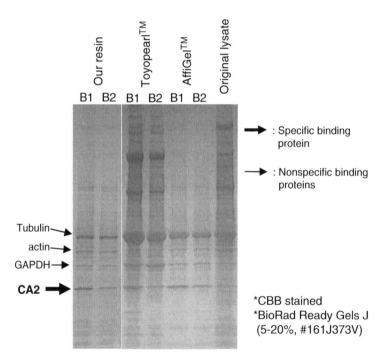

Fig. 5. Compatibility of Binding Proteins on Commercial Available Solid Materials. Each affinity resins bearing benzensulfonamide (10 mL) was mixed with 1 mL of rat brain lysate (total protein; 8 mg/mL, in 0.25 M sucrose, 0.3 mM DDC, 25 mM Tris–HCl 7.6), respectively. Specific binding protein, CA2 in this case, was identified by the SAC method described in **Subheading 3.2** instead of conventional competition method because of low solubility of the compound. After washed with 1 mL of lysate buffer (0.25 M sucrose, 0.3 mM DDC, 25 mM Tris–HCl pH 7.6), the binding proteins were eluted SDS sample buffer (Nacalai's SDS sample buffer (×3), #30566–22), and then analyzed.

more effective affinity resins. Therefore we used Toyopearl™ as solid material in this text. However, these methacrylate polymers bearing bioactive compounds often show high levels of nonspecific binding protein with the target protein due to its hydrophobic property. We have already developed novel solid phases that is chemically stable as poly(methacrylate) derivatives and is hydrophilic enough for elimination of the specific absorption as agarose *(11)*, which is now commercial available (Ieda Chemicals Co., Ltd, http://www.ieda.co.jp/6.html, contact to tsukuba@ieda-group.co.jp).

3. Toyopearl™ is used in this chapter since it is stable in most of synthetic conditions (*see* **Note 2** in details). Toyopearl™ is usually stocked in 20% EtOH. Therefore, resins were washed more than 6 times with 1 mL of NMP before usage, to remove water. Precipitation by flash centrifugation in a microcentrifuge is useful for washes. Dryness of the resins is not recommended, since resins are sometimes irreversibly denatured.

4. Precipitation by flash centrifugation in a microcentrifuge is useful for wash.

5. For Ninhydrin test, small amount of the sample resins was heated in a mixture of 25 mL of 0.28 M Ninhydrin/EtOH solution and 100 mL of pyridine at 100°C for 10 min. The same amount of unused Toyopearl was used for the control. The reaction ratio was estimated based on the OD570 absorption value.

6. Capping of unreacted amines is important to avoid nonspecific interaction between cationic free amine and anionic moieties of proteins like cation exchange resins.

7. Phosgene is highly toxic gas (caution!). Phosgene is a suitable reagent for this method since it can simultaneously activate several functional groups such as amines, carboxylic acids, hydroxyl, etc. Twenty percent of $COCl_2$ in toluene, almost saturated solution, is commercial available from Aldrich (#681776).

8. Excess phosgene will react with amine group on the solid material, which causes decrease in the amount of immobilized ligand.

9. It is thought to avoid unexpected multireactions of activated FK506 with amino groups of solid material because of the hyperdiluted conditions on solid material.

10. Treatment of the resulting resins with an aqueous solution of sodium bicarbonate was carried out to reconvert unreacted and activated functional groups to the original ones.

11. Replacement of organic solvent with aqueous solution should be in a phased manner, since hydrophobic compounds some-

times construct a hydrophobic core on resins with loss of ability to interact with the target proteins.

12. Rotary shaker is one of suitable apparatus. Sixty minutes is usually enough to capture the specific binding proteins by affinity resins. Mixing for longer time sometimes resulted in denaturation of the active proteins in lysate and/or capture of nonspecific binding of denatured proteins.

13. Number of washings is sometime vital for identification of the target protein. When putative binding between compound and protein is not so tight, 1-time washing could be enough.

14. Mixing in SDS sample buffer at 25°C for 10 min is usually enough to elute the entire binding proteins from resins. Mixing at high temperature, such as 100°C often resulted in modifications of amino acids in proteins, which caused decrease of sensitivity of identification of protein.

15. The enzymes are almost inactivated after 1 day.

16. Wash with n-hexane is required for removal of more amount of fatty acids.

17. The same FK506-affinity resins described in **Subheading 3.1** was used. Theoretically 1 μmol of FK506 was immobilized on this 10 μL of FK506-affinity resins. Therefore, the same molar of FK506, 1 μmol in this case, should be added, at least.

18. Incubation with free ligand for 40 min is usually enough. The risk of developing denatured target protein can increase by a prolong time incubation.

Acknowledgments

Author thanks Professor James K. Chen (Stanford University School of Medicine) for critically reading this manuscript, and M. Haramura (Chugai Pharmaceutical), A. Yamazaki, T. Shiyama, T. Takahashi, K. Yamamoto (Dainippon Suitomo), M. Takeuchi (Astellas Pharma.), T. Terada, K. Higashiyama (Nippon Shinyaku), M. Furuya, A. Nakanishi (Teijin Pharma), and T. Tamura (Hitachi Chemical) for their contributions for this work. Financial support from NEDO (The New Energy and Industrial Technology Development Organization) is gratefully acknowledged.

References

1. Harding, MW., Galat, A., Uehling, DE., and Schreiber, S.L. (1989) A receptor for the immunosuppressant FK506 is a cis-trans peptidyl-prolyl isomerase. *Nature* **341**, 758–760.

2. Taunton J, Hassig CA, and Schreiber SL. (1996) A mammalian histone deacetylase related to the yeast transcriptional regulator Rpd3p. *Science* **272**, 408–11.

3. Tamura, T., Terada, T., and Tanaka, A. (2003) A quantitative analysis and chemical approach for the reduction of nonspecific binding proteins on affinity resins. *Bioconjugate Chem.*, **14**, 1222–1230.

4. Talley JJ, Brown DL, Carter JS, Graneto MJ, Koboldt CM, Masferrer JL, Perkins WE, Rogers RS, Shaffer AF, Zhang YY, Zweifel BS, and Seibert K. (2000) 4-[5-Methyl-3-phenylisoxazol-4-yl]- benzenesulfonamide, valdecoxib: a potent and selective inhibitor of COX-2. *J. Med. Chem.* **43**, 775–777.

5. Natarajan AT, Tates AD, Van Buul PP, Meijers M, and De Vogel N. (1976) Cytogenetic effects of mutagens/carcinogens after activation in a microsomal system in vitro I. Induction of chromosome aberrations and sister chromatid exchanges by diethylnitrosamine (DEN) and dimethylnitrosamine (DMN) in CHO cells in the presence of rat-liver microsomes. *Mutat Res.* **37**, 83–90.

6. Siekierka, JJ., Hung, SH., Poe, M., Lin, CS., and Sigal, NH. (1989). A cytosolic binding protein for the immunosuppressant FK506 has peptidyl-prolyl isomerase activity but is distinct from cyclophilin. *Nature* **341**, 755–757.

7. Takahashi, T., Shiyama, T., Mori, T., Hosoya, K., and Tanaka, A. (2006) Isolation of the whole target proteins of FK506 using affinity resins from novel solid phases. *Anal. Bioanal. Chem.* **385**, 122–127.

8. Yamamoto, K., Yamazaki, A., Takeuchi, M., and Tanaka, A. (2006) A versatile method of identifying specific binding proteins on affinity resins. *Anal. Biochem.*, **352**, 15–23.

9. http://www.bio-rad.com/

10. http://www.tosoh.com/EnglishHomePage/tchome.htm

11. Takahashi, T., Shiyama, T., Hosoya, K., and Tanaka, A. (2006) Development of chemically stable solid-phases for the target isolation with reduced nonspecific binding proteins. *Bioorg. Med. Chem. Lett.*, **16**, 447–450.

Part IV

Potential Applicable Techniques for Reverse Chemical Genetics

Chapter 15

Protein Microarrays: Effective Tools for the Study of Inflammatory Diseases

Xiaobo Yu, Nicole Schneiderhan-Marra, Hsin-Yun Hsu, Jutta Bachmann, and Thomas O. Joos

Summary

Inflammation is a defense reaction of an organism against harmful stimuli such as tissue injury or infectious agents. The relationship between the infecting microorganism and the immune, inflammatory, and coagulation responses of the host is intricately intertwined. Due to its complex nature, the molecular mechanisms of inflammation are not yet understood in detail and additional diagnostic tools are required to clarify further aspects. In recent years, protein microarray-based research has moved from being technology-based to application-oriented. Protein microarrays are perfect tools for studying inflammatory diseases. High-density protein arrays enable new classes of autoantibodies, which cause autoimmune diseases, to be discovered. Protein arrays consisting of miniaturized multiplexed sandwich immunoassays allow the simultaneous expression analysis of dozens of signaling molecules such as the cytokines and chemokines involved in the regulation of the immune system. The data enable statements to be made on the status of the disease and its progression as well as support for the clinicians in choosing patient-specific treatment. This chapter reviews the technology and the applications of protein microarrays in diagnosing and monitoring inflammatory diseases.

Key words: Protein microarray, Inflammatory disease, Multiple protein profiling, Biomarker

1. Introduction

Inflammation is a defense reaction of an organism against harmful stimuli such as tissue injury or infectious agents. Upon microbial invasion, an effective immuno-regulatory cascade is activated to protect the body against the intruders. The defense mechanisms that protect an organism against infections can be divided into

Hisashi Koga (ed.), *Reverse Chemical Genetics*, Methods in Molecular Biology, vol. 577
DOI 10.1007/978-1-60761-232-2_15, © Humana Press, a part of Springer Science+Business Media, LLC 2009

cellular defenses, involving monocytes, macrophages, and neutrophils; humoral defense involves antibodies and the complement pathways. The relationship between the infecting microorganism and the immune, inflammatory, and coagulation responses of the host is intricately intertwined *(1)*. The magnitude of the inflammatory response is crucial: an insufficient response may result in immunodeficiency, which can lead to infection and cancer; an excessive response might result in morbidity and diseases such as rheumatoid arthritis, Crohn's disease, atherosclerosis, diabetes, Alzheimer's disease, multiple sclerosis, and cerebral and myocardial ischemia. Local inflammation might lead to sepsis and septic shock syndrome. Such inflammatory responses might be more dangerous than the original stimulus *(2)*. Every day, approximately 1,400 people around the world die from severe sepsis, so it is clear that more effective diagnostic methods and treatments are required *(3)*. Each inflammatory response initiates a series of changes in a variety of signaling pathways via the release of inflammatory mediators such as cytokines, chemokines, matrix metalloproteinases, and soluble receptors. A detailed analysis of these mediators would provide deeper insights into these complex signaling networks *(4–7)*. However, effective tools are needed to study the changes of the inflammatory mediators. Protein microarrays are the tools of choice as the throughput and sensitivity is sufficiently high. Within the last decade, protein microarray technology has made huge progress and research is moving from technological aspects to practical application. High-density microarrays consisting of immobilized recombinant proteins enable the analysis of protein interaction networks, the generation of protein phosphorylation maps, and the identification of disease-specific autoantibodies. Miniaturized multiplexed sandwich immunoassays allow the accurate quantitation of multiple parameters from minimal amounts of sample material *(8–10)*. The number of publications has increased considerably lasting recent months, thus highlighting the increasing use of protein microarrays for studying inflammatory diseases. Biomarker discovery and clinical diagnostics as well as prognosis have now become possible. This chapter summarizes protein microarray technologies and their applications for the study of inflammatory diseases.

2. Protein Micro-array Technology

2.1. Concept

Microarrays are solid phase-based assay systems consisting of an array of miniaturized test sites. This allows many tests to be performed in parallel. Planar protein microarray systems consist of capture molecules immobilized in rows and columns in microspots of about 250 μm in diameter *(11)*. Microscopic glass slides are the most common format. Bead-based systems provide an interesting alternative to planar microarrays, in particular when the number of parameters to be determined in parallel is rather low. Protein microarray technologies allow the generation of an enormous amount of quantitative information from a single experiment. This results in a considerable reduction in reagents, sample volumes, and labor required *(8–10)*.

2.2. Surface Chemistry   In protein microarrays, capture molecules need to be immobilized in a functional state on a solid support. In principle, the format of the assay system does not limit the choice of appropriate surface chemistry. The same immobilization procedure can be applied for both planar and bead-based systems. Proteins can be immobilized on various surfaces **(Fig. 1)** *(12)*. Two-dimensional polystyrene, polylysine, aminosilane, or aldehyde, epoxy- or thiol group-coated surfaces can be used to immobilize proteins via noncovalent or covalent attachment *(13, 14)*. Three-dimensional supports like nitrocellulose or hydrogel-coated surfaces enable the immobilization of the proteins in a network structure. Larger quantities of proteins can be immobilized and kept in a functional state. Affinity binding reagents such as protein A, G, and L can be used to immobilize antibodies *(15)*, streptavidin is used for biotinylated proteins *(16)*, Ni^{2+} chelate for His-tagged proteins *(17, 18)*, anti-GST antibodies for GST fusion proteins *(19)*, and oligonucleotides for cDNA or mRNA-protein hybrids *(20)*.

2.3. Arraying Technologies   Arraying technologies involve contact and noncontact printing. Contact printing arrayers are equipped with sets of tiny pins that position subnanoliter quantities of capture molecules

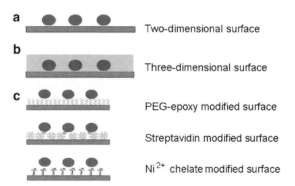

Fig. 1. Different types of surface modification. (**a**) Two-dimensional surface, e.g., polylysine, poly-lysine, aminosilane, or aldehyde, epoxy- or thiol group-coated surface, etc. (**b**) Three-dimensional surface, e.g., nitrocellulose or hydrogel-coated surface. (**c**) Surfaces with a special type of spacer and immobilization procedures such as PEG-epoxy, streptavidin, and Ni^{2+} chelate, etc.

onto the surface. These instruments can be equipped with up to 96 different pins, which increases throughput tremendously, and also allows the generation of high-density protein microarrays. Micropatterned protein arrays can also be produced with photolithographic methods, scanning probe-based lithography *(21)*, or soft-lithography technologies *(22, 23)*. Soft-lithography technologies enable researchers to print delicate biomolecules onto surfaces together with a tiny hydrogel spot *(24)*. The preparation of atomic clusters by physical methods is a nanotechnology-based approach to immobilize and orientate proteins onto distinct surfaces *(25)*. Such approaches might, for example, be used for studying single molecule interactions, where only one specific protein has to be immobilized at a specific location. Non-contact printing is a relatively new technology and involves a greater method spectrum, including photochemistry-based methods, laser writing, electrospray deposition, and inkjet technologies. Nanoliter to picoliter droplets can be deposited on the surface without physical contact between the spotting device and the substrate. This is of particular advantage when preparing many protein microarrays in parallel *(26)*.

2.4. Microarray Detection Systems

A number of different detection technologies have been established, including label-based and label-free detection systems (**Fig. 2**). Fluorescence-based methods are the most commonly

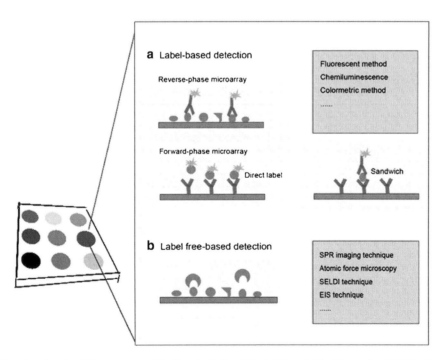

Fig. 2. The principles of protein microarray detection strategies. (**a**) Label-based detection method, (**b**) label-free based detection methods.

used detection system. The fluorescent label of the reporter molecules is determined with confocal laser scanners (**Fig. 2a**). Other high-sensitivity methods involve planar waveguides, chemiluminescence, colorimetry, etc. *(27–30)*. Yu et al. summarized the most important label-free detection methods such as surface plasmon resonance imaging, atomic force microscope, electrochemical impedance spectroscopy, and mass spectrometry *(31)*. Label-free detection systems have a distinct advantage in that no label has to be introduced into the biomolecules, that online monitoring can be performed and kinetic information can be generated. Label-free systems are mainly used to analyze the binding of purified biomolecules to immobilized capture molecules (**Fig. 2b**). The lack of sensitivity, which is generally associated with all label-free detection systems, is not an important issue because well-defined amounts of purified binding molecules can be used.

2.5. Array Formats

Currently, forward-phase protein microarrays (**Fig. 2a**) are the most commonly used assay format. They can be used for the simultaneous analysis of a large number of parameters from distinct samples. Examples of forward-phase protein microarrays include antibody microarrays, which are used to identify and quantify target proteins of interest, and protein affinity arrays, which are used to study the interactions between proteins and immobilized binding molecules such as proteins, peptides, low-molecular weight compounds, oligosaccharides, or DNA *(32, 33)*. Reverse-phase arrays (**Fig. 2b**) immobilize complex samples in a microarray format, which are then screened for the expression of target proteins with highly specific antibodies. Cell lysates, tissue extracts as well as serum samples can be used. In this format, the target proteins, contained in hundreds of samples, can be compared with each other more easily and without the need to label the target proteins. However, an extremely low amount of target protein in the sample spot requires high-sensitivity detection techniques to get a sufficiently strong signal. Tyramide signal amplification and the quantum dot technique are examples of such detection methods *(34–36)*.

2.6. Bead-Based Microarrays

Planar-based microarray systems are perfectly suited for the screening of a large number of target proteins, but their application is limited by the throughput of samples. Bead-based systems have emerged as a very interesting alternative, especially in cases when the number of parameters to be analyzed simultaneously is rather low *(37)*. There is a growing list of commercially available, ready-to-use, multiplexed bead-based assays which can be used to quantify cytokines, cell-signaling molecules, or analyze kinase activity *(38)*. **Figure 3** shows a schematic of the bead-based Luminex system, a sandwich immunoassay of high flexibility and

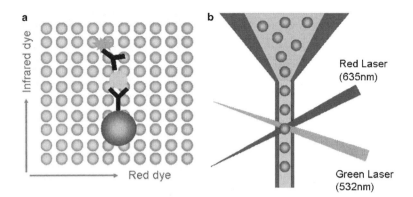

Fig. 3. (**a**) shows a bead set consisting of 100 distinct bead regions. Different bead types are generated using two different classification fluorophores – red and near infrared – in ten distinct concentration ranges. This color code enables the accurate classification of the bead types using a FACS-like instrument. The beads can be immobilized with capture molecules and immunoassays can be performed. (**b**) Once inside the instrument, fluidics leads to the alignment of the microspheres in single file as they pass by two lasers. The *red* laser classifies the color-coded microspheres according to the assay is being carried out on that particle; the *green* laser measures the assay result on the bead surface. The presence and quantity of the reporter tag allows the occurring reactions to be quantified precisely.

sensitivity. The technology performs multiplexed assays on up to 100 different bead sets. Each bead set is encoded with two dyes at a specific ratio and captures a specific analyte that is quantified using a third fluorescent dye coupled to the reporter molecules. Bead-based assays are more flexible, more robust and in a more advanced state of automation than planar microarrays and enable scientists to screen thousands of samples within a very short time *(39–45)*.

3. Applications of Protein Microarray in Inflammatory Diseases

3.1. Molecular Mechanism Analysis

Inflammatory mediators such as cytokines and chemokines are important signaling molecules that play an integral role in the mediation of immune responses. These proteins have important functions in the regulation of pathways that govern inflammatory diseases, angiogenesis, and cellular chemotaxis. Therefore, in order to study the molecular mechanisms underlying inflammatory diseases, the expression of these signaling molecules needs to be studied in great detail. Different cytokine antibody arrays, including planar and bead-based arrays, can be used in such studies. It is possible to detect new cytokine functions by comparing the differential expression of cytokines under different conditions.

For example, Kader et al. studied the role of cytokines and growth factors in dysregulated immune responses occurring in inflammatory bowel disease (IBD). The authors assumed that there were significant differences between pediatric IBD patients with active disease (AD) and those in clinical remission (CR). Planar antibody microarrays were combined with rolling circle amplification. The relative expression of 78 cytokines, growth factors, and soluble receptors were studied in the serum samples of patients with Crohn's disease (CD) and ulcerative colitis (UC) with either active disease or in clinical remission *(46)*. To the surprise of the authors, the proinflammatory cytokine level did not correlate with the severity of disease. Instead, patients with active disease had significantly higher PLGF, IL-7, IL-12p40, and TGF-β1 levels compared to patients in clinical remission. This let the authors assume that these cytokines negatively regulate intestinal inflammation in IBD and also reflect the activity of regulatory T-cells.

Plasmacytoid dendritic cells (pDCs) are professional type 1 IFN-producing cells. Upon activation, the pDCs migrate to the lymphatic organs where they bridge innate and adaptive immunity. The precise cytokine and chemokine networks that account for the role of pDCs in establishing an inflammatory microenvironment are still poorly understood. Decalf et al. mapped the key chemokines and cytokines produced in response to pDCs' activation using multianalyte profiling (MAP) *(47)*. The authors identified four distinct cytokine/chemokine loops that are initiated by TLR signaling pathways. They also found that hepatitis C virus (HCV)-infected patients have fully functional pDCs and produce a broad spectrum of proinflammatory molecules, thus giving rise to an appropriate inflammatory network. This study provides detailed insights into the efficiency of the MAP technology when characterizing cytokine networks and also shows that rare cell types like pDCs affect the activation of other inflammatory cells.

Antibody arrays for the analysis of cytokine and chemokine expression are perfect tools for studying the function of the immune system. Using the yeast two-hybrid system, Tang et al. discovered a regulatory cofactor, signal transducer, and transcription activator (STAT6(B)) that can interact with LPS-induced TNF-α factor (LITAF) *(48)*. The complex formed translocates into the nucleus and upregulates the transcription of different cytokines. The authors demonstrated that co-transfection of LITAF and STAT6 in THP-1 cells upregulates different cytokines such as GRO, IL-1α, RANTES, TNF-α IFN-γ, MCP-2, and IL-10. Most of the genes of these cytokines have a CTCCC sequence upstream of the TATA signal within their promoter. This DNA-binding site is specific for LITAF on the TNF-α promoter. It appears that the LITAF STAT6(B) complex is involved in the regulation of the promoter activity of cytokines.

The same strategy was used to study the molecular mechanisms of the host's innate immunity to human T-cell leukemia virus type I (HTLV-I) *(49)*. Two-hybrid screening showed that HTLV-I p30, which interferes with TLR4 signaling and modulates the release of cytokines from human macrophages, can interact with, and inhibit, DNA binding and transcription activity of PU.1, a unique regulatory protein required for the generation of both the innate and the adaptive immune system. This results in the reduced expression of the Toll-like receptor-4 (TLR4), a transmembrane lipopolysaccharide receptor on the cell surface that provides links between immune stimulants. The bead-based quantification method revealed that the expression of p30 prevented the release of the proinflammatory cytokines MCP-1, TNF-α, and IL-8, and stimulated the release of anti-inflammatory IL-10. Furthermore, p30 regulates IL-10 synthesis by increasing the phosphorylation capacity, which leads to the inactivation of GSK3β. This research suggests that p30 potentially instigates immune tolerance by reducing the activation of the adaptive immunity capacity in adult T cell leukemia (ATL) patients.

Comprehensive insights into the molecular mechanisms of rheumatoid arthritis (RA)-related destruction of cartilage were gained by Andreas et al. who established an in vitro model by combining genome microarrays and antibody-based protein array technology for profiling the key molecules involved in the regulatory of the RA-related destruction of cartilage *(50)*. They found that a synovial cell line obtained from an RA patient released the RA-related soluble mediators IL-6, CCL2, CXCL1–3, CXCL8 following rheumatoid arthritis synovial fibroblast (RASF) stimulation. The genome-wide microarray analysis of RASF-stimulated chondrocytes using marker genes of inflammation, the NF-ΚB signaling pathway, cytokines/chemokines and receptors, cartilage degradation, and suppressed matrix synthesis, revealed a distinct expression profile that was related to the destruction of cartilage. The study provided in-depth insights into regulatory molecular processes occurring in human chondrocytes during the RA-related destruction of cartilage.

3.2. Clinical Diagnostic Research

3.2.1. Biomarker Discovery

Autoimmune diseases include a wide variety of systemic or organ-specific inflammatory diseases that are characterized by the aberrant activation of immune cells. Many autoimmune diseases are characterized by the presence of specific autoantibody types, which can be applied for the diagnosis and classification of autoimmune diseases. The multiplexed analysis of autoantibody responses against a range of antigens represents a powerful screening tool to delineate biomarker signatures in different autoimmune diseases. Hueber et al. used arrays containing 225 peptides and proteins that represented candidate and control synovial antigens in order to identify distinct serum antibody profiles in RA patients *(51)*.

The synovial arrays were incubated with the sera from patients with early and severe RA as well as healthy patients. Hierarchical clustering analysis revealed that autoreactive B-cell responses for citrullinated epitopes were present in a subset of patients with early RA, features which are predictive of the development of severe RA. In contrast, autoantibodies directed against native epitopes including several human cartilage gp39 peptides and type II collagen, were associated with features predictive of less severe RA.

High-density fusion protein microarrays are nowadays available, for example human protein microarrays with more than 8,000 human proteins (Human protein microarray v4.0, Invitrogen, Carlsbad, CA). These fusion proteins are expressed in a baculovirus system, which includes post-transcriptional modifications like glycosylation. Hudson et al. used microarrays with 5,005 human proteins to compare the profile of autoantibodies present in the serum of 30 cancer patients with the profile of autoantibodies present in the serum of 30 healthy individuals *(52)*. Ninety-four antigen candidates were identified, which are recognized by antibodies present in the serum of the cancer patients. Elevated levels of four candidate antigens, lamin A/C, SSRP1, and RALBP1 were found in cancer tissue using immunoblots and tissue microarrays. The combination of antibody reactivity with several antigens enabled a better identification of cancerous ovarian tissue compared to the expression analysis of the cancer antigen 125, a tumor marker elevated in the plasma of people suffering from specific types of cancers. Their specificity makes them interesting markers for tissue diagnostics and targets for therapeutic interventions. Such approaches demonstrate the power of microarrays in identifying proteins that are aberrantly expressed in specific diseases.

Protein arrays based on sandwich immunoassays are used to analyze the expression of secreted proteins and inflammation markers in blood and other body fluids. Celis et al. collected Tumor interstitial fluid (TIF) from small pieces of freshly dissected invasive breast carcinomas and analyzed them by two-dimensional polyacrylamide gel electrophoresis in combination with matrix-assisted laser desorption/ionization time-of-flight mass spectrometry, Western immunoblotting, as well as by planar-based cytokine antibody arrays. Gel-based studies detect mainly high- and medium-abundance proteins whereas antibody-based arrays detect a larger number of low-abundance proteins. This approach identified more than 1,000 different proteins present in TIF. Since these proteins represent the physiological and pathological state of the tissue, TIF provides a new and potentially rich resource for discovering diagnostic biomarkers and for identifying potential targets for therapeutic intervention *(53)*. Kline et al. used membrane-based antibody arrays to screen the aberrantly expressed proteins of bone marrow stromal cells that were stimulated with bone marrow from patients diagnosed with monoclonal gammopathy of undetermined significance (MGUS), smoldering multiple myeloma (SMM), and multiple myeloma (MM). Because the saturation of the membranes made it difficult to evaluate elevated cytokine expression, IL-8 was further quantified with ELISA. The researchers found that IL-8 production is IL-1β induced and correlates with multiple myeloma disease activity and bone marrow angiogenesis. In addition, it also represents a feasible target for current and future therapies *(54)*. These examples highlight the suitability of antibody arrays for biomarker screening.

3.2.2. Clinical Diagnostics   Despite huge advances in the treatment of inflammatory diseases within the last decade, there is still a need for more effective diagnosis. For example, the increasing number of reported sepsis cases requires improved therapies based on better diagnosis. As a result, specific biomarkers are required. A variety of potential sepsis biomarkers have been identified, but it might also be necessary to use panels of biomarkers, reflecting the patient's immune status, and enabling a more detailed understanding of the host immune response, which would finally result in a more patient-specific treatment *(3)*. The most advanced technology to study such panels of biomarkers is the bead-based technology. Bead-based multiplexed sandwich immunoassays have been established under certified conditions for the expression analysis of cytokines, chemokines, immunoglobulins, soluble receptors, MMPs, and growth factors, e.g., cell culture, serum, plasma, tissue homogenate, and cerebrospinal fluid, etc. *(55–61)*. The results obtained demonstrate that bead-based arrays are robust and reliable, and require only minimal amounts of sample, yet providing high throughput.

In order to confirm the combination markers' ability to improve diagnosis and survival compared to single-plex, a 3-plex assay for the soluble urokinase-type plasminogen activator receptor (suPAR), soluble triggering receptor expressed on myeloid cells-1 (sTREM-1), and macrophage migration inhibitory factor (MIF) was employed in parallel with the standard measurements of C-reactive protein (CRP), procalcitonin (PCT), and neutrophils *(62)*. In this experiment, the combination of the three best performing markers and all six markers and the area under the receiver operating characteristic (ROC) curve was used to compare their performance to those of the individual markers. In 98 systemic inflammatory response syndrome (SIRS) patients suffering from bacterial infection, the AUCs (area under the ROC curves) of the composite three-marker test (0.84), and the six-marker test (0.88) were higher than that of the single markers (0.50–0.81). An ideal indicator has a ROC curve with an AUC of 1, and an indicator with poor discriminatory ability has an AUC around 0.5. These results show that combining information from several markers improves diagnostic accuracy in detecting bacterial vs. nonbacterial causes of inflammation.

Being secreted by the components of the innate and adaptive immune systems, inflammatory mediators act as effectors and modulators of an inflammatory response, which in turn plays a prominent role in the development of sepsis *(63, 64)*. Therefore, inflammatory mediators are of great value in diagnosing inflammatory diseases. Bozza et al. used bead-based assays to profile the cytokine concentrations in the plasma of patients with severe sepsis. The cytokine concentrations increased with the severity of inflammation and organ dysfunction. Among the 17 cytokines evaluated, IL-8 and MCP-1 exhibited the best correlation with organ dysfunction on day 1. Elevated IL-6, IL-8, and G-CSF concentrations were found in patients within the first 24 h of measurement and precluded severe organ dysfunction on day 3 (clinical scores did not improve). In terms of predicting mortality, IL-1β, IL-4, IL-6, IL-8, MCP-1, and G-CSF were able to predict early mortality (<48 h), and IL-8 and MCP-1 were most reliable in predicting 28-day mortality (death occurring before day 28 of the investigation). The study shows that the simultaneous analysis of multiple cytokines proved useful in identifying cytokine patterns of inflammatory response associated with the evolution of organ dysfunction as well as early and late mortality in patients with severe sepsis and septic shock *(65)*.

In addition to proinflammatory cytokines, soluble cytokine receptors are also involved in the regulation of inflammatory and immune responses to disease by modulating the systemic effects of cytokines. Compared to cytokine molecules, the determination of their soluble receptors is relative easier to achieve due to higher concentrations and better stability *(66–68)*. Using the bead-based Luminex system, 11-plex soluble receptor assays have been developed in our laboratory. These soluble receptors are sTNF-RI, sTNF-RII, sIL-2R, sgp130, sFas, sRAGE, sE-selectin, sICAM-1, sVCAM-1, sMIF-1, and sFasL. This newly established 11-plex soluble receptor assay demonstrated acceptable intra-assay (4.2–11.52%) and inter-assay (10.31–19.73%) precision, appropriate accuracy, and no cross-reactivity between the analytes. Hundred plasma samples, derived from 36 critically ill intensive care unit (ICU) patients with trauma or sepsis, were analyzed for their plasma concentrations. The patients could subsequently be grouped into a trauma and a sepsis group *(69)*. Four molecules (sFas, sICAM-1, sTNF-RI, and sTNF-RII) show higher concentrations in patients with sepsis than those with trauma, giving the highest discriminatory values for defining the nature of the inflammatory disease originating from pathogen-involved (sepsis) or pathogen-independent inflammation.

The bead-based technology works not only for inflammatory mediators that have diagnostic/prognostic value, but also for others (e.g., C-reactive protein, IL-6). This can make bead-based systems even more powerful. Kofoed et al. combined in-house and commercially available kits and used bead-based Luminex systems to assay biomarkers of potential interest in EDTA-plasma samples *(70)*. A 3-plex assay for suPAR, sTREM-1, MIF was added to a commercially available human cytokine panel, IL-1β, IL-6, IL-8, GM-CSF, and TNF-α. Compared to healthy controls, all eight analytes were significantly higher in plasma from bacterial sepsis patients.

3.2.3. Drug Evaluation

In addition to biomarker discovery and clinical diagnostics, protein microarrays are also effective tools for the identification of potential drug targets, monitoring the effect of a specific therapy, and for studying the molecular mechanisms involved in drug response. In order to investigate the molecular mechanisms associated with vitamin E, Lin et al. developed a planar-based cytokine antibody array system that can detect the presence of 35 cytokines simultaneously *(71)*. Using this technology, the vitamin E-regulated cytokines were analyzed in individuals who had received vitamin E supplements. The cytokine arrays showed that the expression of several cytokines (MCP-1, epithelial cell-derived neutrophil activating-78 (ENA-78), IL-1α, monokine-induced by gamma interferon (MIG), RANTES, TNF-β) were profoundly reduced in individuals that had received the vitamin E supplements. Also, the addition of vitamin E to several cultured cells significantly down-regulated the expression of MCP-1. This is the first time that MCP-1 has been shown to be one of the most important targets of vitamin E. Because of the preventive, antioxidative effects of vitamin E on certain types of cancers and cardiac diseases, this study may provide valuable information about the molecular mechanisms of vitamin E supplementation in chemoprevention and identification of new targets.

Besifloxacin is a new fluoroquinolone being developed by Bausch & Lomb for the topical treatment of ophthalmic infections. Besifloxacin is presumed to have a number of advantages over current therapies due to its structure, unique usage profile, and antimicrobial properties. However, no studies have so far been published on its anti-inflammatory properties. The effect of besifloxacin on LPS-induced cytokine expression in human THP-1 monocytes in vitro was investigated with a 16-cytokine multiplexd assay panel from Luminex, using moxifloxacin, a fluoroquinolone used for the treatment of ophthalmic infections, as the control *(72)*. Compared to moxifloxacin, besifloxacin was far superior in inhibiting LPS-stimulated cytokine production with a significant inhibitory effect at 0.1 mg/L for IL-1a, at 1 mg/L for G-CSF, IL-1ra, and IL-6 and at 30 mg/L for GM-CSF,

IL-12p40, IL-1b, IL-8, IP-10, MCP-1, and MIP-1a. Acting as an anti-inflammatory agent in monocytes in vitro, besifloxacin may enhance its drug efficacy in inflammatory ocular infections. Further investigations are required to substantiate this finding.

4. Prospects

Microarrays have become robust, reliable research tools that enable researchers to screen for a multitude of parameters using minimal amounts of sample material. The acceptance of protein microarrays is growing constantly; they have already been demonstrated to be useful tools in disease-related biomarker discovery. In addition, protein microarrays have been introduced into clinical trials in order to investigate the potential adverse effects of drug candidates. Depending on the number of validated disease-specific biomarkers, as well as on their therapeutic relevance, such assays are performed either on a protein microarray or a bead-based platform.

A lot of effort is being put into using protein microarrays in clinical diagnostics, and some products have already been developed for this market. For example, the Randox Evidence Biochip Array system (Randox Inc.) can perform over 2,700 tests per hour. Multiplexed immunoassay platforms based on the Luminex technology are applied to allergy testing, autoimmune disease, HLA testing, infectious diseases, etc. Several issues have to be resolved before multiple protein profiling technology can be implemented into diagnostics. The first deals with decreasing the costs to a level that potential customers can pay. Secondly, ways have to found to interpret the complicated data obtained from multiplexed immunoassays, and thirdly, the accuracy of the microarrays has to be improved when used in diagnostics and prognosis in order to prevent false-positive results caused by non-specific autoantibodies, especially in autoimmune diseases, as well as false-negatives that might delay therapies *(10, 59, 73)*.

The number of inflammatory mediators used for analyses and studying inflammatory signaling networks is constantly increasing. A more comprehensive knowledge in this field will eventually enable us to understand the molecular mechanisms of inflammation, improve diagnosis, and analyze the response of drugs on a systems biology level. Medical needs and clinical utility, combined with overall cost reductions, have to become the driving forces for protein microarrays to get a substantial share of the in vitro diagnostic market and be able to live up to the high expectations that many people have of this promising new technology.

Acknowledgments

Dr. Xiaobo Yu's research is supported by a Humboldt research fellowship (Alexander von Humboldt Foundation, Germany; fellowship ID: 1126997). Hsin-Yun Hsu is supported by the DAAD (German Academic Exchange Service), Germany (fellowship ID: A/04/07700).

References

1. Lissauer, M.E., et al. (2007) Coagulation and complement protein differences between septic and uninfected systemic inflammatory response syndrome patients. *J Trauma.* **62**, 1082–92; discussion 1092–4.

2. Tracey, K.J. (2002) The inflammatory reflex. *Nature.* **420**, 853–9.

3. Carrigan, S.D., G. Scott, and M. Tabrizian (2004) Toward resolving the challenges of sepsis diagnosis. *Clin Chem.* **50**, 1301–14.

4. Hotchkiss, R.S. and D.W. Nicholson (2006) Apoptosis and caspases regulate death and inflammation in sepsis. *Nat Rev Immunol.* **6**, 813–22.

5. Kemper, C. and J.P. Atkinson (2007) T-cell regulation: with complements from innate immunity. *Nat Rev Immunol.* **7**, 9–18.

6. Lin, W.W. and M. Karin (2007) A cytokine-mediated link between innate immunity, inflammation, and cancer. *J Clin Invest.* **117**, 1175–83.

7. Purwar, R., et al. (2008) Modulation of keratinocyte-derived MMP-9 by IL-13: a possible role for the pathogenesis of epidermal inflammation. *J Invest Dermatol.* **128**, 59–66.

8. Stoll, D., et al. (2005) Protein microarrays: applications and future challenges. *Curr Opin Drug Discov Devel.* **8**, 239–52.

9. Kricka, L.J., et al. (2006) Current perspectives in protein array technology. *Ann Clin Biochem.* **43**, 457–67.

10. Master, S.R., C. Bierl, and L.J. Kricka (2006) Diagnostic challenges for multiplexed protein microarrays. *Drug Discov Today.* **11**, 1007–11.

11. Chipping-Forecast-II (2002) *Nature Genetics*, **32**(supplement), 461–552.

12. Stoll, D., et al. (2002) Protein microarray technology. *Front Biosci.* **7**, c13–32.

13. Liu, Y., et al. (2007) Optimization of printing buffer for protein microarrays based on aldehyde-modified glass slides. *Front Biosci.* **12**, 3768–73.

14. Oh, S.J., et al. (2006) Surface modification for DNA and protein microarrays. *OMICS.* **10**, 327–43.

15. Matson, R.S., et al. (2007) Overprint immunoassay using protein A microarrays. *Methods Mol Biol.* **382**, 273–86.

16. Li, Y.J., et al. (2006) Reversible immobilization of proteins with streptavidin affinity tags on a surface plasmon resonance biosensor chip. *Anal Bioanal Chem.* **386**, 1321–6.

17. Zhu, H., et al. (2001) Global analysis of protein activities using proteome chips. *Science.* **293**, 2101–5.

18. Lauer, S.A. and J.P. Nolan (2002) Development and characterization of Ni-NTA-bearing microspheres. *Cytometry.* **48**, 136–45.

19. Waterboer, T., et al. (2005) Multiplex human papillomavirus serology based on in situ-purified glutathione s-transferase fusion proteins. *Clin Chem.* **51**, 1845–53.

20. Boozer, C., et al. (2006) DNA-directed protein immobilization for simultaneous detection of multiple analytes by surface plasmon resonance biosensor. *Anal Chem.* **78**, 1515–9.

21. Lee, M., et al. (2006) Protein nanoarray on Prolinker surface constructed by atomic force microscopy dip-pen nanolithography for analysis of protein interaction. *Proteomics.* **6**, 1094–103.

22. Wang, Z., T. Wilkop, and Q. Cheng (2005), Characterization of micropatterned lipid membranes on a gold surface by surface plasmon resonance imaging and electrochemical signaling of a pore-forming protein. *Langmuir.* **21**, 10292–6.

23. Rozkiewicz, D.I., et al. (2007) Dendrimer-mediated transfer printing of DNA and RNA microarrays. *J Am Chem Soc.* **129**, 11593–9.

24. Mayer, M., et al. (2004) Micropatterned agarose gels for stamping arrays of proteins and gradients of proteins. *Proteomics.* **4**, 2366–76.

25. Palmer, R.E. and C. Leung (2007) Immobilisation of proteins by atomic clusters on surfaces. *Trends Biotechnol.* **25**, 48–55.

26. Barbulovic-Nad, I., et al. (2006) Bio-microarray fabrication techniques – a review. *Crit Rev Biotechnol.* **26**, 237–59.

27. Pawlak, M., et al. (2002) Zeptosens' protein microarrays: a novel high performance microarray platform for low abundance protein analysis. *Proteomics.* **2**, 383–93.

28. Usui-Aoki, K., K. Shimada, and H. Koga (2007) A novel antibody microarray format using non-covalent antibody immobilization with chemiluminescent detection. *Mol Biosyst.* **3**, 36–42.

29. Guo, H., et al. (2005) Development of a low density colorimetric protein array for cardiac troponin I detection. *J Nanosci Nanotechnol.* **5**, 2161–6.

30. Timlin, J.A. (2006) Scanning microarrays: current methods and future directions. *Methods Enzymol.* **411**, 79–98.

31. Yu, X., D. Xu, and Q. Cheng (2006) Label-free detection methods for protein microarrays. *Proteomics.* **6**, 5493–503.

32. Kingsmore, S.F. (2006) Multiplexed protein measurement: technologies and applications of protein and antibody arrays. *Nat Rev Drug Discov.* **5**, 310–20.

33. Templin, M.F., et al. (2002) Protein microarray technology. *Trends Biotechnol.* **20**, 160–6.

34. Mendes, K.N., et al. (2007) Analysis of signaling pathways in 90 cancer cell lines by protein lysate array. *J Proteome Res.* **6**, 2753–67.

35. Sheehan, K.M., et al. (2008) Signal pathway profiling of epithelial and stromal compartments of colonic carcinoma reveals epithelial-mesenchymal transition. *Oncogene.* **27**, 323–31.

36. Geho, D.H., et al. (2007) Fluorescence-based analysis of cellular protein lysate arrays using quantum dots. *Methods Mol Biol.* **374**, 229–37.

37. Templin, M.F., et al. (2004) Protein microarrays and multiplexed sandwich immunoassays: what beats the beads? *Comb Chem High Throughput Screen.* **7**, 223–9.

38. http://www.biochipnet.de, Biochipnet.

39. Singh, M. and L. Johnson (2006) Using genetically engineered mouse models of cancer to aid drug development: an industry perspective. *Clin Cancer Res.* **12**, 5312–28.

40. Toy, D., et al. (2006) Cutting edge: interleukin 17 signals through a heteromeric receptor complex. *J Immunol.* **177**, 36–9.

41. Perper, S.J., et al. (2006) TWEAK is a novel arthritogenic mediator. *J Immunol.* **177**, 2610–20.

42. Fath, M.A., et al. (2005) Mkks-null mice have a phenotype resembling Bardet–sBiedl syndrome. *Hum Mol Genet.* **14**, 1109–18.

43. Heuer, J.G., et al. (2004) Evaluation of protein C and other biomarkers as predictors of mortality in a rat cecal ligation and puncture model of sepsis. *Crit Care Med.* **32**, 1570–8.

44. Heuer, J.G., D.J. Cummins, and B.T. Edmonds (2005) Multiplex proteomic approaches to sepsis research: case studies employing new technologies. *Expert Rev Proteomics.* **2**, 669–80.

45. Hsu, H.Y., S. Wittemann, and T.O. Joos (2008) Miniaturized parallelized sandwich immunoassays. *Methods Mol Biol.* **428**, 247–61.

46. Kader, H.A., et al. (2005) Protein microarray analysis of disease activity in pediatric inflammatory bowel disease demonstrates elevated serum PLGF, IL-7, TGF-beta1, and IL-12p40 levels in Crohn's disease and ulcerative colitis patients in remission versus active disease. *Am J Gastroenterol.* **100**, 414–23.

47. Decalf, J., et al. (2007) Plasmacytoid dendritic cells initiate a complex chemokine and cytokine network and are a viable drug target in chronic HCV patients. *J Exp Med.* **204**, 2423–37.

48. Tang, X., et al. (2005) LPS induces the interaction of a transcription factor, LPS-induced TNF-alpha factor, and STAT6(B) with effects on multiple cytokines. *Proc Natl Acad Sci U S A.* **102**, 5132–7.

49. Datta, A., et al. (2006) The HTLV-I p30 interferes with TLR4 signaling and modulates the release of pro- and anti-inflammatory cytokines from human macrophages. *J Biol Chem.* **281**, 23414–24.

50. Andreas, K., et al. (2008) Key regulatory molecules of cartilage destruction in rheumatoid arthritis: an in vitro study. *Arthritis Res Ther.* **10**, R9.

51. Hueber, W., et al. (2005) Antigen microarray profiling of autoantibodies in rheumatoid arthritis. *Arthritis Rheum.* **52**, 2645–55.

52. Hudson, M.E., et al. (2007) Identification of differentially expressed proteins in ovarian cancer using high-density protein microarrays. *Proc Natl Acad Sci USA.* **104**, 17494–9.

53. Celis, J.E., et al. (2004) Proteomic characterization of the interstitial fluid perfusing the breast tumor microenvironment: a novel resource for biomarker and therapeutic target discovery. *Mol Cell Proteomics.* **3**, 327–44.

54. Kline, M., et al. (2007) Cytokine and chemokine profiles in multiple myeloma; significance of stromal interaction and correlation of IL-8

production with disease progression. *Leuk Res.* **31**, 591–8.

55. Carson, R.T. and D.A. Vignali (1999) Simultaneous quantitation of 15 cytokines using a multiplexed flow cytometric assay. *J Immunol Methods.* **227**, 41–52.

56. Prabhakar, U., E. Eirikis, and H.M. Davis (2002) Simultaneous quantification of proinflammatory cytokines in human plasma using the LabMAP assay. *J Immunol Methods.* **260**, 207–18.

57. de Jager, W., et al. (2003) Simultaneous detection of 15 human cytokines in a single sample of stimulated peripheral blood mononuclear cells. *Clin Diagn Lab Immunol.* **10**, 133–9.

58. Olsson, A., et al. (2005) Simultaneous measurement of beta-amyloid(1–42), total tau, and phosphorylated tau (Thr181) in cerebrospinal fluid by the xMAP technology. *Clin Chem.* **51**, 336–45.

59. de Jager, W. and G.T. Rijkers (2006) Solid-phase and bead-based cytokine immunoassay: a comparison. *Methods.* **38**, 294–303.

60. Maier, R., et al. (2006) Application of multiplex cytometric bead array technology for the measurement of angiogenic factors in the vitreous. *Mol Vis.* **12**, 1143–7.

61. McDuffie, E., et al. (2006) Detection of cytokine protein expression in mouse lung homogenates using suspension bead array. *J Inflamm (Lond).* **3**, 15.

62. Kofoed, K., et al. (2007) Use of plasma C-reactive protein, procalcitonin, neutrophils, macrophage migration inhibitory factor, soluble urokinase-type plasminogen activator receptor, and soluble triggering receptor expressed on myeloid cells-1 in combination to diagnose infections: a prospective study. *Crit Care.* **11**, R38.

63. Rossi, D. and A. Zlotnik (2000) The biology of chemokines and their receptors. *Annu Rev Immunol.* **18**, 217–42.

64. Zlotnik, A. and O. Yoshie (2000) Chemokines: a new classification system and their role in immunity. *Immunity.* **12**, 121–7.

65. Bozza, F.A., et al. (2007) Cytokine profiles as markers of disease severity in sepsis: a multiplex analysis. *Crit Care.* **11**, R49.

66. Calvano, S.E., et al. (1996) Monocyte tumor necrosis factor receptor levels as a predictor of risk in human sepsis. *Arch Surg.* **131**, 434–7.

67. Pruitt, J.H., et al. (1996) Increased soluble interleukin-1 type II receptor concentrations in postoperative patients and in patients with sepsis syndrome. *Blood.* **87**, 3282–8.

68. Keh, D., et al. (2003) Immunologic and hemodynamic effects of "low-dose" hydrocortisone in septic shock: a double-blind, randomized, placebo-controlled, crossover study. *Am J Respir Crit Care Med.* **167**, 512–20.

69. Hsu, H.Y., et al. (2008) Suspension microarrays for the identification of the response patterns in hyperinflammatory diseases. *Med Eng Phys* **30**, 976–83.

70. Kofoed, K., et al. (2006) Development and validation of a multiplex add-on assay for sepsis biomarkers using xMAP technology. *Clin Chem.* **52**, 1284–93.

71. Lin, Y., et al. (2002) Profiling of human cytokines in healthy individuals with vitamin E supplementation by antibody array. *Cancer Lett.* **187**, 17–24.

72. Zhang, J.Z. and K.W. Ward (2008) Besifloxacin, a novel fluoroquinolone antimicrobial agent, exhibits potent inhibition of pro-inflammatory cytokines in human THP-1 monocytes. *J Antimicrob Chemother.* **61**, 111–6.

73. Joos, T.O. and H. Berger (2006) The long and difficult road to the diagnostic market: protein microarrays. *Drug Discov Today.* **11**, 959–61.

Chapter 16

Preparation of Highly Sensitive Protein Array Using Reactive Polymer

Toshifumi Shiroya, Hiroyuki Tanaka, Minako Hanasaki, and Hisao Takeuchi

Summary

We have discovered a novel protein immobilization method, i.e., a "Three-Dimensional Nanostructured Protein Hydrogel" (3-D NPH), which is composed of protein-reactive polymer hybrid nanoparticles to detect protein–protein interactions. The 3-D NPH can be easily prepared by spotting a protein/reactive polymer mixture on a substrate. The resulting 3-D NPH is characterized by large amounts of immobilized proteins and a novel porous structure.

The 3-D NPH technology was applied to immobilize streptavidin (SA) onto Au-coated surface for surface plasmon resonance imaging (SPRi). By using 3-D NPH method, it was possible to improve the sensitivity of protein–protein interactions drastically comparing to the conventional protein immobilization method.

Key words: Protein microarray, Hydrogel, Immobilization, SPR, Protein–protein interaction

1. Introduction

Chemical genetics is an emerging research field utilizing small molecule intervention, instead of genetic intervention *(1, 2)*. Chemical genetics can be divided into forward chemical genetics and reverse chemical genetics similar to conventional genetics. Reverse chemical genetics discover small molecule partner to the specific target protein identified beforehand, and the phenotypic effect of adding the small molecule is studied *(3)*.

For example, to establish novel drug-screening system for small molecules based on protein–protein interactions using

Hisashi Koga (ed.), *Reverse Chemical Genetics*, Methods in Molecular Biology, vol. 577
DOI 10.1007/978-1-60761-232-2_16, © Humana Press, a part of Springer Science+Business Media, LLC 2009

reverse chemical genetics, it is important to determine the precise interacting modules on each protein molecule and accumulate information about target proteins *(4)*.

Recently, protein microarrays have been widely used to investigate protein–protein interactions on a genome-wide scale *(5–8)*, and protein chips having large numbers of spots have been produced. As the number of spots increases, the amount of immobilized protein per spot decreases. As a general, however, the lower the amount of immobilized protein, the lower the sensitivity of the protein chip. One solution to increase the immobilized proteins per unit area is to use a hydrogel as a three-dimensional (3-D) matrix. There have been various reports about hydrogel matrix using polymer molecules, such as carboxymethyl dextran (CMD) *(9, 10)*, polyacrylamide gel *(11–14)*, agarose thin film *(15)* and hydrogels composed of multifunctionalized polymers *(16)*.

Hydrogel matrices show a superior capacity of immobilization compared to that of planar substrate. However, hydrogel matrices have problems relating mass transfer limitations and reduced accessibility of the hydrogels to analyte proteins *(9, 17)*.

Also, if the substrate is completely covered by the hydrophilic hydrogel, like carboxymethyl dextran, crosscontamination and overflow during microdrop deposition may occur *(18)*.

In our previous study a novel method was developed to prepare a protein-based hydrogel, i.e., a "Three-Dimensional Nanostructured Protein Hydrogel" (3-D NPH), which is composed of protein–polymer hybrid nanoparticles *(19, 20)*. The 3-D NPH could be easily prepared by dispensing a protein and polymer mixture on a substrate. Because the analyte proteins could penetrate into the 3-D NPH, the protein array made by 3-D NPH method has tremendously improved sensitivity in detecting protein–protein interactions compared with that of the direct protein immobilization methods (2-D).

Also, since the 3-D NPH could be formed on specific limited areas of a substrate, a protein array with high protein density can be produced without crosscontamination among neighboring spots and without overflow.

The preparation procedure for the 3-D NPH is shown in **Fig. 1**. A protein/poly(NAM-co-NAS) mixture (protein/polymer = 10/1 (w/w)) was deposited on a substrate having succinimide groups, and amino groups of proteins reacted with succinimide groups of poly(NAM-co-NAS) and/or substrates while the solid components in the mixed solution were concentrated in a drying process. This preparation method for the 3-D NPH includes a process of gelation on substrates between the proteins and the reactive polymers as the components in the mixture become more concentrated during drying.

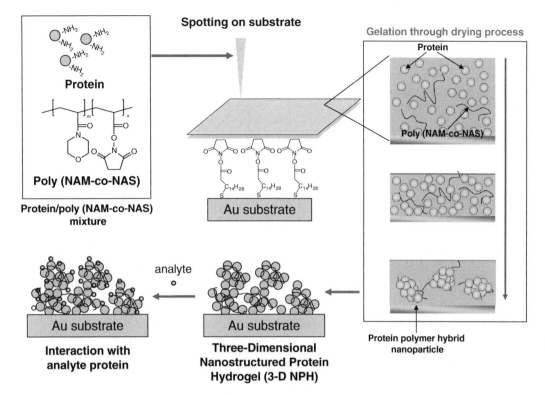

Fig. 1. Schematic representation of the 3-D NPH preparation and analyte interaction with the 3-D NPH.

2. Materials

2.1. Poly(N-Acryloylmorpholine-co-N-Acryloxysuccinimide) (Poly(NAM-co-NAS) Preparation

1. *Monomer.* N-acryloylmorpholine (Sigma-Aldrich, MO, USA). Store at 4°C.

2. *Monomer.* N-acryloxysuccinimide (Acros Organics, NJ, USA). Store at 4°C.

3. Initiator: Azobisisobutyronitrile (Wako Pure Chemical Industries, Ltd, Osaka, Japan). Store at 4°C.

4. *Solvent for polymerization reaction.* Anhydrous dioxane (Wako Pure Chemical Industries, Ltd, Osaka, Japan).

5. *Solvent for polymer purification.* Ethylic ether (Kokusan Chemical Co., Ltd., Japan).

2.2. Characterization of Poly(NAM-co-NAS)

1. N, N-dimethylformamide (DMF, Wako Pure Chemical Industries, Ltd, Osaka, Japan).

2. Lithium Bromide Monohydrate (LiBr, Wako Pure Chemical Industries, Ltd, Osaka, Japan).

2.3. Preparation of 3-D NPH on Substrates

1. 16-mercaptohexadecanoic acid (Sigma-Aldrich, MO, USA).
2. Ethanol.
3. N-ethyl-N'-(3-dimethylaminopropyl) carbodiimide hydrochloride (EDC, Dojindo laboratories, Kumamoto, Japan).
4. N-hydroxysuccinimide (NHS, Wako Pure Chemical Industries, Ltd, Osaka, Japan).
5. Ethanolamine Hydrochloride (Sigma-Aldrich, MO, USA).
6. Sodium Hydroxide.
7. Sodium Hydrogen Carbonate.
8. Streptavidin (SA, Type II, Wako Pure Chemical Industries, Ltd, Osaka, Japan).
9. Bovine Serum Albumin (BSA, Fraction V, Sigma-Aldrich, MO, USA).
10. Tween 20 (polyoxyethylene *(20)* Sorbitan Monolaurate, Wako Pure Chemical Industries, Ltd, Osaka, Japan).
11. Au-coated glass slide (Toyobo, Osaka, JAPAN).

2.4. SPRi Interaction Monitoring

1. *Running buffer.* Phosphate-buffered saline (PBS, pH 7.4).
2. Biotinylated Horse Radish Peroxidase (Pierce, IL, USA).

2.5. Equipment and Supplies

1. *HPLC system.* HLC-8220 GPC(L), (Tosoh, Japan).
2. *Column.* TSK gel GMPWxl (Tosoh, Japan).
3. ¹H-NMR (Avance 500, Bruker, Germany).
4. *SPRi instrument.* MultiSPRinter (Toyobo, Osaka, JAPAN).
5. Microspotter (Omni Grid Accent, Genomic Solutions, U.S.A.).
6. Pin for microspotter (Telechem Inc., U.S.A.).

3. Methods

3.1. Poly(N-Acryloylmorpholine-co-N-Acryloxysuccinimide) (Poly(NAM-co-NAS)) Preparation

Polymerization is performed in a three-necked round-bottomed flask equipped with a condenser, a magnetic stirrer, and a nitrogen inlet. The reaction vessel is loaded with the monomer mixture and anhydrous dioxane as a solvent.

1. 1.13 g of N-acryloylmorpholine, 0.33 g of N-acryloxysuccinimide and 18.03 g of dehydrated dioxane are thoroughly mixed, and the mixture is poured into a 50 mL-four necked flask, which is degassed at room temperature for 30 min under nitrogen.

2. The temperature of this monomer solution is elevated to 60°C in an oil bath.

3. 0.0016 g of azobisisobutyronitrile (a polymerization initiator) which is dissolved in 0.5 g of dehydrated dioxane is added to the monomer mixture to start the polymerization.

4. The polymerization is performed for 8 h under a nitrogen atmosphere.

5. After the polymerization, the solution containing the produced poly(NAM-co-NAS) is added dropwise to 0.5 L of ethylic ether to precipitate the polymer. The supernatant is removed by a decantation and the precipitated polymer is dissolved in 18 g of dehydrated dioxane. The solution is added dropwise to 0.5 L of ethylic ether to precipitate the polymer, again.

6. The solvent was removed under vacuum to give a poly(NAM-co-NAS) as a powder.

7. Store purified polymer in a desiccator before usage (*see* **Note 1**).

3.2. Characterization of Poly(NAM-co-NAS)

Molecular weight of poly(NAM-co-NAS) is determined by size exclusion chromatography (SEC) analysis. The eluent used is a DMF including 50 mM LiBr at a flow rate of 0.5 mL/min (*see* **Table 1**).

The average copolymer composition is determined from ^{1}H-NMR spectra of the copolymer according to ^{1}H-NMR spectrum (200 MHz) of poly(NAM-co-NAS) in CDCl$_3$ *(21)*.

3.3. Preparation of 3-D NPH on Substrates

The following procedures to produce 3-D NPH were carried out at 25°C.

3.3.1. Preparation of the Au-Coated Glass Slide with Reactive Succinimide Esters

1. Immerse an Au-coated glass slide in a 10 mM solution of 16-mercaptohexadecanoic acid in ethanol for 12 h at room temperature.

2. Activate the introduced carboxy groups on the Au surface to form reactive succinimide esters using a solution of 0.1 mol/L EDC and 0.4 mol/L NHS in water for 15 min.

Table 1
Average copolymer composition and molecular weight characteristics of poly(NAM-co-NAS)

Reactive polymer	NAM/NAS molar ratio in the comonomer feed	Average copolymer composition (NAM/NAS molar ratio)	Weight-average molecular weight(g/mol)
Poly(NAM-co-NAS)	80/20	65/35	86,000

3.3.2. Preparation of Streptavidin/poly(NAM-co-NAS) Mixed Solutions

1. Prepare 50 μl of streptavidin (SA) solutions (0.063, 0.13, 0.25, 0.50, 1.0, 3.0 wt.%) using a 100 mM carbonate buffer (adjusted to pH 8.5 by NaOH).

2. Prepare 50 μl of poly(NAM-co-NAS) solutions (0.063, 0.13, 0.25, 0.50, 1.0, 3.0 wt.%) using a 100 mM carbonate buffer (adjusted to pH 8.5 by NaOH).

3. Mix the SA solution and the polymer solution at 10/1 volume (add 5 μl of polymer solution to 50 μl of streptavidin solution) (*see* **Note 2**).

3.3.3 Preparation of the Source Plate

The prepared solutions (SA/poly(NAM-co-NAS), mixed solutions or SA solutions (*see* **Subheading 3.3.2**) are transferred into source plate (384-well) just before the start of the run (*see* **Note 2**). At least 30 μl of solution is added to each well.

3.3.4. Printing

The mixed solutions (SA/poly(NAM-co-NAS)) or SA solutions were contact printed on Au-coated glass slide activated with succinimide esters (*see* **Subheading 3.3.1**) by means of computer-controlled high-speed robotics.

To make a reference for the 3-D NPH-streptavidin (3-D NPH-SA), the solution including no poly (NAM-co-NAS) was dispensed on the Au-coated slide activated with succinimide esters. The product was referred to as 2-D reference (2-D SA).

1. The samples are transferred from 384-well microtiter plates to Au-coated slide activated with succinimide esters by use of stainless steel pins (diameter: about 250 μm) (*see* **Note 2**). The humidity is about 60% and the temperature is 25°C. The pin is estimated to transfer about 3 nl of sample to slide. The six kinds of the mixed SA/poly(NAM-co-NAS) solutions of different concentrations (SA/poly(NAM-co-NAS)=0.063/0.0063, 0.13/0.013, 0.25/0.025, 0.50/0.050, 1.0/0.10, 3.0/0.30 wt.%), and six kinds of the SA solutions (0.063, 0.13, 0.25, 0.50, 1.0, 3.0 wt.%) are dispensed ($n = 2$). **Figure 2** shows the pattern of the 3-D NPH-SA and 2-D SA on the array.

2. After the completion of the printing process, the slide remains inside the microarrayer for at least 1 h. The humidity is about 80% and the temperature is 25°C.

3. Immerse the slide in 1 M ethanolamine solution, 3% BSA (pH 8.5) for blocking nonspotted surface of Au-coated slide and masking the nonreacted succinimide esters at 25°C for 30 min.

4. The Au-coated slide is washed with PBS 0.05% Tween 20 (PBST) 5 times and with MilliQ water 5 times and dried with nitrogen gas flow.

A-F: 3-D NPH-SA

A: SA/polymer
   = 3.0/0.3%
B: SA/polymer
   = 1.0/0.1%
C: SA/polymer
   = 0.5/0.05%
D: SA/polymer
   = 0.25/0.025%
E: SA/polymer
   = 0.13/0.013%
F: SA/polymer
   = 0.063/0.0063%

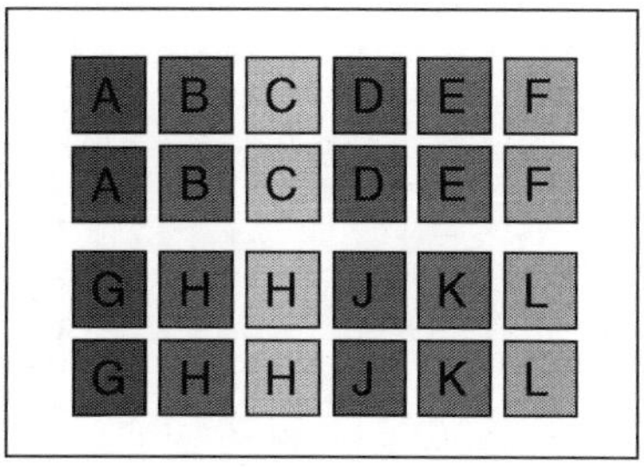

G-L: 2-D SA

G: SA 3.0%
H: SA 1.0%
 I: SA 0.50%
J: SA 0.25%
K: SA 0.13%
L: SA 0.063%

Fig. 2. Description of each spot. (**a–f**) 3-D NPH-streptavidin spots (3-D NPH-SA). (**g–l**) 2-D streptavidin spots (2-D SA). For each SA/polymer concentration for 3-D NPH-SA or SA concentration for 2-D SA, 8 replicate spots of 3-D NPH-SA or SA were dispensed.

3.4. SPRi Interaction Monitoring

The SPRi reader was from Toyobo (Japan). The interactions produce changes in the reflectivity indexes near the gold surface, which result in the changes of the reflectivity recorded by a CCD camera as gray-level contrasts.

3.4.1. SPRi Monitoring of Microarray

The Au-coated glass slide on which the 3-D NPH-SA and 2-D SA were spotted (*see* **Subheading 3.3.4**) was placed in the SPR imaging instrument as described by the manufacturer. Using a pump, the running buffer (PBS) was applied to the array surface at a constant flow rate of 0.5 ml/min.

Figure 3 shows the array image of 3-D NPH-SA and 2-D SA in the running buffer and eight spots of the same concentrations are produced reproducibly (Diameter of the spots: 250 μm).

3.4.2. SPRi Interactions Between 3-D NPH-SA or 2-D SA and Biotinylated Horse Radish Peroxidase (b-HRP)

The inner area of the spot of 3-D NPH-SA should be assayed (*see* **Note 3**). The experiment is started by injection of b-HRP solution (10 μg/ml). It is injected for 15 min. An increase in the signal can be observed in **Fig. 4**, which shows that b-HRP interact with 3-D NPH-SA and 2-D SA. The amount of reacted b-HRP for 3-D NPH-SA (0.13/0.013%) was about 7-times greater than that for 2-D SA (0.13%). **Figure 5** shows the amount of reacted b-HRP with the six kinds of 3-D NPH-SA spots and 2-D SA spots. In the case of 2-D SA, the amount of reacted b-HRP

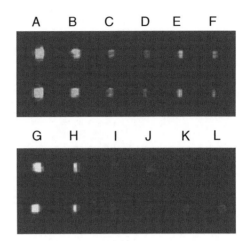

Fig. 3. SPR images of spots on the chip surface. *White spots* in SPR image illustrate 3-D NPH-SA or immobilized SA. The amounts of immobilized 3-D NPH-SA and SA were changed by SA concentrations in feed.

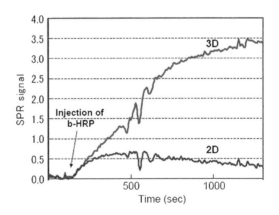

Fig. 4. Sensorgram of injection of biotinylated Horse Radish Peroxidase (b-HRP) (10 μg/ml).

shows the highest value at the spots prepared by 0.5% SA solution in feed. Meanwhile, for the 3-D NPH-SA, the amount of b-HRP shows the highest value around 0.13/0.013% in feed and decreases as the concentrations in feed increase. The reason might be that the thickness of 3-D NPH-SA prepared over the concentration of 0.13/0.013% is too thick to monitor SPR interactions (*see* **Note 4**).

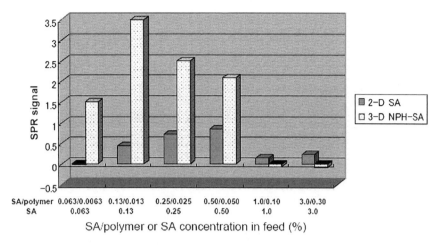

Fig. 5. The effect of SA/polymer or SA concentrations in feed to the amount of reacted biotinylated Horse Radish peroxidase.

4. Notes

1. Because the succinimide esters of poly(NAM-co-NAS) are susceptible to be hydrolyzed during storage, store purified polymer in a desiccator before usage. It is able to be used within 1 year losslessly.

2. The spotting experiment must be finished within 1 h after preparing streptavidin/poly (NAM-co-NAS) mixed solutions. Because the reaction between the succinimide esters of poly(NAM-co-NAS) and the amino groups of SA molecules and hydrolysis of the succinimide esters of poly (NAM-co-NAS) proceed before printing on substrates in 384-well, 3-D NPH-SA is difficult to be made on Au-coated slide activated with succinimide esters.

3. The principle of SPR is based on the evanescent wave phenomenon. The energy of photons is directly absorbed by the free electron constellation of a thin metal layer and converted into an evanescent field, which is propagated through the dielectric medium close to metal for up to 200 nm *(22, 23)*. For SPRi interaction monitoring, the inner areas of the 3-D NPH-SA spots should be assayed. The edge of spots has the shape like a ring which is well known as "Coffee Stain effect" which appears owing to thermodynamic flow. Since the thickness of the edge of the 3-D NPH-SA is over 200 nm, it is not be able to monitor SPRi interaction at the edge of spots.

4. The adequate protein/polymer concentrations in feed for 3-D NPH exist for SPRi, because the evanescent electromagnetic field decays exponentially from the metal surface into the interacting medium as described above. The thickness of 3-D NPH-SA prepared over the concentration of 0.25/0.025% is too thick to monitor SPR interactions even at the center of spots. It is thought that different proteins have each optimum concentration for 3-D NPH immobilization method in the case of SPR measurements.

Meanwhile, in the case of the fluorescence detection, the limitation of the thickness did not exist *(19, 20)*.

Acknowledgments

We thank Dr. Hisashi Koga of Kazusa DNA Research Institute and Haruma Kawaguchi of Keio University for their helpful suggestions.

References

1. Schreiber, S. L., (1998) Chemical genetics resulting from a passion for synthetic organic chemistry. *Bioorg. Med. Chem.*, **6**, 1127–1152.

2. Haggarty, S. J., Mayer, T. U., Miyamoto, D. T., Fathi, R., King, R. W., Mitchison, T. J., and Schreiber, S. L. (2000) Dissecting cellular processes using small molecules: identification of colchicine-like, taxol-like and other small molecules that perturb mitosis. Chem. Biol., 7, 275–286.

3. Koga, H. (2006) Establishment of the platform for reverse chemical genetics targeting novel protein–protein interactions. *Mol. Biosyst.* **2**, 159–164.

4. Spring, D. R., (2005) Chemical genetics to chemical genomics: small molecules offer big insights. *Chem. Soc. Rev.* **34**, 472–482.

5. Macbeath, G., and Schreiber, S. L. (2000) Printing proteins as microarray for high throughput function determination. *Science* **289**, 1760–1763.

6. Stiffler, M. A., Grantcharava, V. P., Sevecka, M., and MacBeath, G. (2006) Uncovering quantitative protein interaction networks for mouse PDZ domains using protein microarrays. *J. Am. Chem. Soc.* **128**, 5913–5922.

7. Michaud, G. A., Salcius, M., Zhou, F., Bangham, R., Bonin, J., Guo, H., Snyder, M., Predki, P. F., and Schweitzer, B. I. (2003) Analyzing antibody specificity with whole proteome microarrays. *Nat. Biotechnol.* **21**, 1509–12.

8. Zhu, H., and Snyder, M. (2003) Protein chip technology. *Curr Opin Chem Biol*, **7**, 55–63.

9. Lofas, S., and Johnsson, B. (1990) A novel hydrogel matrix on gold surfaces in surface plasmon resonance sensors for fast and efficient covalent immobilization of ligands. *J. Chem. Soc. Chem. Commun.*, **21**, 1526–1528.

10. Polzius, R., Schneider, Th., Bier, F. F., Biltewski, U., and Koscinski, W. (1996) Optimization of biosensing using grating couplers: immobilization on tantalum oxide waveguides. *Biosens. Bioelectron.*, **11**, 503–514.

11. Arenkov, P., Kukhtin, A., Gemmell, A., Voloschchuk, S., Chupeeva, V., and Mirzabekov, A. (2000) Protein microchips: Use for immunoassay and enzymatic reactions. *Anal. Biochem.*, **278**, 123–131.

12. Angenendt, P., Glokler, J., Murphy, D., Lehrach, H., and Cahill, D. J., (2002) Toward optimized antibody microarrays: a comparison of current microarray support materials. *Anal. Biochem.*, **309**, 253–260.

13. Charles, P. T., Taitt, C. R., Goldman, E. R., Rangasammy, J. G., and Stenger, D. A. (2004) Immobilization strategy and characterization

of hydrogel-based thin films for integration of ligand binding with staphylococcal enterotoxin B (SEB) in a protein microarray format. *Langmuir*, **20**, 270–272.

14. Brueggemeier, S. B., Wu, D., Kron, S. J., and Palecek, S. P. (2005) Protein-acrylamide copolymer hydrogels for array-based detection of tyrosine kinase activity from cell lysates. *Biomacromolecules*, **6**, 2765–2775.

15. Afanassiev, V., Hanemann, V., and Wolfl, S. (2000) Preparation of DNA and protein micro arrays on glass slides coated with an agarose film. *Nucleic Acids Res.*, **28**, 66e.

16. Dominguez, M. M., Wathier, M., Grinstaff, M. W., and Schaus, S. E. (2007) Immobilized Hydrogels for Screening of Molecular Interactions. *Anal. Chem.*, **79**, 1064–1066.

17. Dai, J., Bao, Z., Sun, L., Hong, S. U., Baker, G. L., and Bruening, M. L. (2006) High-capacity binding of proteins by poly(acrylic acid) brushes and their derivatives. *Langmuir*, **22**, 4274–4281.

18. Y. Zhou, O. Andersson, P. Lindberg and Liedberg, B. (2004) Protein microarrays on carboxymethylated dextran hydrogels: immobilization, characterization and application. *Microchim. Acta.*, **147**, 21–30.

19. Tanaka, H., Shiroya, T., Hanasaki, M., Isojima, T., Takeuchi, H., and Kawaguchi, H., (2008) Preparation of porous protein-based hydrogel for highly sensitive protein chips. *Macromol. Symp.*, **266**, 81–84.

20. Tanaka, H., Isojima, T., Hanasaki, M., Ifuku, Y., Takeuchi, H., Kawaguchi, H., and Shiroya, T. (2008) Porous protein-based nanoparticle hydrogel for protein chips with improved sensitivity. *Macromol. Rapid Commun.*, **29**, 1287–1292.

21. D'Agosto, F., Charreyre, M.-T., Melis, F., Mandrand, B., and Pichot, C., (2003) High molecular weight hydrophilic functional copolymers by free-radical copolymerization of acrylamide and *N*-acryloylmorpholine with *N*-acryloxysuccinimide: Application to the synthesis of a graft copolymer. *J. Appl. Polym. Sci.*, **88**, 1808–1816.

22. Habauzit, D., Chopineau, J., and Roig, B. (2007) SPR-based biosensors: a tool for biodetection of hormonal compounds. *Anal. Bioanal. Chem.*, **387**, 1215–1223.

23. Stenberg, E., Persson, B., Roos, H., and Urbaniczky, C. (1991) Quantitative determination of surface concentration of protein with surface plasmon resonance using radiolabeled proteins. *J. Colloid Interface Sci.*, **143**, 513–526.

Chapter 17

High-Throughput SPR Biosensor

Motoki Kyo, Kimihiko Ohtsuka, Eiji Okamoto, and Kazuki Inamori

Summary

Surface plasmon resonance (SPR) imaging technique is label free, real-time, and high-throughput analysis method for interaction studies with array format. The application of SPR imaging for the small molecule arrays, which were fabricated by photoaffinity crosslinking, can be the first screening step for reverse chemical genomics. The fabrication process of sugar array and sugar–lectin interaction study was demonstrated. The protocol of array fabrication did not require any chemical modifications of sugar chains for immobilizations. The biotinylated sugars were used to investigate signal ratios between lectin and antistreptavidin antibody binding. And it seemed that signal normalization could be achieved, even though the accurate densities of immobilized sugars were unclear.

Key words: Surface plasmon resonance imaging technique, Small molecule arrays, Photoaffinity crosslinking, High-throughput screening, Sugar array, Signal normalization

1. Introduction

Surface plasmon resonance (SPR) technique had become popular in interaction studies between biological molecules (1). It is an optical biosensor, and the interactions can be detected by SPR angle shift or reflection light intensity. In typical SPR measurement, one of pair interacting biomolecules was immobilized on a gold chip, and another was flowed over the chip as its solution. There are two major advantages in SPR assay**; (a) real time evaluations on kinetics studies and (b) label-free measurements.

In last decade, SPR imaging technique, which can analyze biomolecules with array format, has been closed up as a high-throughput

Hisashi Koga (ed.), *Reverse Chemical Genetics*, Methods in Molecular Biology, vol. 577
DOI 10.1007/978-1-60761-232-2_17, © Humana Press, a part of Springer Science + Business Media, LLC 2009

SPR biosensor *(2, 3)*. In SPR imaging measurement, a polarized parallel light and CCD camera were used as light source and detecting device, respectively *(4)*. Recently, several high-throughput analyses with SPR imaging had been reported on oligonucleotides–small molecules *(5, 6)*, oligonucleotides–proteins *(7–10)*, antibodies–proteins *(11, 12)*, peptides–proteins *(13, 14)* and proteins–proteins *(15, 16)*.

Most recently, we reported small molecule arrays on photoaffinity crosslinker coated gold surfaces *(17)*. The small molecule arrays were fabricated by photoreaction, and then analyzed by SPR imaging technique. The small molecules don't have to be modified chemically for immobilization. The small molecules, which can interact with a target protein, can be screened by this methodology. Therefore, the integration of photoaffinity small molecule array and SPR imaging technique can be the first step of reverse chemical genetics.

The integrated technology was applied for sugar array in this chapter. A sugar array was fabricated on gold with photoaffinity crosslinking, and the interaction between a lectin maackia amurensis hemagglutinin (MAH) and a sugar chain sialyl T antigen was analyzed by using SPR imaging technique. Signal normalization was also investigated by using biotinylated sugars.

2. Materials

2.1. Preparation of Sugar Solutions

1. Biotinylated sialyl T antigen with polyacrylamide (PAA) backbone (Sialyl T; Neu5Acα2–3Galβ1- 3GalNAcα-PAA-biotin, Glycotech, USA).

2. Biotinylated sialyl Tn antigen with PAA backbone (Sialyl Tn; Neu5Acα2–6GalNAcα-PAA-biotin, Glycotech).

3. Biotinylated sialyl LacNAc with PAA backbone (Sialyl LacNAc; Neu5Acα2–3Galβ1–4GlcNAcβ- PAA-biotin, Glycotech).

4. 96-well microplate with V-shaped bottoms (Toyobo, Japan).

2.2. Fabrication of Sugar Arrays by Photoaffinity Crosslinking

1. A photoaffinity crosslinker modified gold chip (Toyobo). Store at 6°C. Keep 10 min at room temperature before use.

2. A contact pin type automated spotter with Φ450 μm pin (Toyobo).

3. A UV transmission filter (Sigma-Koki, Tokyo), which can shield UV below 300 nm.

4. A UV crosslinking instrument with 365 nm lamps (Stratagene, USA).

2.3. SPR Imaging Analysis

1. *Tris-based Running buffer.* 50 mM Tris–HCl [pH 7.4], 0.1 mM $CaCl_2$, 0.1 mM $MnCl_2$.
2. Maackia amurensis hemagglutinin (MAH, Vector, CA).
3. Streptavidin (SA, Invitrogen, CA). antistreptavidin antibody (anti-SA, Vector).
4. SPR imaging instrument (Toyobo) with analysis program.

3. Methods

3.1. Fabrication of Sugar Arrays by Photoaffinity Crosslinking

1. Sialyl T was dissolved with distilled water to be 500, 250, 100, 50, and 25 µg/mL (*see* **Note 1**).
2. 500, 250, 100, 50, and 25 µg/mL of Sialyl Tn; Sialyl Lac-NAc were also prepared with distilled water.
3. 10 µL of 15 sugar solutions (three species, five concentrations) were poured into 96-well microplate with V-shaped bottoms.
4. A photoaffinity crosslinker modified gold chip and 96-well microplate with 15 sugar solutions was placed in a contact pin type automated spotter.
5. The spotting pattern was created according to the spotter program.
6. 10 nL drops of sugar aqueous solutions with 500, 250, 100, 50, and 25 µg/mL were delivered by 450 µm pin of the automated spotter on the gold chip, which had photoreactive group (*see* **Note 2**).
7. The chip, on which aqueous drops were aligned, was placed into a vacuum chamber to evaporate water on the spots.
8. The chip with dried spots was covered with a UV transmission filter, and then placed into UV crosslinking instrument.
9. The chip was irradiated with 2.8 J/cm^2 with 365 nm lamps (*see* **Note 3**).
10. The chip surface was repeatedly rinsed with water and ethanol.

3.2. SPR Imaging Analysis

1. The SPR analysis procedures were indicated in **Fig. 1**. The binding of MAH on sialyl T, regeneration with NaOH and the binding of SA and anti-SA were observed.
2. 300 µL of 25 µg/mL MAH, 2.5 µg/mL SA and 2.5 µg/mL anti-SA were prepared with the tris-based running buffer (*see* **Note 4**).
3. The fabricated sugar array was placed into an SPR imaging instrument.

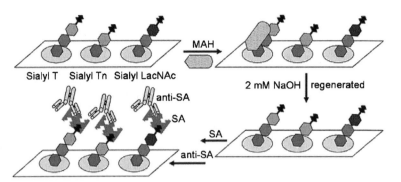

Fig. 1. An analysis procedure of a photocrosslinked sugar array by SPR imaging. A fabricated sugar array with sialyl T, sialyl Tn and sialyl LacNAc were exposed with MAH, regenerated with NaOH and then, exposed with SA and anti-SA.

4. Tris-based running buffer was flowed through SPR instrument with 100 μL/min. SPR experiment was performed at 30°C. The SPR measurement was performed at the angle, which the reflectivities on the sugar spots were approximately 10%.

5. The SPR measuring program was started, and stable base lines were established.

6. 25 μg/mL MAH solution was injected for 10 min with recycling mode, subsequently the running buffer was flowed for 5 min.

7. The chip was regenerated with 2 mM NaOH for 5 min. then the running buffer was flowed for 5 min (*see* **Note 5**).

8. 2.5 μg/mL SA solution was injected for 10 min with recycling mode, subsequently the running buffer was flowed for 5 min.

9. 2.5 μg/mL anti-SA solution was injected for 10 min with recycling mode, subsequently the running buffer was flowed for 5 min.

10. The signal data and images were collected and analyzed with an analysis program.

11. The signal data and image data on the sugars spots, which were prepared with 500 μg/mL sugar solutions, were described in **Fig. 2a, b**, respectively (*see* **Note 6**).

12. The image data on Sialyl T spots, which were prepared with 500, 250, 100, 50, and 25 μg/mL sugar solutions, were shown in **Fig. 3** (*see* **Note 7**).

13. The signals by MAH (S_1) and by anti-SA (S_2) on Sialyl T spots (500, 250, 100, 50, and 25 μg/mL) were summarized in **Table 1**. The signal ratios (S_1/S_2) were calculated (*see* **Note 8**).

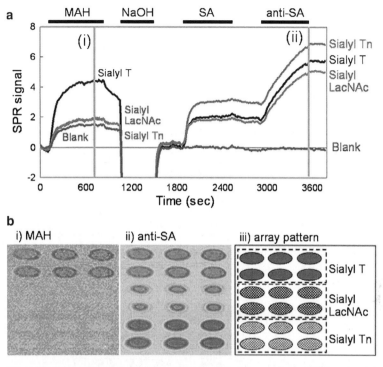

Fig. 2. The interaction analysis of the photocrosslinked sugar array by SPR imaging. (**a**) SPR signal changes on sialyl T, sialyl Tn, sialyl LacNAc and blank spots. (**b**) SPR difference images by exposures of MAH and anti-SA.

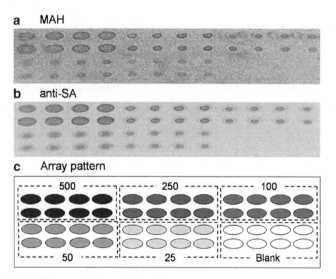

Fig. 3. SPR difference images of the photocrosslinked sugar array fabricated with 25–500 mg/mL sugar concentrations by exposure of (**a**) MAH and (**b**) anti-SA. The array pattern was shown in (**c**).

Table 1
The obtained SPR signals and signal ratios by MAH and anti-SA exposure on sialyl T spots, which were formed with 25–500 μg/mL sugar concentrations

Concentration of spotted sugar solutions (μg/mL)	Signals by MAH (S_1)	Signals by anti-SA (S_2)	Signal ratios (S_1/S_2)
500	3.68 ± 0.68	3.56 ± 0.25	1.03 ± 0.13
250	3.27 ± 0.31	3.11 ± 0.27	1.05 ± 0.05
100	3.01 ± 0.32	2.95 ± 0.19	1.02 ± 0.07
50	2.95 ± 1.06	2.39 ± 0.90	1.25 ± 0.08
25	2.23 ± 0.21	1.99 ± 0.25	1.13 ± 0.05

The average and standard deviation values were calculated from 8 spots ($n = 8$)

4. Notes

1. Distilled water or organic solvents should be used in sample preparations for photoaffinity crosslinking. When detergents or organic salts were contained in diluting solution, the detergents or organic salts molecules might be immobilized preferentially by photocrosslinking. Buffer solutions should not be used for dilution, because precipitation of inorganic salts on spots may weaken UV irradiation.

2. A cylindrical pin with 450 μm diameter was used for spotting. Sharp-edged pins are not preferable, because they may damage gold thin layer on chips. The distance between spots centers were 1 mm.

3. Surface-introduced photoreactive group, aryl diazirine, can generate carbenes by 365 nm UV exposure. However, gold–sulfur bonds, which support photolinker on gold, can be easily broken by UV light below 300 nm. Therefore, UV transmission filter is essential in UV irradiation.

4. The dilution buffer solutions and SPR running buffer must be the same. The lot of buffer should not be changed during the single experiment. Slight component difference of the buffers affect SPR signals, it is so-called "bulk effect."

5. The sugar array could be regenerated with 2 mM NaOH treatment. 0.2 mM was too low to regenerate (not returned to the base lines), and 20 mM might cause hydrolysis of sugars in this experiment (became below zero).

6. The stronger binding of MAH on sialyl T was observed, when MAH was exposed on the array. We thought that the signals

on sialyl Tn and sialyl LacNAc were induced by nonspecific bindings, because the signals were almost same as that of blank spot. SPR signal increases were observed in all sugar spots by exposure of SA and anti-SA. Immobilizations of sugars could be verified by SA and anti-SA.

7. Smaller spots were observed with lower sugar concentrations, even though the same spotting pin was used for all spots. It seemed that the spots of sugar solutions were shrunk and concentrated, during the drying of spots.

8. Higher signals were obtained at the sugar spots, which were prepared with higher concentration solutions. Importantly, the signal ratios (S_1/S_2) were almost constant (around 1.00), and this suggested that lectin binding affinities could be evaluated properly by signal normalization with anti-SA, even though the accurate densities of sugar spots were unclear.

Acknowledgments

We are grateful to Dr. Shigeo Shibatani (Toyobo) and Prof. Hozumi Motohashi (Tohoku University) for critical discussions and advices.

References

1. Homola, J. (2003) Present and future of surface plasmon resonance biosensors. *Anal. Bioanal. Chem.* **377**, 528–539.

2. Jordan, C. E. and Corn, R. M. (1997) Surface plasmon resonance imaging measurements of DNA hybridization adsorption and streptavidin/DNA multilayer formation at chemically modified gold surfaces. *Anal. Chem.* **69**, 1449–1456.

3. Nelson, B. P., Frutos, A. G., Brockman, J. M. and Corn, R. M. (1999) Near-infrared surface plasmon resonance measurements of ultrathin films. 1. Angle shift and SPR imaging experiments. *Anal. Chem.* **71**, 3928–3934.

4. Brockman, J. M., Nelson, B. P. and Corn, R. M. (2000) Surface plasmon resonance imaging measurement of ultrathin organic films. *Annu. Rev. Phys. Chem.* **51**, 41–63.

5. Nishimura, Y., Adachi, H., Kyo, M., Murakami, S., Hattori, S. and Ajito, K. (2005) A proof of the specificity of kanamycin-ribosomal RNA interaction with designed synthetic analogs and the antibacterial activity. *Bioorg. Med. Chem. Lett.* **15**, 2159–2162.

6. Nakatani, K., Hagihara, S., Goto, Y., Kobori, A., Hagihara, M., Hayashi, G., Kyo, M., Nomura, M., Mishima M. and Kojima, C. (2005) Small-molecule ligand induces nucleotide flipping in (CAG)$_n$ trinucleotide repeats. *Nat. Chem. Biol.* **1**, 39–43.

7. Kyo, M., Yamamoto, T., Motohashi, H., Kamiya, T., Kuroita, T., Tanaka, T., Engel, J. D., Kawakami, B. and Yamamoto, M. (2004) Evaluation of MafG interaction with Maf recognition element arrays by surface plasmon resonance imaging technique. *Genes Cells* **9**, 153–164.

8. Egener, T., Roulet, E., Zehnder, M., Bucher, P. and Mermod, N. (2005) Proof of concept for microarray-based detection of DNA-binding oncogenes in cell extracts. *Nucleic Acids Res.* **33**, e79.

9. Yamamoto, T., Kyo, M., Kamiya, T., Tanaka, Y., Engel, J. D., Motohashi, H. and Yamamoto, M. (2006) Predictive base substitution rules that determine the binding and transcriptional specificity of Maf recognition elements. *Genes Cells* **11**, 575–591.

10. Kimura, M., Yamamoto, T., Zhang, J., Itoh, K., Kyo, M., Kamiya, T., Aburatani, H., Katsuoka, F., Kurokawa, H., Tanaka, T., Motohashi, H. and Yamamoto, M. (2007) Molecular basis distinguishing the DNA binding profile of Nrf2-Maf heterodimer from that of Maf homodimer. *J. Biol. Sci.* **282**, 33681–33690.

11. Kyo, M., Usui-Aoki, K. and Koga, H. (2005) Label-free detection of proteins in crude cell lysate with antibody arrays by a surface plasmon resonance imaging technique. *Anal. Chem.* 77, 7115–7121.

12. Lee, H. J., Nedelkov, D. and Corn, R. M. (2006) SPR imaging measurements of antibody arrays for the multiplexed detection of low molecular weight protein biomarkers. *Anal. Chem.* **78**, 6504–6510.

13. Inamori, K., Kyo, M., Nishiya, Y., Inoue, Y., Sonoda, T., Kinoshita, E., Koike, T. and Katayama, Y. (2005) Detection and quantification of on-chip phosphorylated peptides by surface plasmon resonance imaging techniques using a phosphate capture molecule. *Anal. Chem.* 77, 3979–3985.

14. Inamori, K., Kyo, M., Matsukawa, K., Inoue, Y., Sonoda, T., Tatematsu, K., Tanizawa, K., Mori, T. and Katayama, Y. (2008) Optimal surface chemistry for peptide immobilization in on-chip phosphorylation analysis. *Anal. Chem.* **80**, 643–650.

15. Kim, M., Park, K., Jeong, E. J., Shin, Y. B., Chung, B. H. (2006) Surface plasmon resonance imaging analysis of protein-protein interactions using on-chip-expressed capture protein. *Anal. Biochem.* **351**, 298–304.

16. Ha, T. H., Jung, S. O., Lee, J. M., Lee, K. Y., Lee, Y., Park, J. S. and Chung, B. H. (2007) Oriented immobilization of antibodies with GST-fused multiple Fc-specific B-domains on a gold surface. *Anal. Chem.* 79, 546–556.

17. Kanoh, N., Kyo, M., Inamori, K., Ando, A., Asami, A., Nakao, A. and Osada H. (2006) SPR imaging of photo-cross-linked small-molecule arrays on gold. *Anal. Chem.* **78**, 2226–2230.

Chapter 18

Drug Discovery Through Functional Screening in the *Drosophila* Heart

Takeshi Akasaka and Karen Ocorr

Summary

Although advancements in the preventive and therapeutic strategies of cardiac diseases have successfully improved the prognosis of many types of cardiac diseases, they are still challengeable targets because of their high mortality and large medical expenses. Moreover, because heart function is tightly associated with quality of life, it is important to elucidate the genetic and molecular basis of disease progression. One of the recent advances for assessing protein function is reverse chemical genetics, which has the advantages that complement classical reverse genetics and should advance efforts at drug discovery for many diseases. Toward that end an appropriate biological assay system is required to describe specific heart phenotypes.

Resent studies have shown that many aspects of *Drosophila* heart development and function are similar to those observed in the human heart, making *Drosophila* a useful model system with the advantage of a simpler genetic organization and shorter life span. Here we describe several assay systems that can be used to characterize *Drosophila* heart function. The first method is an external electrical pacing assay that is used to assess the response to stress in the adult fly. The incidence of pacing-induced heart dysfunction measured by this method strongly correlates with natural aging and mutation in genes known to be involved in human cardiac dysfunction. Consequently, this method can be used to identify unapparent heart failure phenotypes. This procedure is applicable for both genetic and pharmacological screening. The second method is an image-based heart performance assay. This method provides details of the dynamics of heart contraction in real time similar to clinical echocardiography. This method may be used for secondary drug screening as well as for more detailed analysis of the genetic and pharmacological phenotypes of *Drosophila* hearts.

Key words: *Drosophila*, Genetics, Heart physiology, Electrical pacing, M-mode cardiogram

1. Introduction

Drosophila is a classical and well-studied model organism for genetic analysis. To date many important cellular mechanisms have been successfully elucidated from *Drosophila* studies. The fruit fly

Hisashi Koga (ed.), *Reverse Chemical Genetics*, Methods in Molecular Biology, vol. 577
DOI 10.1007/978-1-60761-232-2_18, © Humana Press, a part of Springer Science+Business Media, LLC 2009

235

offers a number of advantages as a model genetic system. It has a relatively small genome size and while there are often multiple copies of human genes, most homologs in flies exist as a single gene. There are many established genetic tools available including mutant and genetic databases (e.g., FlyBase, http://flybase.bio. indiana.edu/). In addition, double strand RNAi transgenic flies (based on UAS-Gal4 system) *(1, 2)* have been generated for more than 80% of the fly's genes (available from the Vienna *Drosophila* RNAi Center, http://stockcenter.vdrc.at/control/main *(3)* and the National Institute of Genetics, http://www.shigen.nig.ac.jp/fly/nigfly). *Drosophila* also has a relatively short life span and strong reproductive activity, which facilitates genetic manipulation.

The knowledge gained from *Drosophila* studies has been successfully extended to studies of human diseases especially in the field of neural degenerative diseases *(4, 5)*. Recently, studies in flies have been directed at understanding more complex and multifactorial diseases such as heart disease. A better understanding of heart disease and heart failure is critical, not only because heart performance is directly associated with quality of life, but also because mortality associated with heart diseases is rising dramatically in the modern and industrialized world. Therefore, elucidating the cellular and molecular mechanisms responsible for this increased heart disease will be critical for the development of prevention and treatment strategies and reducing the ever rising medical costs *(6)*.

Adult *Drosophila* possesses a tubular heart oriented along the anteroposterior axis **(Fig. 1d)**. This myogenic heart pumps hemolymph and bioactive factors (i.e., neuropeptides) throughout the fly's body through an open circulatory system. The heart consists of an outflow tract or "aorta" and working "heart" that contracts autonomously *(7)*. The heart tube has three sets of valves that form a "chamber-like" structure in each abdominal segment. The heart tube also possesses four pairs of ostia at the middle of each chamber that allows movement of hemolymph between the heart lumen and body cavity *(7)*. Although the anatomical features of *Drosophila*'s simple heart tube are quite different from 4-chamber human heart, heart tube formation from lateral mesoderm during embryogenesis is highly conserved between these organisms. Moreover, these organisms have similar regulatory networks with respect to cell commitment and heart muscle maturation *(8–10)*. The fact that mechanisms underlying cardiogenesis are conserved among these species suggest that cardiac physiology could also be regulated by conserved genetic mechanisms. In fact many ion channels, structural proteins, and contractile proteins seen in mammals also exist in *Drosophila* hearts and data is accumulating that suggests that genetic mutations in the fly produce cardiac phenotypes with pathogenesis similar to that seen in human cardiac disease *(11, 12)*. An additional advantage of using the *Drosophila* model is that compromised heart function is not immediately lethal. This is because it is the tracheal system that

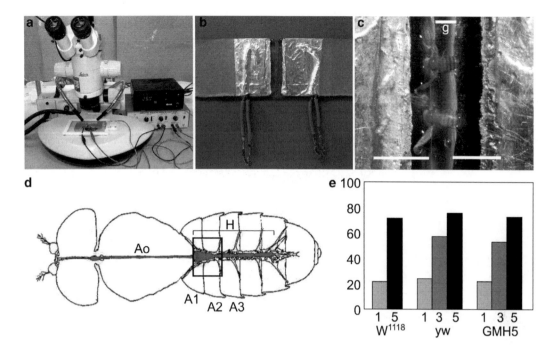

Fig. 1. External electrical pacing assay. (**a**) System used for the pacing assay. The pacing electrodes are connected to an electrical stimulator that supports square wave stimuli at 6 Hz, 30 ms duration, 40 V for 30 s. *Drosophila* heart edges are observed through the cuticle using a stereo microscope. During the experiment flies are kept at a constant temperature by placing the slide, pacing electrode, and flies in electrode gel on a hearting plate at 25°C. (**b**) Image of the pacing electrodes affixed to a glass slide; note 5 mm gap between electrodes. (**c**) Image of fruit flies mounted on the pacing platform. Electrical gel (width of the gel strip is indicated by the *white lines*) is placed along the edge of each metal electrode. Five to ten flies are arranged in the procumbent position between the gel strips with a gel-free gap between the head and the abdomen (*g* gap between the gel strips). The microscope is focused on A2 or A3 segments to observe the heat edge movements. (**d**) Fly heart tube (shown in *gray*), located along the dorsal midline. The heart tube is made up of a thoracic aorta (Ao) and the contractile abdominal heart (H). The observation window is indicated by the *blue rectangle* located at the dorsal part of the first three abdominal segments (A1, A2, A3). (**e**) Overall heart failure rate is measured 30 s following the pacing protocol in 1, 3, and 5-week old flies. Note the threefold to fivefold increase in pacing-induced heart failure with age in two different laboratory wildtype flies and in a heart specific Gal4 driver strain, GMH5 ($n > 100$).

supplies oxygen to peripheral tissues; therefore, genetic and pharmacological manipulation of the *Drosophila* heart can reveal more severe phenotypes than can be observed in mammals.

Recently, reverse chemical genetics has emerged as an important approach to drug discovery. In this approach chemicals that specifically bind known protein targets are screened for their effects on biological function. In comparison with classical reverse genetics by gene locus manipulation, reverse chemical genetics has several advantages; it minimizes the masking of the phenotypes by redundancy and it directly targets specific physiological systems. For this approach to work, it is critical to develop a well-defined assay system.

In this section we review two new experimental methods which assess heart performance in *Drosophila*. The first method is an external electrical pacing assay, which would allow assessment of small molecule function in vivo in different genetic backgrounds. This method could be done relatively quickly and could be applicable for a first screen. The second method is an in situ, image-based heart performance assay. This method is slightly more time consuming than the pacing assay; however, it allows for detailed analysis of a number of heart function parameters in a denervated preparation, which is important because myogenic function can be modulated by neural input. Both methods can be used to assess the effects of pharmacological treatment in vivo. Therefore, we propose that these methods can be used as chemical/genetic assays for drug discovery to treat heart disease and to improve heart performance.

2. Materials

2.1. External Electrical Pacing Assay

1. Signa® gel (Parker Laboratories Inc., NJ) as an electrical conduction gel.
2. Isolated square wave stimulator (Phipps & Bird, VA) for generating the square wave pulse to stimulate the fly hearts.
3. Temperature-controlled platform (Brook Industries IL) for maintaining flies at 25°C.
4. FlyNap® anesthetic (Carolina Biological Supply Co, NC) should be kept in a draft at room temperature.

2.2. Image Based Heart Performance Assay

1. Microscope capable of 10× magnification with a water immersion lens (e.g., Leica DM-LFSA; Leica Microsystems).
2. High-speed video recording camera capable of frames rates greater than 80 frames per second (e.g., Hamamtsu EM-CCD; Hamamatsu Corp.).
3. Simple PCI® (Hamamatsu, Corp) image capture software.
4. *Artificial adult hemolymph without sucrose and trehalose.* $NaCl_2$ (108 mM), KCl (5 mM), $CaCl_2$ (2 mM), $MgCl_2$ (8), NaH_2PO_4 (1 mM), $NaHCO_3$ (4 mM), HEPES (pH 7.1) (15 mM) can be stored at 4°C. Stock solution of sucrose (1 M) and trehalose (1 M) should be added before use.

3. Methods

The following methods were designed to quantify *Drosophila* heart performance in vivo. Because of the molecular and functional similarities it should be possible to use the fly heart to screen for compounds that affect its function. Small compounds that affect the function of specific proteins can be fed to flies and their systemic effects can be assayed using the pacing assay or the image-based heart performance assay. Alternatively, small compounds can be applied directly to hearts during the imaging process to analyze acute actions.

3.1. External Electrical Pacing Assay

Since subclinical heart failure in humans is preferentially recognizable under stress conditions, we have established a challenge test using frequent electrical stimuli to induce a heart failure/dysfunction phenotype in flies *(13–15)*. Flies are placed between two electrodes in contact with electrode gel **(Fig. 1a–c)**. The heart is paced with a square wave stimulator at 40 V and 6 Hz (approximately twice the resting rate) for 30 s and then flies are visually observed for heart dysfunction. Heart failure rate is defined as the percentage of flies that exhibit no heart wall movement (arrest) or unsynchronized heart wall movement (fibrillation) 30 s after the cessation of pacing *(14)*. Using this protocol, we observe a steeply progressive increase in the heart failure rate from about 20 to 30% at young ages (1 week old) to 80% at old age (5–7 weeks old) in a variety of genetic backgrounds considered wildtype **(Fig. 1e)**. We have also observed that orthologs of some human cardiac disease genes show higher heart failure rate in this assay *(16)*. Therefore, this simple and sensitive measurement system for cardiac performance makes it possible to rapidly analyze the effects on heart function as a result of either genetic or pharmacological manipulations.

1. *Anesthesia for flies.* 1 ml of Fly-Nap® (Carolina Biological Supply Co, Burlinton, NC) is added to the foam pad of bottom of the *Drosophila* Anesthetizer® (Carolina Biological Supply Co, Burlinton, NC). Fifty to hundred adult flies are placed into the chamber for 3–5 min until they stop moving (*see* **Note 1**).

2. *Mount the flies to the pacing platform.* Clean up the metal electrodes (made with pieces of aluminum foil) with ethanol if necessary **(Fig. 1b)**. Then put the electrode gel (Parker Laboratories Inc. Fairfield, NJ) along the edges of the metal electrodes **(Fig. 1b, c)** making sure that there is no electrical shunt between two rows of gel (*see* **Note 2**). Using forceps, anesthetized flies are placed in the procumbent position on the gel with the head touching the gel on one electrode and the posterior tip of the abdomen touching the gel on the other electrode **(Fig. 1c)** (*see* **Note 3**). The wings are spread out and placed in the gel near the head; this keeps the heart observation "window" in anterior abdomen clear for viewing heart contractions **(Fig. 1d** rectangle).

3. *Device setting.* We use the Isolated Square Wave Stimulator (Phipps & Bird #7092–611 Richmond, VA) as an external electrical pulse generator. Overdriving is performed by applying a

continuous square pulse at 6 Hz, 30 ms duration, 40 V for 30 s at 25°C (*see* **Note 4**).

4. *Electrical over-drive pacing.* Both an inverted microscope (10× objective lens) and a dissecting microscope are suitable for monitoring the heart movements through the abdominal cuticle. In the many cases the most anterior part of the abdomen (conical chamber in A1–A2 region, **Fig. 1d**) is the optimal location for observing heart movements. It is also sometimes possible to visualize the heart in the next abdominal segment (A3 region, **Fig. 1d**) (*see* **Note 5**). Importantly, the flies should be scanned during the pacing procedure to ensure that the pacing occurs as expected and that no short circuits occur (identified by erratic and continuous twitching of appendages).

5. *Scoring pacing-induced heart failure.* 30 s after the pacing, the heart movement is evaluated and scored according to three possible outcomes: *Recovered* – the hearts recover their regular heart rhythms with substantial and concerted contractility, *Arrest* – the hearts show no movement, *Fibrillation* – the heart walls move but show no coordinated contraction (*see* **Note 5**). In the recovered heart both edges of the heart tube come together at the same time resulting in productive pumping, whereas fibrillating hearts show a kinetic movement of the heart walls. The pacing induced heart failure rate is defined by the percentage of flies exhibiting either arrest or fibrillation (*see* **Note 6**).

3.1.1. Pacing Induced Heart Failure in Wildtype Flies

We observe a steeply progressive increase in heart failure rate from about 20 to 30% at a young age (1 week) up to 80% at old age (5–7 weeks) in a variety of genetic backgrounds considered wildtype (**Fig. 1e**). This measure in cardiac performance has made it possible to analyze the age-dependent functional changes of heart in response to manipulating genes (i.e., insulin receptor) as well as the human cardiac disease genes *(15, 17)*.

3.1.2. Drug Application and Example for Pacing Assay (K_{ATP} Channel)

It is possible to administer chemicals to the adult flies orally. For short treatments (1–2 days) we use a glass filter paper soaked with drug containing grape juice (0.5–1.0 ml) (**Fig. 2b, c**). The glass filter is placed at the bottom of regular vials. For longer drug application we mix the chemicals into a yeast paste that is placed on the regular fly medium.

K_{ATP} channels are thought to sense the intracellular metabolic state (the intracellular ATP and ADP ratio), which can be affected by various important metabolic stresses. K_{ATP} channels are inhibited by ATP binding and are thought to be involved in tolerance against metabolic stresses *(18–20)*. Interestingly, human K_{ATP} channel-associated mutations (in SUR2) have been found in two independent families and were shown to cause dilated cardiomyopathy and refractory ventricular tachycardia suggesting that K_{ATP} channels are also involved in human heart development and adult heart function *(21)*.

Drosophila has a single gene *dSUR*, which is a homologue of the SUR gene and a subunit of the K_{ATP} channel in mammals. Remarkably, flies in which dSUR is knocked down in the mesoderm using the Gal4-UAS system exhibit a higher heart failure rate compared to the outcrossed controls **(Fig. 2a)**. Additionally when we applied tolbutamide, a K_{ATP} channel inhibitor, to young adult flies (using a glass filter for 18 h), they also exhibited an increased incidence of heart failure compared to the nontreated controls **(Fig. 2b)**. On the other hand when adult flies were exposed to pinacidil, a K_{ATP} channel activator, measures of the heart failure rate showed a significant reduction in older flies (3–4 weeks) compared to the control group **(Fig. 2c)**. This provides an example

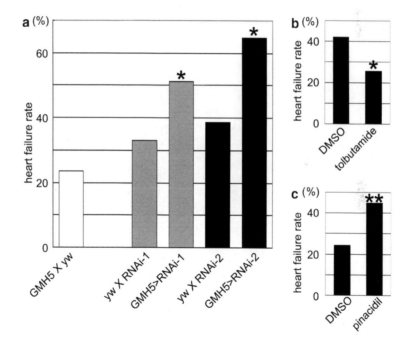

Fig. 2. dSUR contributes a protective role against both pacing induced heart failure and aging heart phenotype. (**a**) Heart failure rate after 30 s pacing regimes in young, 1-week-old flies. Progeny of crosses between the heart specific Gal4 driver GMH5 and UAS-dSUR-RNAi lines (GMH5 > RNAi-1 or GMH5 > RNAi-2) were tested. Transgenic RNAi-mediated knock down of the dSur potassium channel resulted in an increase in pacing-induced heart failure compared to that of the outcrossed controls (GMH5 X yw and yw X RNAi-1 or yw X RNAi-2). (**b**) 1-week-old flies treated with the dSUR inhibitor tolbutamide showed a higher pacing-induced heart failure rate than control flies treated with vehicle (DMSO). (**c**) Older, 3.5-week-old flies treated with the dSUR activator pinacidil exhibited lower pacing-induced heart failure rate than did control flies treated with vehicle (DMSO, *p* value * < 0.01, ** < 0.02.), suggesting that loss of K_{ATP} channel activity may contribute to the observed age-dependent increases in pacing-induced heart failure and heart aging. Adapted from Ref. 17.

where in vivo heart performance in response to stress is altered in different genetic backgrounds and in response to chemical application. Moreover, this pacing assay will be useful for evaluating drug efficacy and unexpected effects in various genetic backgrounds.

3.2. Image Based Heart Performance Assay

Real-time imaging of heart movements using high-speed digital video recording system provides a more detailed analysis of cardiac performance and pathology. In this system a semi-intact heart (a heart exposed by microsurgery which removes inputs from the central nervous system) is visualized at speeds up to 200 frames per second. Movies are analyzed using two movement detection algorithms that can accurately track movement of the heart. In addition edge tracings can be obtained from the movies creating movement traces called M-modes. These M-modes are similar to those prepared from clinical echocardiographs. Using this image-based analysis heart period, rhythmicity, heart size, and fractional shortening can be quantified *(22, 23)*. The observed age-dependent changes in cardiac rhythmicity and performance are reminiscent of the increased incidence of atrial fibrillation and heart failure seen in elderly humans *(24–26)*. Also fractional shortening (% FS), an index of contractility, declines with age in flies as it also does in response to mutations that underlie some human cardiac diseases. We have now firmly established this assay as a sensitive method for examining the relationships between gene mutations, protein structure/function, and heart performance *(12, 22, 23)*.

1. *Anesthesia for flies.* Flies should be maintained at low density in culture vials at 25°C. Flies are anaesthetized with FlyNap® in the same manner as described above.

2. *Semi-intact heart preparation.* Flies are dissected ventrally using irridectomy scissors to make a diagonal cut across the thorax (from postero-ventral to anterodorsal) which removes the head, legs, and ventral nerve cord. Dissections are performed in oxygenated artificial adult hemolymph (108 mM $NaCl_2$, 5 mM KCl, 2 mM $CaCl_2$, 8 mM $MgCl_2$, 1 mM NaH_2PO_4, 4 mM $NaHCO_3$, 15 mM HEPES (pH 7.1), 10 mM sucrose, 5 mM trehalose) (*see* **Note 7**). The terminal tip of the abdomen is removed with a cut using irridectomy scissors and this cut provides access for making additional lateral cuts along the abdominal cuticle. Then ventral parts of the abdominal cuticle as well as the all internal organs are removed. Adipose tissue surrounding the heart can be removed by gentle suction using fine glass pipettes (*see* **Note 8**).

3. *Equilibration.* The semi-intact preparations are allowed to equilibrate with oxygenation for approximately 30 min prior to recording (*see* **Note 9**).

4. *Image acquisition.* Image analysis of heart contractions is performed using a Hamamatsu EM-CCD digital camera mounted

on a Leica DM LFSA microscope with a 10× water immersion lens. Heart movement movies are typically taken at rates of 100–150 frames per second. All images are acquired and contrast enhanced using Simple PCI® imaging software (Compix, Inc. Lake Oswego, OR).

5. *Data analysis.* We use a combination of two movement detection algorithms *(23)* written in Matlab® environment (The MathWorks, Inc.) to accurately track movement of the heart edges (*see* **Note 10**). Measurements of diastolic and systolic diameters as well as diastolic and systolic intervals, % fractional shortening (% FS), arrhythmicity index, and contraction direction and velocity are obtained as output from this analysis program. Heart rate is calculated as the inverse of the heart period where one period corresponds to a single diastolic interval plus subsequent systolic interval. % FS is quantified based on diameter measurements and is calculated as ((diastolic diameter-systolic diameter)/diastolic diameter) × 100 (%). Heart beat rhythmicity is quantified based on the standard deviation of the mean heart period normalized to the median heart period for each fly providing a dimensionless arrhythmicity index.

3.2.1. Image Based Heart Performance Assay in Wild Type Flies

Heart period (HP) and arrhythmic phenotype. HP increases significantly with age in wildtype flies (**Fig. 3f**). This increase is disproportionately due to an increase in the diastolic interval compared to the systolic interval. Arrhythmic events also increase significantly with age as evidenced by significant increases in the arrhythmia index. Typically the arrhythmias observed in older flies include episodes of tachycardia/fibrillation as well as bradycardia or prolonged diastolic intervals.

Heart size. Heart size is dimorphic with the female having a slightly wider heart tube than the male in proportion to the differences in their body size. The heart size can be quantified during relaxation (diastolic diameter, DD) and contraction (systolic diameter, SD); measured at the end-diastolic and systolic phases, respectively (**Fig. 3e**). In *Drosophila* the heart tube is a single cell thick, so it is not possible to discern a heart wall. The tube itself is fairly uniform in diameter in the third and fourth abdominal segments and the heart edges are more reliably visible in the third segment (**Fig. 3a**). Consequently we make measurements on the outside edge of the heart tube muscle at two points, one on each side of the ostea in the third abdominal segment (**Fig. 3b**). There is a tendency for heart size to decrease with age.

Contraction index. We have observed that %FS declines with age in wildtype flies *(12, 23)* as it does in some human cardiac diseases and with gene mutations, suggesting that this index could be a reliable marker of heart performance similar to its use in mammals. Representative values for wildtype hearts are shown in **Table 1** and the details are described in *(23)*.

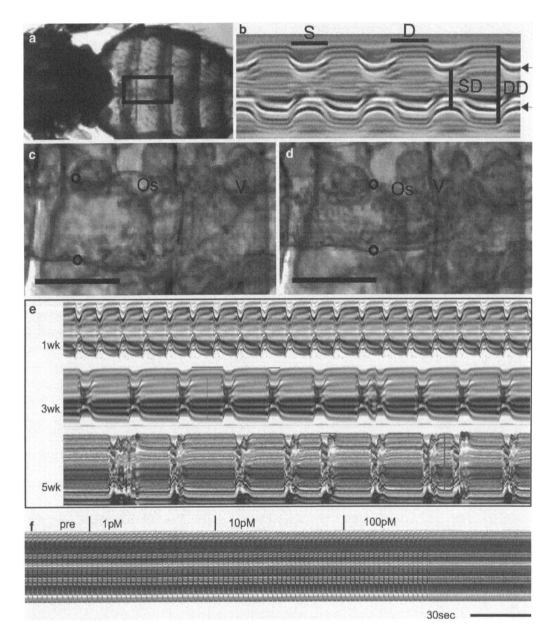

Fig. 3. Image based heart performance assay. (a) Typical view of the semi-intact fly preparation. Head, ventral thorax, ventral nerve cord, and all abdominal organs have been removed. Optically opaque adipose tissue has been removed by gentle suction, which also severs residual peripheral nerve trunks. The portion of the heart that is typically filmed is located in abdominal segment 3 (indicated by a rectangle). (b) For M-modes, a vertical strip of pixels that spans the outer edges of the heart wall is selected and electronically excised. Strips taken from the identical location in each frame of the movie are aligned horizontally to create the M-mode edge tracing. *S* systolic phase, *D* diastolic phase, *SD* systolic diameter, *DD* diastolic diameter. Heart tube edges are indicated by *arrows*. (c–e) Heart kinetics. Edge tracing is indicated by the *arrow head* at systolic (c) and end-diastolic phase (d). (*O* ostea, *V* valve.) (e) Typical M-mode record. Position of the heart wall is indicated by arrow head. (f) Representative 10 s M-modes of 1-week, 3-week, and 5 week-old laboratory wildtype flies. Note the increase in heart period and arrythmicity with age. (e) The effect of acute octopamine application on fly heart function. Continuous M-mode showing serial application of 1 pM, 10 pM, and 100 pM octopamine in artificial adult hemolymph. A chronotropic effect is observed in a dose dependent manner similar to the effect of norepinephrin on mammalian heart.

Table 1
Representative index of young and old wildtype flies from image based heart performance assay

	1-week-old	7-week-old
Heart rate (beats/s)	2.20	1.56
Heart period (s)	0.50	1.01
Diastolic interval (s)	0.30	0.60
Systolic interval (s)	0.20	0.41
Diastolic diameter (μm)	72.3	63.0
Systolic diameter (μm))	43.6	39.5
Fractional shortening (%)	40	36
Retrograde contraction (%)	51	58
Retrograde velocity (cm/s)	0.99	0.87

Adapted from Ref. 23

3.2.2. Drug Application and an Example of the Semi-intact Optical Heartbeat Analysis (Voltage Dependent K+ Channel)

Pharmacological manipulation of heart function can be achieved in two ways in the semi-intact heart preparation. Flies can be fed various agents in their food followed, at some later time point, by an analysis of heart function. Alternatively, it is possible to apply the chemicals via the artificial hemolymph used to bathe the heart during the image capture. This latter method permits an assessment of acute effects on heart performance and a determination of the dose dependence of the effect (**Fig. 3f**).

Long QT syndrome is characterized by a prolonged QT interval that is the result of a delayed repolarization of the myocardium. This syndrome frequently shows noncoordination of action potential duration in ventricles and this sometimes induces ventricular tachycardia by a re-entry mechanism. Prolonged QT may also be a trigger of lethal arrhythmia (i.e., torsade de pointes). Mutations in the gene *KCNQ1*, encoding a potassium channel α subunit, have been linked to long QT syndrome in humans. As a first test of the similarity of heart function between flies and humans, we examined heart function in flies mutant for the *KCNQ* gene (a homologue of human KCNQ1). One *KCNQ* mutant generated by P-element hop out (KCNQ[186]) exhibits a high incidence of tachycardia/fibrillation and other arrhythmic events even at young ages (1-week old flies, **Fig. 4a, b**). This increased incidence of arrhythmia is dramatically rescued with mesodermal overexpression of the *KCNQ* gene using the Gal4-UAS system suggesting that the *KCNQ* potassium channel plays an important role in normal heart function in the fly (**Fig. 4c**).

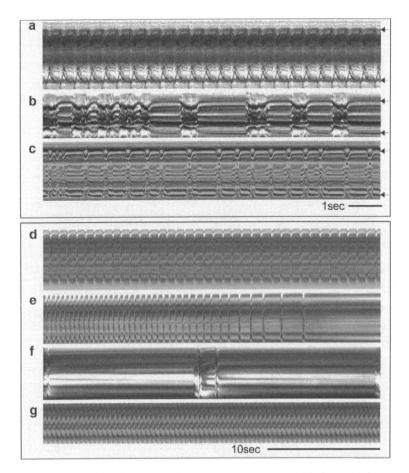

Fig. 4. Representative M-modes illustrating the effects of altered KCNQ channel function. (**a–c**, Adapted from Ref. 22) The effects of a mutation in the single KCNQ gene in
Drosophila. All records are from 1-week old flies. Heart tube edges at the end-diastolic
phase are indicated by *arrows*. (**a**) Wildtype control showing regular contractions as
evidenced by the regular vertical deflections of the heart tube edge overtime. (**b**) KCNQ
mutant fly with a deleted transmembrane domain shows multiple premature contraction with prolonged heart period. (**c**) Mesodermal overexpression of wildtype KCNQ in the
KCNQ mutant background partially rescues the arrhythmic phenotype. (**d–g**) The effects
of pharmacological manipulation of the KCNQ channel. (**d**) M-mode from a 3-week
old wildtype fly prior to treatment with the KCNQ inhibitor chromanol. (**e**) M-mode
from the same wildtype fly at 1 min following application of artificial hemolymph containing 5 μM chromanol. (**f**) M-mode at 10 min in 5 μM chromanol. (**g**) M-mode at 10 min
after washout of chromanol. (Data unpublished).

The effects seen in response to mutations in potassium channels
can be mimicked by application of an inhibitor of *KCNQ* channel
function, chromanol. Acute application of this drug on exposed fly
hearts resulted in an increase in arrhtyhmicity (**Fig. 4d–g**). These
data suggested that *KCNQ* potassium channel plays a role in regular
heart contraction in *Drosophila* that is similar to its role in the
human heart. In addition to the pacing assay, this method can provide
detailed information on the cardioactive compounds which may

be informative as to their effects in human heart. Therefore, the two methods discussed here should provide effective and efficient models for drug development, especially in the initial phases.

4. Notes

1. Flies should be collected on the day they eclose, separated by sex, and kept in low density (25–30 flies per 30 ml vial) at a constant temperature and humidity until performing either the pacing assay or the image-based heart assay (see the next section). This is because environmental stressors such as extremes of heat, overcrowding, and mate competition negatively impact heart performance. Exposure to Fly-Nap® for less than 5 min Fly-Nap treatment appears to have no negative effects on heart failure rate or on heart performance as assessed by the image-based assay but longer exposures should be avoided. Immobilization by ether or carbon dioxide is not recommended because both affect heart rate. The presence of a balancer chromosome often causes heart irregularities. Therefore, non-balancer line should be prepared for both experiments and control lines.

2. Electrodes are made using heavy duty foil affixed to both ends of a microscope slide with a small (5 mm) gap in between. Wire loops are sandwiched between layers of each foil electrode. The wire loops can then be connected to the pulse generator.

3. Flies are placed in contact with the foil electrodes using a conductive electrode gel. Two rows of gel are applied using a 3 ml syringe (without a needle) taking care to ensure that all gel residue in the central gap is removed. It is necessary to replace the gel after 2–4 pacing sessions because bubbling and gel dry out affect the conductivity and fly contact, respectively.

4. The number of the flies that can be paced at one time is limited by electrode size and the experimenter's experience; usually less than ten flies per session. To maintain a constant temperature throughout the experiment, a heating plate (Brook Industries, Lake Villa, IL) that can rest on the microscope stage is used (**Fig. 1a**).

5. The conical chamber, visible just under the dorsal cuticle in the first and second abdominal segments (A1 and A2) as well as the heart tube in the third abdominal segment (A3) are monitored for heart contractions (**Fig. 1c**).

6. Thirty seconds recovery after pacing is usually a sufficient time for the recovery of "healthy" young fly hearts in this assay. However this timing should be optimized for each application. For optimization 1-week-old wild type adult flies are scored

at 15, 30 45, 60, 90, and 120 s after the pacing; the time that shows a 20–30% failure rate for young witldtype flies provides the best conditions for detecting effects of genetic manipulation or drug application. At least 50 flies are required for each genotype or treatment. Statistical analysis is performed by using a nonparametric Chi-squared test.

7. Adult hemolymph without sucrose and trehalose can be stored at 4°C. Aliquots of 1 M sucrose and 1 M trehalose stock solutions are added just before use. Artificial hemolymph is bubbled with air (or oxygen) for least 30 min at room temperature.

8. We use 100 μl glass capillary tubes (VWR international #53432–921) pulled by a horizontal micropipette puller (Sutter Instrument Co. Model P-97) for suctioning of adipose tissue. Suction strength is controlled by tip size which is typically 10–20 μm.

9. An equilibration period is critical as the dissection procedure can affect heart contraction rates for the short term. However, measurements of heart parameters usually stabilize after 15–30 min and remain stabile for up to 4 h (23). Typically, recordings are made between 30 and 60 min following dissection.

10. This imaging system can monitor the entire heart tube in real-time similar to two-dimensional echocardiograms (B-mode). Both qualitative measures (e.g., M-mode) and quantitative measures (e.g., heart size, pace maker activity, diastolic and systolic intervals, % fractional shortening, and contraction velocities) are obtained. An advantage of this system is that measurements are made for every heart beat in a record (typically 60–120) providing statistical power. Finally, the indicies measured in flies of similar ages and/or genotypes are highly reproducible. M-modes are generated by specifying a vertical, one-pixel wide column in a movie frame that spans both edges of the heart tube. This strip is then electronically "cut" from the same position in every frame of the movie. Strips are aligned horizontally producing an M-mode like image with heart wall movement displayed in the y-axis overtime in the x-axis.

Acknowledgments

The authors would like to thank Professor Rolf Bodmer for his critical advice and encouragement. TA is a Sanford Fellow, supported by a fellowship of the Sanford Child Health Center at BIMR. KO is supported by a grant from the American Heart Association.

References

1. Brand AH, Perrimon N. (1993) Targeted gene expression as a means of altering cell fates and generating dominant phenotypes. *Development* **118**, 401–15.

2. Kennerdell JR, Carthew RW. (2000) Heritable gene silencing in *Drosophila* using double-stranded RNA. *Nat Biotechnol* **18**, 896–8.

3. Dietzl G, Chen D, Schnorrer F, et al. (2007) A genome-wide transgenic RNAi library for conditional gene inactivation in *Drosophila*. *Nature* **448**, 151–6.

4. Bilen J, Bonini NM. (2005) *Drosophila* as a model for human neurodegenerative disease. *Annu Rev Genet* **39**, 153–71.

5. Marsh JL, Thompson LM. (2006) *Drosophila* in the study of neurodegenerative disease. *Neuron* **52**, 169–78.

6. Bier E, Bodmer R. (2004) *Drosophila*, an emerging model for cardiac disease. *Gene* **342**, 1–11.

7. Curtis NJ, Ringo JM, Dowse HB. (1999) Morphology of the pupal heart, adult heart, and associated tissues in the fruit fly, *Drosophila melanogaster*. *J Morphol* **240**, 225–35.

8. Bodmer R, Venkatesh TV. (1998) Heart development in *Drosophila* and vertebrates: conservation of molecular mechanisms. *Dev Genet* **22**, 181–6.

9. Cripps RM, Olson EN. (2002) Control of cardiac development by an evolutionarily conserved transcriptional network. *Dev Biol* **246**, 14–28.

10. Olson EN. (2006) Gene regulatory networks in the evolution and development of the heart. *Science* **313**, 1922–7.

11. Ocorr K, Perrin L, Lim HY, Qian L, Wu X, Bodmer R. (2007) Genetic control of heart function and aging in *Drosophila*. *Trends Cardiovasc Med* **17**, 177–82.

12. Cammarato A, Dambacher CM, Knowles AF, et al. (2008) Myosin transducer mutations differentially affect motor function, myofibril structure, and the performance of skeletal and cardiac muscles. *Mol Biol Cell* **19**, 553–62.

13. Paternostro G, Vignola C, Bartsch DU, Omens JH, McCulloch AD, Reed JC. (2001) Age-associated cardiac dysfunction in *Drosophila melanogaster*. *Circ Res* **88**, 1053–8.

14. Wessells RJ, Bodmer R. (2004) Screening assays for heart function mutants in *Drosophila*. *Biotechniques* **37**, 58–60, 62, 64 passim.

15. Wessells RJ, Fitzgerald E, Cypser JR, Tatar M, Bodmer R. (2004) Insulin regulation of heart function in aging fruit flies. *Nat Genet* **36**, 1275–81.

16. Qian L, Liu J, Bodmer R. (2005) Neuromancer Tbx20-related genes (H15/midline) promote cell fate specification and morphogenesis of the *Drosophila* heart. *Dev Biol* **279**, 509–24.

17. Akasaka T, Klinedinst S, Ocorr K, Bustamante EL, Kim SK, Bodmer R. (2006) The ATP-sensitive potassium (KATP) channel-encoded dSUR gene is required for *Drosophila* heart function and is regulated by tinman. *Proc Natl Acad Sci USA* **103**, 11999–2004.

18. Peart JN, Gross GJ. (2002) Sarcolemmal and mitochondrial K(ATP) channels and myocardial ischemic preconditioning. *J Cell Mol Med* **6**, 453–64.

19. Gross GJ, Fryer RM. (1999) Sarcolemmal versus mitochondrial ATP-sensitive K⁺ channels and myocardial preconditioning. *Circ Res* **84**, 973–9.

20. Hanley PJ, Daut J. (2005) K(ATP) channels and preconditioning: A re-examination of the role of mitochondrial K(ATP) channels and an overview of alternative mechanisms. *J Mol Cell Cardiol* **39**, 17–50.

21. Bienengraeber M, Olson TM, Selivanov VA, et al. (2004) ABCC9 mutations identified in human dilated cardiomyopathy disrupt catalytic KATP channel gating. *Nat Genet* **36**, 382–7.

22. Ocorr K, Reeves NL, Wessells RJ, et al. (2007) KCNQ potassium channel mutations cause cardiac arrhythmias in *Drosophila* that mimic the effects of aging. *Proc Natl Acad Sci USA* **104**, 3943–8.

23. Fink M, Callol-Massot C, Chu A, et al. (2009) A new method for Detection and Quantification of Heartbeat Parameters in *Drosophila*, Zebrafish, and Embryonic Mouse Hearts. *BioTechniques* **46**, 101–113.

24. Wolf PA, Abbott RD, Kannel WB. (1991) Atrial fibrillation as an independent risk factor for stroke: the Framingham Study. *Stroke* **22**, 983–8.

25. Lakatta EG, Levy D. (2003) Arterial and cardiac aging: major shareholders in cardiovascular disease enterprises: Part II: the aging heart in health: links to heart disease. *Circulation* **107**, 346–54.

26. Olivetti G, Giordano G, Corradi D, et al. (1995) Gender differences and aging: effects on the human heart. *J Am Coll Cardiol* **26**, 1068–79.

Chapter 19

Permeable Cell Assay: A Method for High-Throughput Measurement of Cellular ATP Synthetic Activity

Kiyotaka Y. Hara

Summary

"Permeable Cell Assay" is an efficient method to measure cellular activity of ATP synthesis. Although ATP is a major energy source for biological reactions, it has been difficult to measure cellular ATP synthetic activity quantitatively. In this assay, bioluminescence from the luciferin–luciferase reaction is used for the quantitative measurement. Under the assay condition, bioluminescence from standard ATP solution showed no attenuation within several minutes, and the intensity corresponded proportionally to ATP concentrations of the standards. To measure cellular ATP synthetic activity, combination of osmotic shock and detergent, Triton X-100 treatment is used to make bacterial cells permeable. ATP is discharged from permeable cells and reacted with external luciferase. Because permeable cells used glucose to synthesize and accumulate ATP without further growth, intensity of bioluminescence is increasing during the cellular consumption of glucose. Cellular ATP biosynthetic activity is calculated from the slope of linearly increasing bioluminescence.

Key words: ATP, ATP synthesis, Glycolysis, Luciferin, Luciferase, Luminescence, Rapid screening, High-throughput, Permeable cell, Semi-intact cell

1. Introduction

ATP (Adenosine 5′-triphosphate) plays a critical role in all living beings as an energy source for various enzyme activities and as a direct precursor in RNA synthesis. ATP is rapidly regenerated mainly by the glycolytic pathway and oxidative phosphorylation. A conventional luciferin-luciferase method was established *(1, 2)*, and many investigators have been using it to measure static ATP concentration *(3)*. However it has been difficult to measure cellular ATP synthetic activity *(4)*. Recently, we developed

Hisashi Koga (ed.), *Reverse Chemical Genetics*, Methods in Molecular Biology, vol. 577
DOI 10.1007/978-1-60761-232-2_19, © Humana Press, a part of Springer Science+Business Media, LLC 2009

"Permeable Cell Assay" for high-throughput measurement of cellular ATP synthetic activity *(4)*. In this assay, osmotic shock and Triton X-100 treatment made bacterial cells permeable for ATP. Discharged ATP reacted with external luciferase and is detected as bioluminescence. An increased bioluminescence is observed with permeable cells, whereas it is not observed with standard ATP solution and heat-inactivated permeable cells. The cellular ATP synthetic activity is calculated from the slope of increasing bioluminescence. Permeable Cell Assay is simple and rapid with a small amount of cell culture for quantification of ATP synthesis.

Permeable Cell Assay has potential to apply to 'Reverse Genetics' using target gene knockout mutants and designed mutant collections. Schematic illustration of this assay is shown in **Fig. 1**. In the last few years, it has become possible to undertake systematic genome-wide functional screening using genome information and genetic tools for perturbation of gene function. Collections of nearly complete sets of single-gene mutants have been constructed in some organisms *(5)*. In fact, by using the Permeable Cell Assay, we determined the cellular ATP synthetic activity in the stationary-phase of a complete set of single-gene deletion strains of *Escherichia coli (6)*. We also applied this result for ATP-driven glutathione production *(7)*. Furthermore, the Permeable Cell Assay also has potential to apply to 'Reverse Chemical Genetics' using chemical libraries and specific inhibitors for target gene products (*see* **Fig. 1**). Application of Permeable Cell Assay to Reverse Chemical Genetic approaches takes some advantages: first, many inhibitors can access to their target proteins in permeable cell, even if their permeability for cell

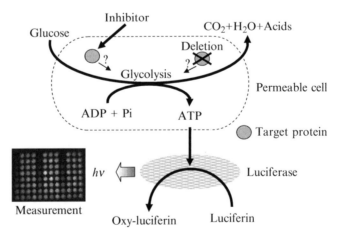

Fig. 1. Schematic illustration of the method for quantitating cellular ATP synthetic activity. ATP is generated mainly by the glycolytic pathway in the permeable cell during the cellular consumption of glucose. ATP molecule permeates the membrane and reacts with external luciferase to produce luminescence with luciferin. The effect of target protein for cellular ATP synthetic activity can be investigated by using the inhibitor of the target protein or by using the target gene deletion strain. The image of luminescence from the assay plate was captured with LumiVision Pro HSII (AISIN, Tokyo, Japan).

membrane is very low, because very hydrophobic compounds, ATP, can pass through the permeable cell. Second, the starting time of inhibition can be changed. Reverse Genetic approach cannot be applied for essential genes because of their genes cause no growth. However, addition of inhibitor after growing makes us possible to measure the cellular ATP synthetic activities of essential gene deletion strains. Third, controllable inhibitory level depending on inhibitor concentration is a further advantage of Reverse Chemical Genetics for analyzing relationship between cellular ATP synthetic activities and target gene products.

2. Materials

2.1. Bacterial Strains

1. The *E. coli* K-12 strain BW25113 [*lacIq rrnBT14 ΔlacZWJ16 hsdR514 ΔaraBADAH33 ΔrhaBADLD78*] and its derivatives of F_1-ATPase mutants were a courtesy gift from Dr. H. Mori and Dr. T. Baba at the Nara Advanced Institute of Science and Technology *(8)*.

2. Mutants were constructed by replacing one of *atp* genes with a selectable antibiotic-resistant gene (*kan*) as reported by Datsenko and Wanner *(9)*.

3. All other bacterial species were type strains as follows. *Corynebacterium ammoniagenes* ATCC6871, *Corynebacterium glutamicum* ATCC21171, *Pseudomonas fluorescens* ATCC13525, and *Pseudomonas putida* ATCC12633 (*see* **Note 1**).

2.2. Cell Culture

1. *LB agar plate.* Luria–Bertani (LB) medium (Difco, NJ, USA) and Bacterial agar (Difco).

2. *LBG medium.* LB medium supplemented with 2.8% Glucose (Nacalai, Kyoto, Japan). Store at room temperature.

3. 96-deep-well plate (Master Block; Greiner Bio-One, Kremsmuenster, Austria) covered with an AirPore® Tape Sheet (Qiagen, Hilden, Germany).

4. N-704 plate shaker (Nissin Rika, Tokyo, Japan).

2.3. Permeable Cell Assay

1. *Pretreatment Solution.* 40% [w/v] glucose (*see* **Note 2**), 0.8% [v/v] Triton X-100 (Nacalai) (*see* **Note 3–5**). Store at room temperature for up to 2 months. Mix well before using.

2. *Assay Buffer (5×).* 25 mM $MgSO_4$, 500 mM ethylenediaminetetraacetic acid, and 125 mM Tricine buffer, pH 7.8. Store at 4°C for up to 2 months.

3. *Luciferase Solution.* Addition of 1 mM dithiothreitol (DTT, Wako, Osaka, Japan), 0.5 mM firefly D-luciferin (Roche, Basel, Switzerland), 1.25 µg/ml firefly luciferase (Promega,

WI, USA) to Assay Buffer. Store all materials in aliquots at −20°C.

4. *Assay Solution*. Addition of 1/20 volume of 8% Triton X-100 and 300 mM potassium phosphate (*see* **Note 6**) to Luciferase Solution. Make immediately before measurement.

5. Black 96-well microplate (Multiplate 96FII; Sumitomo Bakelite Co., Osaka, Japan).

3. Methods

3.1. Culture

1. Streak glycerol-stocks of bacterial strains on LB plate by 1 µl loop.
2. Incubate the LB agar plate at 30°C for 24 h.
3. Pick up bacterial cells from the LB agar plate by wide side of teeth pick and rinse them into 1 ml of LBG medium in 96-deep-well plate covered with an AirPore® Tape Sheet.
4. Shake the plate with N-704 plate shaker at 30°C for 24 h.

3.2. Preparation of Cell Suspension

1. Harvest cultured bacterial cells by centrifugation ($3,000 \times g$, 4°C for 5 min).
2. Wash the harvested cells by ice-cold 100 mM Tris–HCl (pH 7.4).
3. Suspended the washed cells into appropriate volume of ice-cold 100 mM Tris–HCl (pH 7.4).
4. Measure the OD of cell suspension at 595 nm by microplate reader.

3.3. Permeable Cell Assay

1. Mix the cell suspension with equal volume of Pretreatment Solution and incubate at room temperature for 20 min.
2. Prepare Luciferase Solution. Keep in dark and incubate at room temperature for 15 min.
3. Prepare Assay Solution immediately before using.
4. The reaction was initiated by addition of 10 µl of cell suspension into 90 µl of Assay Solution in a 96-well black microplate.
5. Measure the time-course of luminescence for several minutes using microplate reader.
6. The static ATP concentration (nM ATP/OD) was given in the simplest calculation, by $Lo/\alpha d$. The ATP synthetic activity (nM ATP/min/OD) was given by $\Delta/\alpha d$. Lo, intercept of luminescence (RLU, Relative Luminescence Unit); Δ, velocity

Table 1
Cellular ATP synthetic activities of F$_1$-ATPase deletion mutants

Mutant	Subunit	Activity (µM ATP/min/OD)	s.d.
Parent	–	0.23	0.010
ΔatpH	δ	0.91	0.106
ΔatpA	α	1.02	0.074
ΔatpG	γ	0.95	0.087
ΔatpD	β	0.93	0.039
ΔatpC	ε	0.60	0.055

It was supposed that permeable cells should lose the activity of oxidative phosphorylation for ATP synthesis because detergents could uncouple F$_o$F$_1$-ATP synthase *(13)*. We assumed that measured ATP synthetic activity by this method should depend on mainly glycolytic activity for ATP synthesis. To demonstrate this issue, we tested F$_1$-ATPase mutants that were reported to show up-regulated glycolytic activity *(14, 15)*. All single gene deletion mutants of each subunit consisting of F$_1$-ATPase, ΔatpA, ΔatpC, ΔatpD, ΔatpG, and ΔatpH were grown until the stationary phase and assayed for their ATP synthetic activities consistently in a 96-well format. Mutants showed poor growth, and final ODs of Δatp mutants were about half of the parental strain. However, ATP synthetic activities per OD of Δatp mutants were more than 2 times higher than that of the parent. This result proved that this assay mainly detect glycolytic ATP synthesis. Activities were the mean ($n = 4$)

of luminescent increasing (RLU/min); *d*, OD of cell; α, conversion value of luminescence into ATP concentration obtained from an ATP standard curve (RLU/nM ATP). Examples of the cellular ATP synthetic activities are shown in **Table 1**.

4. Notes

1. The Permeable Cell Assay was optimized for *E. coli* K-12 (BW25113) *(4)*. To investigate applications of this assay, *P. fluorescens, P. putida, C. ammoniagenes,* and *C. glutamicum* were tested. All bacteria were grown in LBG medium at 30°C for 24 h. The final OD of each bacterium was adjusted to 0.1, and the intensity of luminescence was measured. The intensity of luminescence from all bacteria tested with various concentrations of Triton X-100 showed saturated luminescence with 0.4% Triton X-100 *(4)*. Both species of *Corynebacterium*

Table 2
Cellular ATP synthetic activities of various bacterial species

Cell types	Activity (nM ATP/min/OD)	s.d.
P. putida	48	10
P. fluorescens	85	22
E. coli K-12	230	10
C. ammoniagenes	163	21
C. glutamicum	361	14

All bacteria were cultivated in a 96-deep-well plate, and their ATP synthetic activities were assayed using a 96-well format. Cellular ATP synthetic activity of C. glutamicum was highest among the bacteria tested. Activities were the mean ($n = 3$)

showed the highest intensity of luminescence, which suggests relatively higher intracellular ATP concentration among bacteria tested. This result indicates that the Permeable Cell Assay could apply to gram-positive bacteria. We also measured ATP synthetic activities of these species (**Table 2**).

2. Osmotic shock by rapid dilution of glucose makes ATP permeate through the bacterial membrane and glucose also acts as carbon source for ATP synthesis. The osmotic shock showed better reproducibility than authentic freeze-thaw treatment. Glucose could be replaced with other sugars when it is required.

3. The used detergent condition for this assay should not inhibit luciferase activity. Therefore, several following detergents were tested for their effect on luminescence from luciferin-luciferase; benzalkonium chloride, SDS, Nymeen S-215 dissolved in xylene, and Triton X-100. SDS inhibited luciferase activity most strongly. In the case of using benzalkonium chloride, luciferase was inhibited when its concentration was higher than 0.002%. A combination of 4 g/l Nymeen S-215 and 10 ml/l xylene was used to permeate bacterial cells in the previous reports *(10, 11)*. When this combinatorial mixture was added to the luciferin-luciferase reaction mixture, the intensity of luminescence was initially very high but rapidly attenuated within several minutes. Triton X-100 gave the highest and most stable luminescence among detergents tested. Triton X-100 is a nonionic micelle-forming solvent, and its enhancement of activity of luciferase was reported *(12)*.

4. You can optimize the condition for permeation of your target strain under procedure; harvest your target strain by

centrifugation and wash by Preparation Buffer and suspended into the same buffer. Mix the cell suspension with equal volume of pretreatment solution [40% (w/v) glucose, various concentration of Triton X-100] for 20 min at room temperature (mixture A). Preincubate Luciferase Solution for 15 min at room temperature. Add Triton X-100 to Assay Solution at the final concentration equal to mixture A (mixture B). The reaction is initiated by addition of 10 μl of mixture A into 90 μl of mixture B and measure the luminescence by microplate reader. Determine the best concentration of Triton X-100 which shows maximum luminescence as an optimized condition for your target strain.

5. In this assay, Triton X-100 is a critical chemical. Triton X-100 permeates ATP through the *E. coli* membrane, enhances bioluminescence from luciferase, and suppresses the attenuation of the luminescence. Even in the standard luciferin-luciferase method, addition of Triton X-100 must be helpful to amplify luminescence and keep its stability. The stability of luminescence is an important factor for high-throughput measurements.

6. The Permeable Cell Assay is a simple method to measure the cellular ATP synthetic activity. ATP should be synthesized from domestic ADP and externally added inorganic phosphate mainly by the glycolytic pathway with consumption of glucose. High concentration of inorganic phosphate inhibits luciferase. The used concentration of inorganic phosphate (1.5 mM) was determined that it does not inhibit the activity of luciferase too much.

Acknowledgments

The author is grateful to Dr. Hirotada Mori and Dr. Tomoya Baba at the Nara Advanced Institute of Science and Technology for providing us *BW25113* and *atp* mutant strains. This study was carried out in Biofrontier Laboratories, Kyowa Hakko Kogyo Co. Ltd. The author would like to thank many supports from the members of this laboratory, especially Dr. Hideo Mori for his management and Natsuka Shimodate for her technical assistance. This work was carried out as a part of The Project for Development of a Technological Infrastructure for Industrial Bioprocesses on R&D of New Industrial Science and Technology Frontiers by the Ministry of Economy, Trade, & Industry (METI) and was supported by the New Energy and Industrial Technology Development Organization (NEDO).

References

1. McElroy, W. D., Seliger, H. H., and White, E. H. (1969) Mechanism of bioluminescence, chemiluminescence and enzyme function in the oxidation of firefly luciferin. *Photochem Photobiol.* **10**, 153–170.

2. DeLuca, M., and McElroy, W. D. (1974) Kinetics of the firefly luciferase catalyzed reactions. *Biochemistry.* **26**, 921–925.

3. Schneider, D. A., and Gourse, R. L. (2004) Relationship between growth rate and ATP concentration in *Escherichia coli*: a bioassay for available cellular ATP. *J Biol Chem.* **279**, 8262–8268.

4. Hara, K.Y., and Mori, H. (2006) An efficient method for quantitative determination of cellular ATP synthetic activity. *J Biomol Screen.* **11**, 310–317.

5. Carpenter, A. E., and Sabatini, D.V. (2004) Systematic genome-wide screens of gene function *Nat Rev Genet.* **5**, 11–22.

6. Hara, K.Y., Shimodate, N., Ito, M., Baba, T., Mori, H., and Mori, H. (2009) Systematic genome-wide scanning for genes involved in ATP generation in *Escherichia coli. Metab. Eng.* **11**, 1–7.

7. Hara, K.Y., Shimodate, N., Hirokawa, Y., Ito, M., Baba, T., Mori, H., and Mori, H. (2009) Glutathione production by efficient ATP-regenerating *Escherichia coli* mutants. *FEMS Microbiol Lett.* (in press).

8. Baba, T., Ara, T., Hasegawa, M., Takai, Y., Okumura, Y., Baba, M., Datsenko, K.A., Tomita, M., Wanner, B.L., and Mori, H. (2006) Construction of *Escherichia coli* K-12 in-frame, single-gene knockout mutants: the Keio collection. *Mol Syst Biol.* **2**, 0008 (doi:10.1038/msb4100050).

9. Datsenko, K. A., and Wanner, B. L. (2000) One-step inactivation of chromosomal genes in *Escherichia* coli K12 using PCR. products *Proc Natl Acad Sci USA.* **97**, 6640–6645.

10. Fujio, T., and Furuya, A. (1985) Effect of magnesium ion and chelating agents on enzymatic production of ATP from adenine. *Appl Microbiol Biotechnol.* **21**, 143–147.

11. Mori, H, Iida, A., Fujio, T., and Teshiba, S. (1997) A novel process of inosine 5'-monophosphate production using overexpressed guanosine/inosine kinase. *Appl Microbiol Biotechnol.* **48**, 693–698.

12. Kricka, L. J., and DeLuca, M. (1982) Effect of solvents on the catalytic activity of firefly luciferase. *Arch Biochem Biophys.* **217**, 674–681.

13. Tsunoda, S. P., Aggeler, R., Noji, H., Kinosita, K. Jr., Yoshida, M., and Capaldi, R. A. (2000) Observations of rotation within the $F_{(o)}F_{(1)}$-ATP synthase: deciding between rotation of the $F_{(o)}c$ subunit ring and artifact. *FEBS Lett.* **470**, 244–248.

14. Ford, S. R., Hall, M. S., and Leach, F. R. (1992) Carbon and energy metabolism of atp mutants of *Escherichia coli. Anal Biochem.* **204**, 183–191.

15. Yokota, A., Terasawa, Y., Takaoka, N., Shimizu, H. and Tomita, F. (1994) Pyruvic acid production by an F_1-ATPase-defective mutant of *Escherichia coli* W1485lip2. *Biosci Biotechnol Biochem.* **58**, 2164–2167.

Chapter 20

Novel Methodology for Immobilization of Biomolecules on the Surface of a Photoresponsible Polymer Containing Azobenzene Moiety

Osamu Watanabe

Summary

We have introduced the principles of a newly created photoimmobilization technology using photoresponsive azopolymers and reviewed its application to the fabrication of immunochip. We can consider two important factors in our approach, the deformation process that is induced by interaction between the micro-objects and the azopolymer surface, and the immobilization process that resulted from the deformation process. We believe that there is further potential to develop this technique more widely; for instance, applications involving biological molecules are an intriguing field with high potential for future growth, including aspects of molecular orientation and the formation of organized structures. This novel approach would serve as a stepping stone for further development. The research field could enlarge by considering how to use the immobilized surface such as biochip and bioreactor.

Key words: Photoirradiation, Immobilization, Azopolymer, Immunochip, Biomarker, Chemiluminescence

1. Introduction

A large number of methods for immobilizing biomolecules on the surface of solid substrate have been proposed in the past few decades, in which the molecules are immobilized on a carrier using covalent bonds *(1)*, ionic bonds *(2)*, physical adsorption *(3)*, cross-linkage of the biomolecules *(4)*, or by microencapsulation *(5)*. Immobilizing techniques are indispensable to treat biomolecules in an experiment. The provision of an immobilization process is one of the most essential processing steps that are required in order to obtain practical biomolecule carriers such as

Hisashi Koga (ed.), *Reverse Chemical Genetics*, Methods in Molecular Biology, vol. 577
DOI 10.1007/978-1-60761-232-2_20, © Humana Press, a part of Springer Science + Business Media, LLC 2009

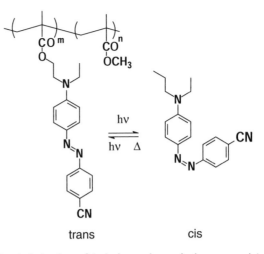

Fig. 1. The chemical structure of typical azopolymer. Azobenzene moiety isomerizes between *trans* and *cis* form.

biosensors, bioreactors, or biochips. In this section, we introduce an immobilizing method on the basis of novel principle by using photoresponsible polymer containing azobenzene moiety (azopolymer) *(6–11)*.

Figure 1 shows the chemical structure of a typical azopolymer. When exposed to light of a certain wavelength, the *trans* form can be isomerized to the *cis* form. *Cis–trans* back-isomerization can occur thermally or/and photochemically. This property of azobenzene moiety leads a drastic change in physical properties of the polymer matrix. One of an intriguing property is that azopolymer is a photoinduced deformable polymer; it deforms slowly during light irradiation and stays deformed after ceasing light irradiation. We have applied the phenomenon of azopolymer to the immobilizing biomolecules and developed an immunochip for detecting a biomarker in the body.

Figure 2 shows the principle of photoinduced immobilization, which represents a very simple technique. First, the microobject (immunoglobulin in the case shown in **Fig. 1**) is set on the surface of the azopolymers, which is then photoirradiated from above. The surface of the azopolymer deforms in the presence of the immunoglobulin because the viscoelastic properties of azopolymer surfaces change during photoirradiation. The deformation occurs such that it enfolds the immunoglobulin, and so the contact area between the surfaces of the immunoglobulin and the azopolymer increases. The surface of the azopolymer glaciates again and maintains the deformed shape after ceasing the irradiation, as shown in **Fig. 2** (right-hand side). As a result, the immunoglobulin is effectively immobilized on the surface of the azopolymer without chemical modification.

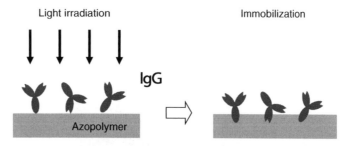

Fig. 2. Schematic Illustration of the photoimmobilization of biomolecules (immunoglobulin) on the surface of an azopolymer. The surface of the azopolymer is deformed to the shape of the immunoglobulin after photoirradiation.

2. Photoinduced Immobilization

First, we demonstrate the immobilization of polystyrene microspheres on the surface of azopolymer using the photoinduced immobilization technique. An aqueous solution with 1 μm diameter polystyrene microspheres (5100A, Duke Scientific Corp., Palo Alto, CA) was dropped on to the flat surface of the polymer film, and the solution was then sucked with a pipette to form self-organized colloidal crystals. Area-selective photoimmobilization was performed by moving the irradiation site using a confocal laser-scanning microscope with a wavelength of 488 nm (OLS1100, Olympus Corp., Tokyo, Japan). The sample was washed by ultrasonic cleaning to remove the unimmobilized and multilayered spheres, and then examined with the microscope after drying. **Figure 3a** shows checker board designed 2D colloidal spheres crystals immobilized on the polymer films. The microspheres were immobilized only in the irradiated region. Furthermore, multilayered colloidal spheres were easily removed. Although the microspheres have relatively large diameter of 1 μm, they were fixed firmly to the polymer film in a monolayer structure. The patterned colloidal crystals on the film remained even after a 3-min ultrasonic treatment in water with a power of 125 W. Photoinduced immobilization provides a simple method by a patterned monolayer of spheres that can be easily and optionally immobilized on the substrate.

Second, we tried the immobilization of DNA molecules as a potential target material for the immobilization of biological macromolecules. An aqueous solution of 1 mg/mL λ-DNA was spotted onto the surface of an azopolymer and covered with a cover glass, where the λ-DNA was stained with a fluorophore (YOYO-1 iodide, Molecular Probes Inc., Eugene, OR) in advance and the surface was then irradiated with the linearly shaped laser beam for 5 min, as shown in **Fig. 3b**. The surface was washed for 5 min in an aqueous solution and was then observed using

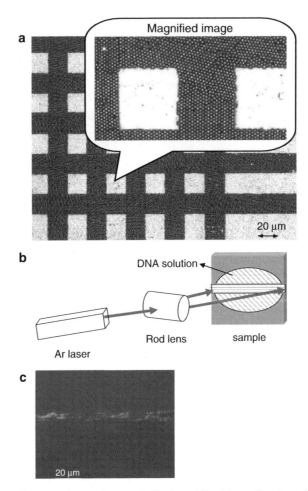

Fig. 3. **(a)** Microscope image of area-selective immobilized 1 μm diameter polystyrene microspheres on the flat surface of an azobenzene-containing polymer film. The irradiated area was controlled by moving the sample stage. **(b)** Experimental set up for patterned immobilization using a linearly-shaped laser beam. **(c)** Fluorescence image of the immobilized λ-DNA molecules.

a conventional fluorescence microscope. **Figure 3c** confirms that the labeled λ-DNA was only immobilized in the irradiated region. Unimmobilized DNA molecules were easily removed by washing. The same experiment using Green Fluorescent Protein (GFP) also indicates the immobilization of protein in the irradiated region. In this way, we could demonstrate that an azopolymer can capture micrometer- to nanometer-scaled micro-objects, including synthetic polymers and biological molecules, on the photoirradiated area. Azopolymers can immobilize micro-objects that possess a variety of surface characteristics, including negatively charged DNA, charged proteins, and hydrophobic polystyrene. This versatility in terms of immobilization is a significant advantage of this technique. Chemically induced immobilization methods require optimized processes depending on the structures and properties of the individual biomolecules, which in turn requires some complicated procedures *(12)*, yet these techniques have become widely used. The characteristics of the azopolymer make it possible to immobilize a wide variety of biological molecules on the same substrate through a one-step photoirradiation process.

In order to take advantage of the functionality of these biomolecules, identifying an immobilization process that does not lead to deactivation of the molecules is important. In particular, biomolecules such as proteins show sensitive behavior in terms of changes in environment, as shown by the denaturing of proteins when the surrounding temperature increases even slightly. Since it is possible that damage to biomolecules following photoinduced immobilization could trigger functional degradation, we first examined the activity of an immobilized enzyme. An aqueous solution of 1 mg/mL bacterial protease (subtilsin; 27.5 kDa, Sigma-Aldrich, St. Louis, MO) was spotted onto the surface of an azopolymer, and the surface was irradiated with a laser beam of 488-nm wavelength and 80 mW/cm^2 optical power density for 5 min to immobilize the enzyme. As a control experiment, a similar specimen was prepared without photoirradiation. The activity of the subtilisin was verified as the hydrolysis of the artificial substrate (*tert*-butoxycarbonyl-Gly-Gly-Leu-*p*-nitroanilide, Mw = 465.5, Merck Inc., Whitehouse Station, NJ). The artificial substrate solution was spotted onto the azopolymer surface in the same area where the subtilsin had been immobilized, and then the specimen was maintained at 37°C and 85% relative humidity for 1 h. The hydrolysis of the artificial substrate was determined spectroscopically by immediately measuring the absorbance of the reactant at a wavelength of 410 nm. The conversion ratio of the reaction was about 10% for the subtilsin-immobilized sample, whereas it was about 1% for the control sample (without photoirradiation). These results clearly show that biomolecules immobilized on an azopolymer surface can maintain their enzyme functionality during and after the immobilization process.

We also checked immune reaction on the surface of azopolymer. Phosphate buffered saline (PBS) solutions of human serum albumin (HSA) and bovine serum albumin (BSA) with different concentrations were spotted onto azopolymer surfaces. After evaporating the spotted solution, photoirradiation was performed over the entire surface using an array of blue light-emitting diode (LED), and was then washed with PBS containing 0.01 wt% Tween 20 in order to remove the unimmobilized albumins. After drying the sample again, the obtained sample was reacted with anti HSA monoclonal mouse antibodies and then the washed sample was reacted with Cy-5 labeled antimouse polyclonal goat antibodies as a secondary antibody to detect albumins. Fluorescence emission was only observed from the spot on which the HSA had been immobilized, which means that a reaction which was selective to the HSA had occurred on the antigen-immobilized surface of the azopolymer and then was detected.

Next, we investigated how deformation of an azopolymer surface can be induced by biomolecules as well as by microspheres. Changes in the azopolymer surface topography with λ-DNA before and after photoirradiation were observed by atomic force microscopy (AFM) An aqueous solution of 1 mg/mL λ-DNA was spin-coated onto the azopolymer surface, and the surface was irradiated with laser light of 488-nm wavelength and 10 mW/cm^2 optical power density for 10 min. A surface image was obtained by tapping-mode AFM (Digital Instruments, Dimension 3100) using a sharp silicon cantilever with a tip radius of less than 5 nm. The fibrous object in **Fig. 4a** is considered to be a bundle of λ-DNA (the diameter of bundle is about 50 nm), which has been immobilized on the azopolymer surface by spin-casting and subsequent photoirradiation. By increasing the applied force of the AFM tip **(Fig. 4b)**, the fibrous objects wiped away by the tip, and it can be seen that the shape of the fibrous object is clearly imprinted as a fibrous valley on the surface. The findings lead to the conclusion that the azopolymer surface recognize molecules shape and deforms along the contour of the molecules upon photoirradiation. The result also suggests that the increase in contact area between azopolymer and the biomolecules after photoirradiation enhances the adsorption force, and inhibits their desorption from the azopolymer surface.

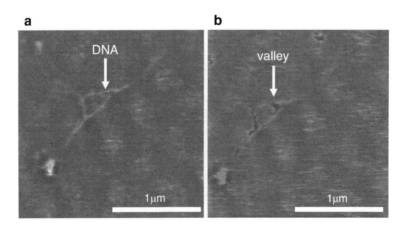

Fig. 4. (**a**) AFM image of azopolymer surface covered with λ-DNA. (The image heights from 0 to 20 nm). (**b**) AFM image at the same position after wiping the λ-DNA molecules.

3. Application for Immunochips

In the next phase, we applied the photoimmobilization method to try to obtain protein chips, and more specifically, an immunochip. Enzyme-linked immunosorbent assay (ELISA) systems are commonly used *(13, 14)* as a popular method for detecting small amounts of protein in sample solutions such as serums. Although the ELISA system is an excellent method for the detection of proteins, it still has some problems; it is comparatively expensive, and it is difficult to detect proteins when using small quantities of the sample solution. We might be able to realize an immunochip that could act as a micro-ELISA system with the capability to deal with small quantities of sample solutions if we could succeed in immobilizing the antibodies on the substrate. Such an immunochip could be used to measure multiple target proteins on the same substrate simultaneously, so it has the potential to become a novel method of replacing conventional ELISA systems in the fields of biochemical indexes, diagnostic agents, and clinical inspection *(15)*. We can say that the photoimmobilization method is one of the most promising prospects for immunochip applications because it can provide immobilization on the substrate surface irrespective of the surface states of the biomolecules.

We first examined specific reactions of photoimmobilized antibodies on azopolymer surfaces for the immunochip application. Solutions of antigoat antibodies (left-hand side) and antirabbit antibodies (right-hand side) were spotted onto an azopolymer surface at different concentrations, the layout of which is shown in **Fig. 5a**. After photoimmobilization and washing, the sample was reacted separately with Cy-5 labeled antigens (goat

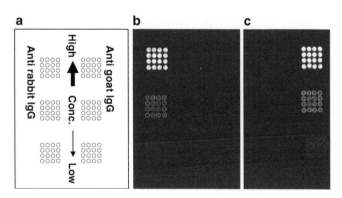

Fig. 5. (**a**) Layout of a slide that was spotted and immobilized using the anti goat IgG rabbit antibody and the anti rabbit IgG goat-antibody. (**b**) Fluorescent image after incubation of a Cy5-labeled goat IgG. (**c**) Fluorescent image after incubation of a Cy5-labeled rabbit IgG.

IgG and rabbit IgG). The antigoat IgG antibody recognized goat IgG when Cy-5 labeled goat IgG was introduced onto the sample, while on the other hand, antirabbit IgG recognized rabbit IgG when Cy-5 labeled rabbit IgG was introduced, as shown in **Figs. 5b, c**. The specific reactivity of the antibodies was realized by fixing photoimmobilized antibodies on the surface of the azopolymer.

We also examined the preservation stability of the photoimmobilized antibodies. Although the reactivity of the antibodies dropped away over a period of 10 days when they were stored at room temperature, it was maintained for about 2 months when stored at 4°C. This result is acceptable in terms of commercial viability, though further increase in stability would be preferable. We next examined the sensitivity for the immunochips. An immunochip usually has a two-dimensional surface, so the detection limit for antigens can be estimated from the amount of immobilized antibodies that are present. It was difficult to increase the sensitivity of a detection system which uses a photoluminescence probe. However, we succeeded in obtaining higher sensitivity for an immunochip in which we adopted a chemiluminescence detection system using an enzyme reaction.

We selected adiponectin, which is a biologically active agent that is excreted from adipose cells and which prevents arteriosclerosis, as the intended biological marker, and we tried to assay it using an enzyme sandwich immunoassay on the azopolymer surface. Antiadiponectin antibodies were photoimmobilized on the azopolymer surface and then a solution including adiponectin was reacted on the fabricated immunochip. Subsequently, the sample that had captured the adiponectin on its surface using the immobilized antibodies was treated with biotin-labeled antiadiponectin antibodies (first sandwich process), and was then treated with alkaline phosphatase (ALP) labeled streptoavidin (second sandwich process) *(16)*. After introducing the chemiluminescent substrate onto the surface, the intensity of the chemiluminescence was measured to determine the concentration of adiponectin. We measured the intensity of the chemiluminescence against the concentration of adiponectin using samples with predetermined concentrations. **Figure 6** exhibits the calibration curve that was obtained in the region of low concentration, and it shows that a linear relationship exists between intensity and concentration. We can detect adiponectin in a sample solution down to a concentration of at least 0.1 ng/ml, which is almost the same sensitivity as that obtained with ELISA. We compared a conventional ELISA system and the IgG chip system using mouse adiponectin of culture supernatant. **Figure 7** shows the correlation between the immunochip and conventional ELISA. A high degree of correlation exists ($r^2 = 0.97$) indicating that the use of an immunochip with an azopolymer film is a promising candidate for practical use.

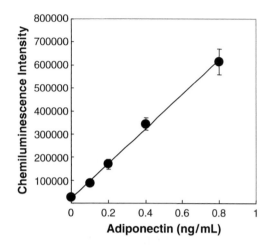

Fig. 6. Calibration curve for quantifying mouse adiponectin. Each *error bar* indicates the standard deviation for each data point.

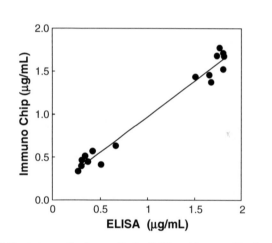

Fig. 7. Correlation between the two methods, ELISA and immunochip, for quantifying mouse adiponectin at a level of 16 culture supernatant.

References

1. Feng CL, Zhang Z, Forch R, Knoll W, Vancso GJ, Schonherr H. (2005) Reactive thin polymer films as platforms for the immobilization of biomolecules. *Biomacromolecules* **6**, 3243–51.

2. Lee Y, Lee EK, Cho YW, et al. (2003) ProteoChip: a highly sensitive protein microarray prepared by a novel method of protein immobilization for application of protein–protein interaction studies. *Proteomics* **3**, 2289–304.

3. Ouyang Z, Takats Z, Blake TA, et al. (2003) Preparing protein microarrays by soft-landing of mass-selected ions. *Science* **301**, 1351–4.

4. Levy I, Shoseyov O. (2004) Cross bridging proteins in nature and their utilization in bio- and nanotechnology. *Curr Protein Pept Sci* **5**, 33–49.

5. Hartmann M. (2005) Ordered Mesoporous Materials for Bioadsorption and Biocatalysis. *Chem Mater* **17**, 4577–93.

6. Ikawa T, Hoshino F, Matsuyama T, Takahashi H, Watanabe O. (2006) Molecular-shape imprinting and immobilization of biomolecules on a polymer containing azo dye. *Langmuir* **22**, 2747–53.

7. Ikawa T, Hoshino F, Watanabe O, Li Y, Pincus P, Safinya CR. (2007) Molecular scale imaging of F-actin assemblies immobilized on a photopolymer surface. *Phys Rev Lett* **98**, 018101.

8. Narita M, Hoshino F, Mouri M, Tsuchimori M, Ikawa Y, Watanabe O. (2007) Photoinduced immobilization of biomolecules on the surface of azopolymer films and its dependence on the concentration and type of the azobenzene moiety. *Macromolecules* **40**, 623–9.

9. Narita M, Ikawa T, Mouri M, Tsuchimori M, Hoshino F, Watanabe O. (2008) Aminoazopolymers with the capability of photoinduced immobilization developed for protein arrays with low photoluminescence. *Jpn J Appl Phys* **47**, 1329–32.

10. Watanabe O. (2004) Molecular recognition and immobilization of biomolecules induced by photoirradiation on the surface of an azopolymer. *R&D Review of Toyota CRDL* **39**, 46.

11. Watanabe O, Ikawa T, Kato T, Tawata M, Shimoyama H. (2006) Area-selective photoimmobilization of a two-dimensional array of colloidal spheres on a photodeformed template formed in photoresponsive azopolymer film. *Appl Phys Lett* **88**, 204107.

12. Peluso P, Wilson DS, Do D, et al. (2003) Optimizing antibody immobilization strategies for the construction of protein microarrays. *Anal Biochem* **312**, 113–24.

13. Voller A, Bartlett A, Bidwell DE. (1978) Enzyme immunoassays with special reference to ELISA techniques. *J Clin Pathol* **31**, 507–20.

14. Karlsson R, Michaelsson A, Mattsson L. (1991) Kinetic analysis of monoclonal antibody-antigen interactions with a new biosensor based analytical system. *J Immunol Methods* **145**, 229–40.

15. Kambhampati D. (2003) Protein Microarray Technology. 1 ed. Weinheim: Wiley-VCH.

16. Kendall C, Ionescu-Matiu I, Dreesman GR. (1983) Utilization of the biotin/avidin system to amplify the sensitivity of the enzyme-linked immunosorbent assay (ELISA). *J Immunol Methods* **56**, 329–39.

INDEX